OCCUPATIONAL THERAPY AND OLDER PEOPLE

Edited by

Anne McIntyre and Anita Atwal

Lecturers in Occupational Therapy
School of Health Sciences and Social Care
Brunel University
London
UK

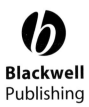

Blackwell
Publishing

© 2005 by Blackwell Publishing Ltd

Editorial offices:
Blackwell Publishing Ltd, 9600 Garsington Road, Oxford OX4 2DQ, UK
  Tel: +44 (0)1865 776868
Blackwell Publishing Inc., 350 Main Street, Malden, MA 02148-5020, USA
  Tel: +1 781 388 8250
Blackwell Publishing Asia Pty Ltd, 550 Swanston Street, Carlton, Victoria 3053, Australia
  Tel: +61 (0)3 8359 1011

First published 2005 by Blackwell Publishing Ltd

Library of Congress Cataloging-in-Publication Data is available
Occupational therapy and older people / edited by Anne McIntyre and Anita Atwal.
    p. ; cm.
  Includes bibliographical references and index.
  ISBN-13: 978-1-4051-1409-7 (pbk. : alk. paper)
  ISBN-10: 1-4051-1409-6 (pbk. : alk. paper)
    1. Occupational therapy for older people.   I. McIntyre, Anne.   II. Atwal, Anita.
  [DNLM: 1. Occupational Therapy–Aged.   2. Rehabilitation–Aged.
  WB 555 O14117 2005]

  RC953.8.O22O22 2005
  615.8′515′0846–dc22
                                                                         2004023191

ISBN-13 978-14051-1409-7
ISBN-10 1-4051-1409-6

A catalogue record for this title is available from the British Library

Set in 10/12.5pt Sabon
by Graphicraft Limited, Hong Kong
Printed and bound in India
by Replika Press Pvt. Ltd, Kundli

The publisher's policy is to use permanent paper from mills that operate a sustainable forestry
policy, and which has been manufactured from pulp processed using acid-free and elementary
chlorine-free practices. Furthermore, the publisher ensures that the text paper and cover board
used have met acceptable environmental accreditation standards.

For further information on Blackwell Publishing, visit our website:
www.blackwellnursing.com

OCCUPATIONAL THERAPY AND OLDER PEOPLE

CONTENTS

ACKNOWLEDGEMENTS

We would like to thank our parents for being an inspiration to us, and our long-suffering families for their unstinting support.

We would also like to thank Caroline Dunkin, Steven Rice, Harry Thompson, and David and Elizabeth McIntyre for their technical support.

LIST OF CONTRIBUTORS

Stephen Ashford, MSc BSc MCSP PGCE
Former course leader for the MSc in Neurorehabilitation at Brunel University.
Now clinical specialist in physiotherapy and research physiotherapist, The
Regional Rehabilitation Unit, Northwick Park Hospital, London.

Anita Atwal, PhD MSc DipCOT
Lecturer in Occupational Therapy, School of Health Sciences and Social Care. Brunel
University, Middlesex.

Helen Barrett, BA(Hons) BSc(Hons)
Senior I Occupational Therapist, The Royal Marsden Hospital, Surrey.

Wendy Bryant, MSc DipCOT
Lecturer in Occupational Therapy, School of Health Sciences and Social Care., Brunel
University, Middlesex.

Alexandra Farrow, PhD MSc BSc MRSC
Course director: MSc Occupational Health & Safety Management, School of
Health Sciences and Social Care, Brunel University.

Linda Gnanasekaran, MSc BSc(Hons) DipCOT ILTM
Lecturer in Occupational Therapy, School of Health Sciences and Social Care, Brunel
University, Middlesex.

Mary Grant, MSc DipCOT
Postgraduate research student, School of Allied Health Professions, University of
East Anglia, Norwich.

Wendy Gregson, BSc(Hons) Occ Therapy
Senior 1 Occupational Therapist in Respiratory Medicine, Royal London Hospital,
London.

Zoe Harvey-Lee, BSc(Hons)OT SROT
Occupational Therapist.

Anna Kittel, BSc(Hons) Dip COT
Senior I Occupational Therapist, Marie Curie Hospice, Surrey.

Kee Hean Lim, MSc Dip COT
Lecturer in Occupational Therapy, School of Health Sciences and Social Care, Brunel
University, Middlesex.

Jill Lloyd, BA MCSP
Senior Lecturer in Physiotherapy, School of Health Sciences and Social Care, Brunel University, Middlesex.

Alice Mackenzie, MSc, BSc OT (C), Dip COT
Lecturer in Occupational Therapy, School of Health Sciences and Social Care, Brunel University, Middlesex.

Anne McIntyre, MSc PGcertTLHE DipCOT
Lecturer in Occupational Therapy, School of Health Sciences and Social Care, Brunel University, Middlesex.

Trudi Minns, MSc BSc
Chief Speech and Language Therapist, The Regional Rehabilitation Unit, Northwick Park Hospital, London.

Frances Reynolds, PhD Dip.Psych.Couns. AFBPsS BSc(Hons)
Senior Lecturer in Psychology, School of Health Sciences and Social Care, Brunel University, Middlesex.

Marcus Sivell-Muller, MPhil PGDipOT BA(Hons). FRAI.
Lecturer in Occupational Therapy, School of Health Sciences and Social Care, Brunel University, Middlesex.

Kirsty Tattersall, BSc Occ. Therapy
Senior Occupational Therapist, Hounslow Primary Care Trust.

Lindy van den Berghe, BMedSci BM BS
Editor and Managing Director, First Line Medical Communications Ltd
Marlow, Bucks.

Lesley Wilson, MSc BSc DipCOT CMS PGCertTLHE
Lecturer in Occupational Therapy, School of Health Sciences and Social Care, Brunel University, Middlesex

Alison Warren, MSc, Dip COT
Lecturer in Occupational Therapy, School of Health Sciences and Social Care, Brunel University, Middlesex.

Ann A Wilcock, PhD(Adel), GradDipPublicHealth(Adel), BAppScOT(UniSA), DipCOT(UK)
Professor of Occupational Science and Therapy, School of Health and Social Development, Deakin University, Waterfront Campus, Geelong, Victoria, Australia.

HOW TO USE THIS BOOK

Working with older people is a rapidly developing and exciting area of practice for occupational therapists. In response to government policies and legislation around the world, occupational therapists are changing how and where they work to serve the needs of older people. Older people themselves have different expectations of services, with the 'baby-boomers' entering older age with very different experiences and attitudes, expecting a quality of life that their parents and grandparents would not have dreamed of.

It is hoped that this book will both inspire and be a working reference for students of occupational therapy and those who are new to working with older people. The drivers for this book are international and national changes in social policy and legislation; emphasis on public health and wellbeing; proposed radical changes in the occupational therapy profession; and the introduction of the World Health Organisation's International Classification of Functioning, Disability and Health (2001) (ICF) as a universal model to promote health and wellbeing. These drivers will lead occupational therapists to radically change their practice with older people.

Many older people are referred to occupational therapy services with multiple difficulties in their occupational performance, and not all of these are caused by a pathological process. The move away from a medical model of ageing, disability and illness is therefore necessary. To this purpose this book uses the ICF (WHO 2001) as a framework to help the reader consider the issues impacting upon an older person, irrespective of a diagnostic 'label', and the ICF (WHO 2001) is discussed in Chapter 1.

This book is problem focused as opposed to condition focused and therefore steers away from being a 'pathology' based text. The book also wishes to reflect the biological, psychological and social elements of health and wellbeing and therefore the chapters of this book follow the framework of the ICF and the domains provide the operational definitions within the chapters. However Chapter 5 does consider some of the more common pathologies of older age. Chapter 1 introduces core issues that impact on practice – such as theories and concepts of ageing, the challenges for occupational therapists working with older people, as well as discussing the ICF. The emergence of occupational science as a new discipline enables us to consider the core values of occupational therapy within the contextual factor of occupational justice and deprivation, and these are discussed in Chapter 2. Chapters 3, 4 and 10 consider other contextual factors such as the social, legislative, natural and human made environment. As most of the authors live and work in England, their experience mostly derives from English settings. However, the themes discussed in this book have a broader national and international context. Examples from an international setting are introduced where appropriate, as is the international literature. Chapters 6–9 consider the body functions and structures and activity and participation issues of older people.

Whilst considering the challenges of working with older people, this book will encourage practitioners to view the strengths of older people and the ageing process. Fictitious case studies have been used to provide examples and these have been presented in boxes, along with further information and some suggested activities for the reader. Key words have been highlighted in bold to identify links between chapters.

Reference

World Health Organisation (2001) *The International Classification of Functioning Disability and Health*. Geneva: WHO.

Chapter 1

INTRODUCTION

Anne McIntyre and Anita Atwal

Ageing is a process that occupational therapists cannot ignore, for globally there will be 1.2 billion people over the age of 60 by the year 2025, and by 2050 these figures will have doubled, with 80% of older people living in developing countries (WHO 2002). However, instead of considering increasing life expectancy as a success story it is commonly viewed with doom and gloom, often associated with the belief that old age equals dependency, requiring more money to pay for additional health and social care. Yet healthy older people should be considered a precious resource, making important contributions to their families, communities and the economy at large, by either paid or voluntary employment (WHO 2002). Butler (1975:12) who first used the term 'ageism' suggests that we have a 'deep and profound prejudice against the elderly. Such attitudes need to be challenged and eradicated.' This is of particular importance to occupational therapists, for as a profession, we have a core role to enhance occupational performance utilising client-centred rehabilitation and health promotion techniques.

The 'doom and gloom' approach to older people can be traced to relative unglamorous background of older people's medicine. The original role of the geriatrician was to manage the patients of the chronic long-stay institutions, with no access to the general hospital. This changed following the work of Marjory Warren in the 1930s, who demonstrated that older people who resided in workhouses had treatable diseases that responded well to rehabilitation. In 1947 the British Medical Association recommended that specific geriatric units should be set up to treat older people. The word 'geriatric' was created by Igantz Nascher in 1906 whose initiatives inspired social and biological research on ageing (Grimley-Evans 1997). Since then different names have been used for older people's services, such as 'care of the elderly' or 'geriatrics'. These terms are seen as demeaning and imply that older people need to be cared for. Consequently throughout this book the term 'older people' will be used to reflect the spirit of current health and social care background.

Indeed the unglamorous and low prestige of older people's services has resulted in many professionals (including occupational therapists) not wanting to work within this speciality. This book aims at moving away from depicting old people as a problem and from the attitude that society gains little from older people. This ethos is reflected in the term 'active ageing' adopted by the World Health Organisation (WHO 2002). Active ageing signifies an important paradigm shift: that is away

Box 1.1

> **What is active ageing?**
> 'The process of optimising opportunities for health, participation and security in order to enhance quality of life as people age.'
>
> (WHO 2002:12)

from a needs-based approach to a rights-based approach, which support the rights and continued participation of older people both in the community and the political process (WHO 2002). One document which reflects the ethos of active ageing in the United Kingdom (UK), is the National Service Framework (NSF) for Older People (DH 2001a). This document has helped to revolutionise the way in which older people's health is managed and the way in which the occupational therapist will work for the next ten years.

What is ageing?

Describing a person as old because they are 65 is simplistic and convenient, when clinical experience and research tells us that older people vary considerably in their abilities and outlook, with many 75-year-olds having a younger attitude than those years their junior. The NSF for Older People (DH 2001a) has also recognised that older people are not a homogenous group and suggest that older people could belong to three broader groups –

- Those entering old age.
- Those in transition between healthy old age and frailty.
- Frail older people.

However chronological age is commonly used as a basis for entry into or exit from many services, screening and investigations and it is considered that such age discrimination should not continue.

Ageing is inevitable and how and why we age has been scrutinised by many over the centuries. More recent theories are of interest as they will impact on how older people perceive themselves and how they are perceived by their families, health and social care professionals and society. Biological ageing could be said to begin at conception (*in utero*) or from the age of 30 when physiological decline becomes more apparent. Past theories of biological ageing have considered that an organism is programmed to live for a set period of time (for example four score years and ten), with an 'ageing' gene that determines when we will die (Hayflick & Moorhead, 1961). However not all structures and functions deteriorate at the same time or rate. The more recent evolution theory considers that organisms are genetically programmed to live rather than die (Kirkwood 2002). Kirkwood (2003) suggests that our survival is determined by 25% genetic inheritance and 75% by lifestyle, such as nutrition, physical activity, freedom from disease and trauma, as well as living and working in **healthy environments**. Evolution theory considers that ageing occurs because of an accumulation of mutations within cells because of oxidative stress caused by the presence of free radicals. The speed at which cells become defective will be affected by our genetic inheritance, lifestyle, or environment (Kirkwood 2002). This theory suggests that ageing is to some extent malleable and within our control. Such malleability is also considered with the co-existence of disability with older age. Other theories consider that disability is not caused by ageing, but strongly associated with it, and that healthy lifestyles can delay the onset of disability, compressing morbidity into fewer and later years (Fries 1980).

Not all theories are concerned with biological ageing. Psychological ageing is considered to occur at any time, involving the concepts of maturity, wisdom and senility. Not all functions are said to deteriorate with age, with experience and acquisition of knowledge increasing whilst reaction times decline (Woodruff-Pak 1997). Aspects of social ageing also vary. It is evident that many older people are disadvantaged by social class inequalities, in terms of life expectancy and successful ageing, in both the UK, and elsewhere in the world (WHO 2003). Changes can be experienced by the individual in terms of change of role and relationships within the family and work, in terms of both positive and negative attitudes within their social environment. Sociological theories encompass:

- Erikson's theory of psychosocial development (1950). Older people reach the stage of 'integrity versus despair', where they are able to accept their past life and prepare for death.
- Disengagement theory (Cumming & Hurry 1961). Older people turn inward, withdrawing from society and family in preparation for death. This eases the way for the eventual loss of the older person and leaves the way free for younger people. This is more noticeable in terminal illness and also 'abandonment' of the older person in residential care far away from family and friends.
- Activity theory (Neugarten *et al.* 1968). Successful ageing, happiness and fulfilment occur as a result of participation in social and family activities.

Professional and personal attitudes to older people's **activity** and **participation** will vary according to the theoretical stance on ageing adopted. For example, if we view ageing as an inevitable decline in all functions from our 40s onwards, the expectations of activity and participation in a 70-year-old will be less than that of a 50-year-old. However, as many older people (including those considered as 'the oldest old') live highly active lives – in sport, in full-time employment, as volunteers, carers and in lifelong education, their lifestyles support evolution, compression of morbidity and activity theories in that body functions and systems can be maintained and optimised by regular physical, cognitive and social activity. The following chapters reinforce that a great variability (or heterogeneity) in occupational performance can be observed in older people. It is therefore important not to assume a decline in functioning in all older adults of the same age, but

Box 1.2

> 'The word *active* refers to continuing participation in social, economic, cultural, spiritual and civic affairs, not just the ability to be physically active or participate in the labour force.'
>
> WHO (2002:12)

to consider each person as an individual, as dictated by core occupational therapy client-centred values.

Active ageing

Current thinking considers that client- (or person)-centred policies and services should focus on **active ageing** (WHO 2002), otherwise described as 'successful ageing and living well in later life' (Wistow *et al.* 2003), with successful ageing entailing control and interdependence (empowerment) rather than choices and independence.

Research of successful ageing points to a proactive and promotional approach, rather than a slowing down of inevitable decline. These approaches mean that occupational therapists need to be more aware of the health promotional aspects of their interventions and reinstate rehabilitation programmes. Older people give successful ageing a multidimensional definition, including physical and psychological health (being disease-free), functional health and social health (active engagement with life) (Phelan *et al.* 2004). What is of overriding interest and should have impact on occupational therapy, is that social and productive activities in older life reduce mortality risks as much as fitness activities (Glass *et al.* 1999). The evidence for such behavioural interventions continues to strengthen, with Cassel (2002) suggesting that continued social, physical and mental activities should be combined with biomedical and pharmacological interventions to enhance physical and mental health and capacity, thus changing how health care is organised and delivered.

It is therefore important that old age is not medicalised and treated as a disease. However many older people do see disability in older age as inevitable, having more negative perceptions of themselves and older age. Such negativity leads them to have low expectations of themselves and services, dismissing declining body functions and activity participation as part of old age, rather than part of a new and treatable disability (Sarkisian *et al.* 2002). These negative attitudes of older people and society need to be carefully monitored and altered as part of a wider prevention scheme.

Another aspect of successful ageing and living well in later life is that of 'dying well' or a 'good death' (Wistow *et al.* 2003). Person-centred care is just as necessary in dying as it is in life and it has been argued that death has been medicalised in the same way as old age has been, so that death is seen as a failing of medical science rather than as a certainty (Smith 2000).

Box 1.3

> Age Concern produced a Policy Position Paper titled *'End of Life Issues'* (Age Concern 2002). This discusses death and dying in older age, including current public policy, and can be accessed on:
> http://www.ageconcern.org.uk/AgeConcern/media/EndoflifepppSept2002.pdf

Challenges for occupational therapy

Health promotion

Much of what determines successful or active ageing fits perfectly within the occupational therapy philosophy of Occupation; that is the 'doing' to enable health and wellbeing. However, the role of occupational therapy within health promotion still needs to be further developed. In the UK, this role has been directly influenced by Wilcock (1998, 2002) who sets out strong arguments for the role of occupational therapists as health promoters in the public health arena. Her main proposition is that occupational therapy must extend beyond the amelioration of illness and become directly involved with the promotion of optimal states of health in line with health-promoting philosophies (see also Chapter 10).

The term 'health promotion' was used for the first time in the mid-1970s (Lalonde 1974). An early influence on the thinking of health promotion was a story by McKinlay (1979) (see Box 1.4).

Box 1.4

> A man rescues a drowning man from the river and gives him artificial respiration, as this man begins to breathe, another drowning man appears, he is pulled out and artificial respiration is given and then another cry, and another, is heard. The first man is too busy downstream giving artificial respiration to be able to see upstream why these people are falling in the river.
>
> McKinlay (1979)

Here McKinlay (1979) describes the different types of health promotion which are commonly known as primary, secondary and tertiary health promotion, which therapists may not have appreciated before:

- Primary health promotion (upstream activity) – targeting the well population and aiming at preventing ill health and disability. For occupational therapists this means working with well older people (see Clark *et al.* 1997).
- Secondary health promotion (midstream) – directed at individuals or groups to change health-damaging habits and/or to prevent ill health evolving to a chronic or irreversible stage and, where possible, to restore people to their former state

of health. For example, teaching accident prevention techniques in falls prevention programmes.

- Tertiary health promotion (downstream) – takes place with individuals who have chronic conditions and/or who are disabled, to make the most of their potential. With older people, occupational therapists are already actively involved in rehabilitation and the provision of assistive products and technology.

It is evident that occupational therapists are already involved in different types of health promotion with older people. However a recent study by Flannery & Barry (2003) concluded that the greatest perceived barrier to occupational therapists making a praxis shift to becoming health promoters were limited resources, including time, staffing levels and funds.

Interprofessional working

Occupational therapy older people's services have grown rapidly since the introduction of the National Health Service and Community Care Act in 1990 and are now seeing more change since the arrival of the NSF for Older People (DH 2001a). Multidisciplinary teamwork is a key mechanism through which care to older people especially is managed in health and social care services throughout the world. Consequently, it is important that occupational therapists are comfortable and competent with interprofessional, interagency and multisector working. The occupational therapy literature offers very little evidence as to how therapists collaborate with their health and social care colleagues. Furthermore, the effectiveness of this policy is still a matter for debate, and hard research evidence as to the impact of interprofessional collaboration on patient care is lacking (Zwarenstein & Reeves 2000). However, interprofessional practice brings with it many challenges. Caldwell & Atwal (2003) have outlined these in relation to fundamental ideological differences existing between the health care professions; unequal power relations between the members of the hospital team can be seen to constrain effective teamwork. Communication within and between health care professionals is often complex and ineffective, with role overlap and confusion. In order to resolve these difficulties it is essential that the profession consider how it will enable occupational therapists to not only be skilled team players, but also how it will manage issues such as interprofessional education, role boundaries, evidence-based practice and the image of the profession.

Evidence-based practice

Occupational therapists working in older people services face several challenges if they are to contribute to and promote active or successful ageing. A major challenge is to ensure that practice is evidence-based, for there is little research available that demonstrates the effectiveness of occupational therapy with older people. This in turn will mean more randomised control trials to complement qualitative research. Grimley-Evans (1997:1066) in the *British Medical Journal* states that the most pressing problem that faces older people's medicine is 'how to ensure both clinical

Box 1.5 Methodological issues in research with older people.

Subject selection

Even though chronological age is considered *not* to be a good determinant of ageing this is often used for subject selection.

How old is old? Is it 55 and upwards or 75 and upwards?

Are all older people considered as one group?

There is greater variability between 70-year-olds in activity performance than there is between 40 to 50-year-olds (Rabbitt 1997).

Have subjects been fully screened for absence or presence of pathology in studies of normal ageing?

What is the definition of frail? Or mild, moderate or severe disability?

Choice of design

Surveys of client satisfaction are often skewed with older people often reluctant to express criticism (Atwal and Caldwell, in press).

Involving older people in the construction of satisfaction questionnaires would however enhance reliability and validity (Sixma *et al.* 2000).

Cross sectional designs are favoured in quantitative methodology but are affected by heterogeneity of the sample.

Longitudinal studies eradicate the possible bias of heterogeneity but suffer from participant attrition and repeated measures effect.

Outcome measures

Many standardised outcome measures of activity and participation are based on what a client can do (capacity) rather than what they do do (performance), with evidence of significant differences between older people's capacity and performance. It is therefore important to ensure the method of assessment is fully described (Bootsma-van der Wiel *et al.* 2001).

A definition of 'with help' is also important, as this often means taking over of an activity rather than assistance.

and research excellence without threatening the essential link between them; [this] is now perhaps the single most important issue for geriatrics'. There are many methodological issues in current research, and it is important to consider these when reading and analysing it (see Box 1.5).

Older people are often excluded from research because they are considered a vulnerable group (DH 2001b) or more worryingly, are excluded for no apparent reason (Bayer & Tadd 2000). Older people with dementia are excluded even more so from research (Wilkinson 2002). Such exclusion feeds the negative stereotype of old age, disempowering and marginalising older people from the benefits of research. The exclusion of 'normal' older people from clinical trials means that there is a lack of baseline data for many tests and investigations of body functions and structures, impacting upon their response to medication as well as surgical intervention, for example. It is important that occupational therapy research and that of other disciplines, take these issues on board, and more importantly involve older people in the planning and carrying out of the research process.

Use of the ICF

The International Classification of Functioning, Disability and Health (ICF) is a member of the WHO's group of classifications devised to provide a global language and classification. It can be linked with the ICD-10, which considers diagnosis and disease, whereas the ICF considers health and wellbeing, in terms of the way we function in the context of our lives. The ICF supersedes the ICIDH (1980) and was also known as the ICIDH-2 until November 2001.

Box 1.6

> The ICF can be accessed and explained in more detail on:
> http://www.who.int/classifcation/icf and also in the *Guidance for the Use of the International Classification of Functioning, Disability and Health* and the *Ottawa Charter for Health Promotion in Occupational Therapy Services* produced by the College of Occupational Therapists (COT 2004).

The ICF has been adopted by occupational therapy associations and bodies in the UK, Canada, USA, Australia and Scandinavia as a model of health and disability, because of its person–context interaction. It is not an occupational therapy specific model, but is a universally devised and accepted tool, involving many professions, organisations and user groups from around the world in its construction. It was devised for all agencies and not just health and social care. It therefore considers itself a bio-psycho-social model of functioning, applying to all people throughout the world. Even though it is used as a means of collecting data it also provides a framework to consider the occupational performance of individuals and how this is impacted by extrinsic factors. It therefore fits in with the ideals of client-centred practice. It is useful for interprofessional and interagency working as a 'common ground' or language for communication and intervention planning.

In the past the consequences of health conditions were considered in terms of mortality rates, however the ICF provides us with an opportunity to collect evidence of what older people can and cannot do. It enables us to consider the links between intrinsic factors from a health condition and also the contextual barriers or facilitators that impact upon their functioning. The ICF considers that the different elements within the classification can interact to a lesser or greater degree, rather than having a causal or hierarchical effect (see Figure 1.1). For example, an older person may not have any **impairment** or **activity limitation** but may have **participation restriction** because of the attitudes of the society in which he lives (**environmental factor**).

The main components of the ICF are **body functions** and **structures, activity, participation** and the personal and **environmental contextual factors**. This fits easily with OT thinking of the person–environment–occupation interaction described in models of **occupational performance** (Christiansen & Baum 1991). Each component can be described and defined in a positive or negative way (e.g. impairment

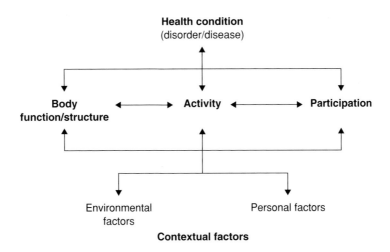

Figure 1.1 The World Health Organisation's International Classification of Functioning, Disability and Health (WHO 2001:18). Permission to use this figure kindly granted by the WHO.

of body structure or function). Each of the **body functions** and **structures** are considered by systems rather than organs, because of overlapping functions of many structures. **Activity** and **participation** can be considered in terms of **activity limitation** and **participation restriction**, with **environmental factors** described in terms of potential facilitators or barriers for the client's **activity** or **participation**. For example, an older person may be facilitated in going to their adult education classes by using the dial-a-ride service, but the barrier of a waiting list means that they cannot get to use this on a regular weekly basis.

Each of the components is subdivided into separate domains and these are defined within the ICF providing much needed universal definitions of self-care and mobility for example. The reader is advised to explore these on the ICF website mentioned above in Box 1.5.

Use of the ICF as a framework

For many of our older clients, the interaction of the normal ageing process, pathological processes and the environment impact on functioning causing disability. Consider Mrs Anand's story in Box 1.7.

Mrs Anand's problems have been identified using the ICF as a framework in Figure 1.2. The ICF codes have also been included so that the reader can consult the classification and definitions on the ICF website.

Using the ICF as a framework to identify Mrs Anand's problems helps to establish the most appropriate intervention and outcome measurement. The choice of intervention can be determined by the occupational therapist and the organisation's beliefs, philosophy and theoretical model. For example, the occupational therapist may have a rehabilitation approach and be concerned about Mrs Anand's activity limitations that are related to her impairments – such as fatigue, endurance and energy levels, so that the outcome measure may consider Mrs Anand's capacity to

Box 1.7

Mrs Anand started attending her local day hospital whilst recovering from tuberculosis. Before her illness, Mrs Anand liked cooking for her grandchildren, but afterwards became too fatigued and apprehensive with all kitchen activities. As a result, Mrs Anand's busy daughter cooked meals for her and her husband.

The occupational therapist took Mrs Anand into the OT kitchen and was able to observe and talk to Mrs Anand whilst they make a cup of tea together. The occupational therapist identified those tasks that Mrs Anand found problematic and considered how these could be resolved. Initially the occupational therapist provided Mrs Anand with a perching stool and advised her of other compensatory and energy saving techniques, so that she could work safely in her own kitchen and start cooking again. As Mrs Anand's fatigue lessened and confidence grew, the occupational therapist continued to take Mrs Anand into the OT kitchen gradually encouraging Mrs Anand to stand for longer, both with and without support, by altering the demands of the kitchen tasks, using them as a means of addressing her impaired performance skills. Eventually Mrs Anand was able to cook for her grandchildren safely and confidently, returning the equipment the occupational therapist had provided, as she no longer needed them.

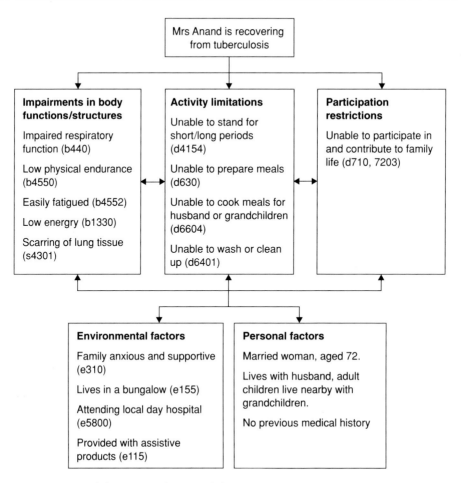

Figure 1.2 Use of the ICF as a framework for practice.

prepare a meal in relation to how long it is before she becomes fatigued, or even the length of time she can stand for. As Mrs Anand's impairments diminish, the activity demands increase and the environmental facilitators may be gradually removed to encourage Mrs Anand's capacity within any environment. Mrs Anand's family will also need to be involved so they can assist her in carrying out kitchen activities – working alongside her and recognising how her impairments may limit her activity, instead of taking the task over. If a compensatory approach is utilised, then Mrs Anand's activity limitations will be considered in terms of her environmental facilitators and barriers. The outcome measure and intervention will account for these issues – such as a well-organised kitchen with easily accessible cupboards and space for a perching stool, the amount or type of help that Mrs Anand may get from her anxious daughter or husband with no domestic skills. The intervention will be directed at providing the appropriate assistive products and services, which will either allow Mrs Anand to make meals independently or with the assistance of others, or will provide Mrs Anand and her husband with meals so that Mrs Anand does not have to attempt to prepare them.

Using the ICF as a framework not only highlights the areas of importance for the client and therapy services but also can clarify roles, identify areas of overlap and discrepancies in service provision when working in interprofessional and interagency teams where roles seem to be blurred. Using the ICF can avoid two services working at odds with each other – one with a rehabilitative approach (working on activity capacity) and another with a compensatory one (working on activity performance) with the same client.

Summary

This chapter has sought to provide the reader with an introduction to theories and concepts of ageing which will influence occupational therapy practice. Current challenges to the profession have been discussed – such as interprofessional and interagency working, the emerging role of occupational therapy in health promotion, evidence-based practice and the use of the WHO's International Classification of Functioning, Disability and Health (ICF) as a universal model and language for practice. Many of these aspects will be referred to in later chapters and the reader is reminded of the use of keywords highlighted in bold to facilitate cross-referencing.

References

Age Concern (2002) *End of Life Issues. A Policy Position Paper*. London: Age Concern.
Age Positive (2003) Tackling age discrimination and promoting age diversity in employment. Accessed 11.01.2004. Http://www.agepositive.gov.uk/template2.cfm?sectionid=55.
Atwal A & Caldwell K (2005) The enigma of satisfaction surveys. *Australian Occupational Therapy Journal* (in press).
Bayer A & Tadd W (2000) Unjustified exclusion of elderly people from studies submitted to research ethics committee for approval: descriptive study. *British Medical Journal* 321, 992–993.

Bootsma-van der Wiel A, Gussekloo J, de Craen AJM *et al.* (2001) Disability in the oldest-old: can do or 'do do'? *Journal of the American Geriatrics Society* 49(7), 909–914.

Butler RN (1975) *Why Survive? Being Old in America.* New York: Harper and Row.

Caldwell K & Atwal A (2003) The problems of interprofessional health care practice in the hospital setting. *British Journal of Nursing* 20(12), 1212–1218.

Cassel CK (2002) Use it or lose it: activity may be the best treatment for aging. *Journal of the American Medical Association* 288(18), 2333–2335.

Christiansen C & Baum C (1991) *Occupational Therapy: Overcoming Human Performance Deficits.* Thorofare, NJ: Slack Inc.

Clark F, Azen SP, Zemke R *et al.* (1997) Occupational therapy for independent-living older adults: a randomised controlled trial. *Journal of the American Medical Association* 278(16), 1321–1326.

College of Occupational Therapy (2004) *Guidance for the use of the International Classification of Functioning, Disability and Health and the Ottawa Charter for Health Promotion in Occupational Therapy Services.* London: College of Occupational Therapists.

Cumming E & Hurry WE (1961) *Growing Old: The Process of Disengagement.* New York: Basic Books Inc.

Department of Health (2001a) *National Service Framework for Older People.* London: HMSO.

Department of Health (2001b) *Seeking Consent: Working with Older People.* London: HMSO.

Erikson E (1950) *Childhood and Society.* Middlesex: Penguin.

Flannery G & Barry M (2003) An exploration of occupational therapists' perceptions of health promotion. *The Irish Journal of Occupational Therapy* Winter.

Fries JF (1980) Aging, natural death and the compression of morbidity. *New England Journal of Medicine* 303(3), 130–135.

Glass TA, de Leon CM, Marottoli RA, Berkman LF (1999) Population based study of social and productive activities as predictors of survival among elderly Americans. *British Medical Journal* 319, 478–483.

Grimley-Evans J (1997) Geriatric medicine: a brief history. *British Medical Journal* 315, 1075–1077.

Hayflick L & Moorhead PS (1961) The serial cultivation of human diploid cell strains. *Experimental Cell Research*, 25(3), 585–621.

Kirkwood TBL (2002) Evolution of ageing. *Mechanisms of Ageing and Development* 123(7), 737–745.

Kirkwood TBL (2003) The most pressing problem of our age. *British Medical Journal* 326, 1297–1299.

Lalonde M (1974) *A New Perspective on the Health of Canadians.* Ottawa: Information Canada.

McKinlay JB (1979) A case for refocusing upstream: the political economy of health. In: Javco EG (ed.) *Patients, Physicians and Illness.* Basingstoke: Macmillan.

Peto R & Doll R (1997) There is no such thing as ageing. *British Medical Journal* 315, 1030–1032.

Neugarten BL, Havinghurst RJ, Tobin SS (1968) Personality and patterns of aging. In: Neugarten BL (ed.) *Middle Age and Aging.* Chicago: University of Chicago Press, pp. 173–177.

Phelan EA, Anderson LA, LaCroix AZ, Larson EB (2004) Older adults views of 'successful ageing'. How do they compare with researchers definitions? *Journal of the American Geriatrics Society* 52(2), 211–216.

Rabbitt P (1997) Ageing and human skill: a 40th anniversary. *Ergonomics* 40(10), 962–981.

Sarkisian CA, Hays R, Mangione CM (2002) Do older adults expect to age successfully? The association between expectations regarding aging and beliefs regarding healthcare seeking among older adults. *Journal of the American Geriatrics Society* 50(11), 1837–1843.

Sixma HJ, van Campden C, Kerssens JJ, Peters L (2000) Quality of care from the perspective of elderly people: the QUOTE-Elderly instrument. *Age and Ageing* 29(2), 173–178.

Smith R (2000) A good death. *British Medical Journal* 320, 129–130.

Wilcock AA (1998) Occupations for health. *British Journal of Occupational Therapy* 61(8), 340–345.

Wilcock AA (2002) *Occupation for Health, Volume 2: A Journey from Prescription to Self Health*. London: College of Occupational Therapists.

Wilkinson H (2002) Including people with dementia in research: methods and motivations. In: Wilkinson H (ed.) *The Perspectives of People with Dementia: Research Methods and Motivations*. London: Jessica Kingsley.

Wistow G, Waddington E, Godfrey M (2003) *Living Well in Later Life: From Prevention to Promotion*. Leeds. Nuffield Institute for Health.

Woodruff-Pak DS (1997) *The Neuropsychology of Aging*. Malden USA: Blackwell Publishing.

World Health Organisation (1986) *Ottawa Charter for Health Promotion*. 1st International Conference on Health Promotion Ottawa, 21st November 1986. (WHO/HPR/95.1). Accessed 05.04.2004. http://www.who.int/hpr/NPH/docs/ottawa_charter_hp.pdf.

World Health Organisation (2001) *The International Classification of Functioning Disability and Health*. Geneva: WHO.

World Health Organisation (2002) *Active Ageing. A Policy Framework*. Geneva: WHO.

World Health Organisation (2003) *Social Determinants of Health: The Solid Facts*, 2nd edn. Wilkinson R & Marmot M (eds). Geneva: WHO.

Zwarenstein M & Reeves S (2000) What's so great about collaboration? We need more evidence and less rhetoric. *British Medical Journal* 320, 1022–1023.

Chapter 2
OLDER PEOPLE AND OCCUPATIONAL JUSTICE

Ann A. Wilcock

Introduction

Occupational therapists, from early in the profession's twentieth century history, have held views that resonate with a largely unarticulated belief in people's right to engage in occupations of meaning to them. This idea, whilst bound up for occupational therapists in concepts of health and the remediation or adaptation to illness and disability, embodies the notion of the right to such occupations being a matter of justice. That right is encapsulated in the emerging term – occupational justice. It will be considered with respect to older people in this chapter.

From an occupational perspective, two vastly different visions of older people provide a snapshot of western views of ageing. One is of a seated row of sleepy, unresponsive men and women wrapped in crocheted blankets, isolated and alone in front of a blaring unwatched television. The other is of energised vibrancy as older performers strut their 'stuff' in front of bemused audiences at arts festivals ready to take to the road again towards another performance. The latter occupationally dynamic vision suggests that the world is still the potential oyster for those who dare. The former occupationally empty vision, is a much more common reality and one that many people fear may be their ultimate fate. Such disparate realities lead to questions about whether or not either is a matter of choice, a matter of cultural expectations, a matter of economic necessity, a matter of health or illness, a matter of access or, even, a matter of justice. Either extreme or the range of possibilities between them conjure up a number of questions about what enables or empowers older adults to maintain or invent a lifestyle that allows them to continue to grow and develop in ways meaningful to each of them.

This chapter will introduce the notion of occupational justice in terms of older people being able to engage in the occupations of their need and choice. It is an important concept to bear in mind in any text that addresses intervention strategies to enable older people to lead satisfying and healthy lives that facilitate exercise of capacities and continuing growth. This is particularly so because occupation is intimately related with health, wellbeing, morbidity and mortality. Indeed this is the premise upon which occupational therapy exists. It is a premise that is only now becoming recognised within advanced health and social care research.

With such recognition, not to provide opportunities for health-giving occupations can be considered a matter of injustice.

It is not just any occupation or activity that is **health-promoting** in an ultimate sense. Occupations can lead to both negative and positive health outcomes (Wilcock 1998). The effects can differ from person to person, and be socially and contextually linked. It is imperative to give consideration to what, why and how the occupations of older people provide them with physical, mental and social exercise in a way that has meaning for each and every one of them. Additionally, for individuals to reach towards their potential as part of an **active ageing** process, occupations must also provide them with opportunity to meet unique occupational wants and needs.

It is easy to marginalise the occupational wants and needs of people beyond paid employment years. Commonly and patronisingly this can be in the name of risk management. There is general acceptance that risk management is a necessary and admirable objective within advanced western societies despite the fact that, in many ways, it encourages restrictive, externally imposed strategies that can disempower recipients. Risk management strategies fail in many respects to recognise individual experience or potential, or the morbidity and mortality links between what people do or do not do. In that way it does not appreciate that lack of balanced, health-maintaining, and satisfying occupation can be a risk in itself, and that restriction of occupational aspirations can be viewed as a matter of discriminatory practice and occupational injustice. It is becoming an issue more and more imperative to address because of the increasing numbers of older people in comparison to the world's population as a whole. As the United Nations explained, the ageing of populations is a 'pervasive, unprecedented and enduring process with profound social and economic implications' (Gordon 2001:1002). Justice with regards to opportunities for occupations of need, meaning and choice has both profound social and economic implications.

To address concerns such as these, the chapter will consider several key global concepts with particular reference to older people living in post-industrial western societies. To substantiate the claims that occupational justice is an issue worthy of occupational therapists pursuing, the links between occupation, morbidity, mortality and health promotion will be discussed briefly. Those considerations will highlight common attitudes and approaches that are antithetical to occupational justice at legislative, societal and personal levels. However the place to start is with consideration of personalised occupational engagement as a right, and reflection about that as a matter of social justice.

Occupation as a right

In Vienna in 1982 the United Nations (UN) held the first World Assembly on Ageing. A report that followed of the Resolutions taken by the General Assembly of the UN included recognition that:

'. . . the aged are an asset not a liability to society because of the invaluable contribution they can make by virtue of their accumulated wealth of knowledge and
experience' (UN 1982:1186).

The Assembly reaffirmed that the Universal Declaration of Human Rights:

'. . . apply fully and undiminished to the ageing and recognised that the quality
of life was no less important than the longevity, and that the ageing should
therefore, as far as possible, be enabled to enjoy in their own families and communities a life of fulfillment, health, security and contentment, appreciated as
an integral part of society' (UN 1982:1186).

Such statements support the need for those who are older being able to continue
to fulfill their occupational needs and wants in ways that enhance each person's
potential and growth.

Continuing in that theme, by 1989 the UN was recommending the growth of
policies and programmes for and by older people that reflect biological, social,
and economic aspects of ageing as well as demographics and epidemiology. They
argued for the establishment or strengthening of national machinery to 'ensure that
the humanitarian needs and developmental potential of the aged' were adequately
addressed, and that older people themselves were encouraged and supported to put
into place 'self-help initiatives' (Flynn-Connors 1989:688–689). Not only that, it
was recommended that, where necessary, income-generating projects for and by
older people should be used to enhance their income security (Flynn-Connors 1989).

Ten years on, 1999 saw the 'International Year of Older Persons', when 80 Nations
explored or celebrated in some way the theme 'A Society for All Ages'. The UN
reports stressed a growing consciousness that the ageing of the world's population
presents major challenges to governments around the world. Despite that, meeting older people's occupational needs remained a focus. Issues raised that have
bearing on this subject were:

- Recognition of their human resource potential to society.
- Involvement and consultation with them about their needs.
- Consciousness that discrimination and stereotyping constitutes and leads to
  violations of human rights.
- Encouragement of governments, press and media to play a central role in elim-
  inating stereotypes and discrimination of older persons (Gordon 1999:1125).

By 2001, the UN Year Book continued to centre some of its recommendations
about older people towards women as it had some twelve years earlier. It did so
with the awareness that they constitute the majority of older populations world-
wide. Reports focused on their importance as a human resource that was not fully
recognised. The lack of recognition was partly because few statistics are available
about the situation of older women, and because older women in particular, like
women of all ages, 'continue to suffer from discrimination and lack opportunities'
(Gordon 2001:1086). Positive action was recommended to attend to those issues.

Emphasis was placed on the role of governments in creating enabling environments for the social and economic development of citizens that ensured equal rights and 'full enjoyment for women of all ages' (Gordon 2001:1086). In cooperation with civil societies, governments were also urged to promote the development of programmes for healthy, **active ageing**. These, it was argued, should ensure quality of life and full enjoyment of human rights through active engagement that addressed needs for independence, equality, **participation**, and security.

The World Health Organisation (WHO) picked up on the theme of **active ageing** when it provided a contribution to the second UN's World Assembly on Ageing held in Madrid in 2002. The Organisation developed a Policy Framework for discussion and action to promote healthy ageing (WHO 2002:2). This pointed out that there can be dramatic differences in health status, participation and levels of independence amongst older people of the same age and recommended that policies and programmes for older people needs to take such variations into account, in order to:

- Prevent discriminatory action that can be counterproductive to wellbeing.
- Enable those who are able to continue to contribute to society in important ways (WHO 2002:4).

Also posed were some important questions that could be relevant to issues of human rights and justice from an occupational point of view. These are:

- How do we help people remain independent and active as they age?
- How can we strengthen health promotion and prevention policies especially those directed to older people?
- As people are living longer, how can the quality of life in old age be improved?
- How do we acknowledge and support the major role that people play as they age in caring for others? (WHO 2002:5).

Two other questions that were posed related to economic concerns of the increasing number of older people being seen as likely to overburden health and social welfare systems, and the perceived balancing act between family and state care for people who need assistance as they age.

One further question that arises from this overview of occupation as a human right concerns why there appears to be so little emphasis in health and social welfare literature on encouraging older people to engage in the **active ageing** process. Literature and funded programmes appear to focus on mundane self-care tasks, sedentary occupations that may or may not hold interest for recipients, and risk management to prevent accidents. This may well be because of the increasing litigious nature of western societies or economic concerns about the cost of institutional care. Family members and caregivers, too, are often restrictive or discouraging of active pursuits apparently fearful of detrimental effects on health that may lead to increasing dependence. Whether institutionally or privately constituted such limitations can be viewed as discriminatory and, potentially, as a matter of injustice.

Occupation as a matter of social justice

Justice has been an accepted part of both ancient and modern societies, although its nature has differed somewhat through the ages, often in accord with what people do to obtain the requirements of life. In the post-modern world it visions societies as fair, ethical and moral, holding civic principles that enable the experience of freedom of expression and liberty to go about individual lives, responsibly, without interference but in tune with culturally bound ideas (Rawls 1975; Botes 2000; Metz 2000). Justice is seen as more than measures taken to prevent or protect from abuse, violence or crime. It is also about the right to vote for and participate in civic governance, and the fair allocation and distribution of opportunities, rights, and services as well as goods and resources (Daniels *et al.* 1999; Armstrong 2000). It is usually considered a 'given' from the state – a political and institutional background on which people play out the daily grind as well as their talents and aspirations. Indeed, underlying political decisions that determine justice are seldom obvious in day-to-day discourse. In that regard, justice provides a major part of the underlying and often unstated determinants that guide what people are not allowed to do within societies, how people express themselves and how they are able to go about the lawful occupations they need and want to do.

The concept of social justice is of more recent origin, but it has become an accepted part of post-modern societies. It centres on social relations and conditions that are just regardless of difference in class, income, race, gender, disability, health status, and such like factors. Advocates for social justice work towards social change to decrease discrepancies between those who have more than most and those seen to not have as much as the norm. This is largely achieved by focusing on ethical ways to distribute and share resources, rights, and responsibilities between people.

In the United Kingdom during the early 1990s, Member of Parliament John Smith, set up the Commission on Social Justice. It was an independent body established under the auspices of the Institute for Public Policy Research. Its report stated that the values of social justice are concerned with:

> '. . . the equal worth of all citizens, their equal right to be able to meet basic needs, the need to spread opportunities and life chances as widely as possible, and finally the requirement that we reduce and where possible eliminate unjustified inequalities' (Commission on Social Justice 1994:1).

Four propositions ran through the policies proposed, namely:

- The transformation of 'the welfare state from a safety net in times of trouble to a springboard for economic opportunity'.
- The radical improvement of 'access to education and training' and investment 'in the talent of all our people'.
- The promotion of 'real choices across the life-cycle for men and women in the balance of employment, family, education, leisure and retirement'.
- The reconstruction of the 'social wealth of our country. Social institutions, from the family to local government, must be nurtured to provide a dependable

social environment in which people can lead their lives' (Commission on Social Justice 1994:1–2).

The report argued that taking such a focus would result in social renewal built upon an inclusive society. In an inclusive society rights would carry responsibilities, and individuals would experience opportunities to realise their potential (Commission on Social Justice 1994:3).

Despite the applicability of the propositions to occupational aspects of social justice for all people, the Commission centred discussion about them on people of working age. With regard to older people issues addressed were limited to comments about economic concerns such as pensions. Similarly the OECD in 1988 had responded to the prediction that the number of people over the age of 65 would double by 2040 with concern about the intensification of 'demand for retirement pensions, health services, and social care' (Gilbert 1995:76). Whilst to be applauded, in some regard such responses presume that older people are an inevitable drain rather than possible contributors to the economic fabric of the State. It also suggests that the provision of opportunities to enable older people to continue towards realising their potential is not of prime concern.

Despite systems of social protection endorsed in mainstream political quarters being transformed from welfare to enabling states (Gilbert 1995:151), the omission of strategies to enable older people to play an active role in active societies was, and still is, common in the western world. Like the British Commission on Social Justice, the diplomatic language of other international organisations encouraged the development of active societies by enabling employment and thereby restricting the concept to people under traditional retirement ages (OECD 1989; Kalisch 1991; Gilbert 1995). A Progressive Policy Institute 'blueprint for a new America' to the Clinton administration, for example, recommended:

'. . . the enabling state be organised around the goals of work and individual empowerment . . . Above all, it should help poor Americans develop the capacities they need to liberate themselves from poverty and dependence . . . An enabling strategy should see the poor as the prime agents of their own development, rather than as passive clients of the welfare system' (Marshall & Schram 1993:228).

Noteworthy is the lack of reference to older people, despite the fact that many of them would rate as poor. This can be seen as a reflection of common views that older people are entitled to rest on their laurels, a reflection of post-modern societies' obsession with youth or, simply, a natural oversight. Whatever the cause it is also a matter of both economic oversight and social injustice, particularly when the statistics relating to poverty and illness are revisited.

The relationship between social justice and health has been the subject of numerous investigations, because ill health can result from the inequitable distribution of resources and power. In 1977, the Black Report on 'Inequalities in Health' in Britain, for example, presented a landmark account of the inverse relation between social location and health status and called for a radical overhaul of health services (Hart 1982). Similar results have been found in other western countries such as

Australia (Martin 1976; Broadhead 1985). There, in the same period, approximately 15% of the population suffered from poverty, lack of autonomy or power, with subsequent depression, anxiety, risk-taking, excessive alcohol consumption, and premature death. The old were amongst those suffering most (Opit 1983). Appropriately, the rhetorical commitment to social justice in most liberal economies was challenged at that time. Similar challenges could be made in the present day, often with regard to health and social welfare strategies for older people whether ill or not in a medically defined way.

Occupational therapy is one health profession that assists older people to deal with health and social difficulties. Although social justice issues are implicit in occupational therapy's philosophical base, they have not been well-documented, despite more clients from socially disadvantaged than affluent groups being recipients of its therapy services. In the 1993 Muriel Driver lecture, Townsend advanced the idea that 'enabling people to participate as valued members of society despite diverse or limited potential' is central within the vision of social justice. She worried, though, that it could be 'narrowed to comply with dominant community, managerial and medical approaches to disability and ageing' (Townsend 1993:174–184). At about the same time I was identifying a social justice model of occupational therapy practice, suggesting that issues relating to occupational justice might be their particular focus (Wilcock 1998). In the last few years Townsend and Wilcock have combined their interests to concentrate on exploration of the concept of occupational justice (Wilcock & Townsend 2000; Townsend & Wilcock 2004).

Occupational justice

Occupational justice juxtaposes moral, ethical and political ideas of justice such as rights, fairness, empowerment, and equity with recognition that people are occupational beings who 'be and become' through what they do. It calls for understanding and action by national, civic, institutional, political and organisational systems as well as individuals to enable occupation for both personal and the common good. Closely aligned with social justice to the extent that some people regard them as indivisible, it takes a particular focus that is about all people being able to engage regularly in meaningful and health-giving occupations according to their different needs and talents. Additionally it calls for sociocultural recognition and valuing of different contributions to the fabric of society, without prejudice.

An occupationally just society would be one that provides opportunity for older people as well as younger ones to continue to develop their distinct talents, not straitjacketed by societal or familial expectations. Occupational injustice is possible because the organisation and privileging of occupations is not naturally determined but socially constructed, and taken for granted. Legislative changes that reduce risks can also reduce individuality, freedom of expression or experimentation. Quite frequently occupational opportunity, choice and satisfaction can also be reduced, and that can result in occupational alienation, deprivation or imbalance.

To create occupationally just societies for older people is not without difficulty in capitalist economies. Despite rhetoric to the contrary, such economies embrace social relations and occupational opportunities that sustain inequalities. Political and organisational processes are largely driven by monetary considerations in preference to the enabling or enhancement of human capacities. The importance of individual and community achievement is rarely recognised except in economic or heroic terms largely because the central role of occupation in personal and community development, health and wellbeing is seldom carried through into real life.

Occupational therapists who have participated in workshops that explored the notion of occupational justice have used a variety of words and concepts to express their ideas. These are applicable to older as well as younger people. Words used have included **participation**, empowerment, sharing, choice, fulfillment, growth, satisfaction and opportunity. Concepts used have been concerned with enabling equal opportunity for meaningful, purposeful and diverse occupations, the right to satisfying occupations specific to individual needs, the linking of rights to responsibilities, the nourishment of body, mind and spirit of communities as well as individuals, and attention to the participatory and cultural nature of occupations. They have also included ideas about the accessibility of **environments** that promote occupational development, facilitation and empowerment so that adaptation to changing occupational demands is possible. Along with those have been notions of acceptable or unacceptable occupations, social and ethical standards of communities, the transformation of **systems**, redefinition of the way resources are shared, dilemmas of simultaneous seeking of justice for individuals and the common good, and the encouragement of political strategies aimed at equity in living by reducing disadvantage (Starbuck *et al.* 1999).

Such concepts interweave ideas about a justice that recognises older people's need for fulfillment and empowerment through engagement in diverse occupations and that difference and diversity will be the norm for people of any age (Young 1990). At the same time issues about the equitable distribution of services, resources and opportunities have to be attended to.

On that latter point, Piachaud, at the National Social Policy Conference held in Sydney, in 1993, argued that social policies need to move beyond issues of redistribution. In ways similar to occupational therapy rhetoric, suggested instead is a need to consider people's capabilities including how those with limited mental, physical or social capabilities may be empowered to help themselves (1993:13). Occupational therapists as health practitioners could be more aggressive about this particular aspect of justice. However, as well as centering on overcoming an individual's difficulties that result from disability, they could be more proactive in terms of helping all people to appreciate the connections between occupation, morbidity, mortality, and good health.

Occupation, morbidity and mortality and the promotion of health

My own historical research into the relationship between occupation and health has revealed a close association between them (Wilcock 1998). That association is in tune with Ornstein & Sobel's explanation in *The Healing Brain*, that the integrative nature of the central nervous system is related to health and healing. Indeed, they claim, 'the major role of the brain is to mind the body and maintain health' (1988:11–12).

As part of that inbuilt health system the central nervous system develops, responds and adjusts as people go about their daily occupations to meet the multiple requirements of life. It is one of Nature's provisions for health that is largely ignored and poorly understood. That has not always been the case. Sensible regimes concerned with what people do – physically, mentally, and socially, the activity–rest continuum, what they eat and drink, all within healthy natural environments, have been regarded as important in protecting good health for centuries. Indeed, six such rules for health, which were based on classical Greek medicine and known as the 'Regimen Sanitatis', formed the basis of modern western medicine after they were reintroduced into Europe via Arabia during the early middle ages (Daremberg 1870; Risse 1993).

Whilst occupational therapy can be seen to have adopted much of that philosophy, it has been largely left to recent research to justify occupation as a potential health source for older people. Two American randomised controlled trials are of particular note. Glass and colleagues in a 13-year study of 2761 male and female older Americans found:

'. . . social and productive activities (occupations) that involve little or no enhancement of fitness lower the risk of all cause mortality as much as fitness activities do. This suggests that in addition to increased cardiopulmonary fitness, activity may confer survival benefits through psychosocial pathways. Social and productive activities that require less physical exertion may complement exercise programmes and may constitute alternative interventions for frail elderly people' (Glass et al. 1999:478–483).

Occupational scientists and therapists from the University of Southern California conducted the second study. This affirmed the connection between occupation and wellbeing for older people living in community housing in Los Angeles. Benefits were shown across health, function, and quality of life domains for subjects engaged in a programme that enabled older people to consciously articulate and gain appreciation of the importance of occupations in affecting health and successfully employ occupationally based principles of healthy living (Clark et al. 1997:111).

At the start of the twenty-first century, the United Nations Commission on Human Rights reaffirmed 'the right of everyone to the enjoyment of the highest standard of physical and mental health' (2001:574). This inclusive policy suggests that occupational therapists need to consider closely what constitutes physical and mental health for older people, and what occupation based interventions can enable their enjoyment of its highest standard.

That fits well with the call for the reorientation of all health professionals towards the pursuit of health as well as the absence of illness made by the WHO in the 1986 Ottawa Charter for **Health Promotion**. It appears that occupational therapists along with many other health professionals have found it difficult to reorient. Most remain centred on illness models of practice despite rhetoric to the contrary. Consideration of the health needs of older people in terms of a justice approach may be helpful in turning them towards a health driven practice in addition to being a useful tool for programmes aimed at enabling older people with disability to meet their unique occupational needs.

Occupational justice and older people

Older people living in post-industrial societies commonly face attitudes and approaches that are antithetical to occupational justice at legislative, societal and personal levels.

At legislative level for example, compulsory retirement **policies**, pension provision, limited resource allocation as well as lack of provision of professional expertise about occupation as a fundamental requirement for health and wellbeing, are often problematic. They can restrict access to the multiple of occupations that enable older people to shape their daily life in ways that have meaning to them. Occupational therapists working in aged care or with older people leading ordinary lives in the community could become more proactive in examining and assessing policies for potentially damaging **legislation**. They could join in debates as policies are discussed and enacted, and articulate and publish views about occupational justice for older people.

At societal level common and patronising expectations of older people's lack of physical or mental acuity can often diminish belief that they can continue to develop their own occupational potential, shape communities or participate in the world in ways that are valued. The case was often different in pre-industrial times when the ideas, experiences and life knowledge of older people was sought to contribute wisdom to public decisions. This remains the case in some pre-capitalist societies. Community expectations about the limitations that can affect the occupational experiences of older people often fail to appreciate simple initiatives and strategies that would benefit the well older people. More often, societal initiatives are aimed at action for people with obvious disability, but even those, if over helpful, can have detrimental effects on occupational health. Because occupation is so fundamental to individuals functioning in societies, at this level occupational therapists need to put forward ideas about how societies can be organised so that the occupational experiences of all older people are considered as a matter of social justice. They need to become more articulate about what older people can and should be able to do to achieve meaning, quality of life, health, happiness and wellbeing and empowerment within the societies in which they live. A starting point is the obvious questions of occupational justice raised by one of the scenarios given at the start of the chapter. What can be done to improve the lives of older people sitting isolated in a group of similarly lonely people in nursing homes? How can occupational therapists effectively promote the need to resource environments in which the order of the day is to provide personal encouragement to find a way forward for older people that has meaning and purpose to them?

At personal levels older people are often lovingly restrained from over-exertion or participation in continuing with occupations that have been central to their previous sense of self, even by caring families. Occupations are most health-giving if they are embedded with purpose and meaning, and enable the expression of a sense of individual pleasure, vocation, or spirit. Physical, mental or social occupations that are imposed upon older people by circumstances or others can lead to unhealthy consequences, even if they are suggested or demanded with the good of the person in mind. Active or passive denial of opportunities and resources for older people's continued engagement in meaningful occupation are forms of occupational injustice despite goodly intent. It is such restraint, limited resources or opportunity, plus situations of isolation that are major sources of occupational dysfunction and forms of occupational injustice in the western world. Without someone to do things with occupation often loses its purpose and health-giving potential. For older people in western societies where single occupancy housing is increasing, this is particularly relevant.

Occupational therapists could be more proactive in raising awareness of the relationship between occupation, health and wellbeing, the need for meaning and purpose, the need for older people's growth and development to continue throughout the life course, and the need for what they do having some social value. They need to ask questions about how it feels to older people if their only experience is as a receiver rather than a provider of help, if their occupations are limited to using the toilet, bathing or dressing independently, or if social interactions are reduced to expressing thanks to people providing food and meeting hygiene needs.

The questions that have been raised are related to enabling older people to make life worth living through what they do and about recognising individual difference and diversity from an occupational justice perspective. Meeting such occupational needs and wants are related to experiences of positive health. As Ornstein and Sobel explain, the brain minds the body and maintains health through making countless adjustments which preserves stability between social worlds, our mental and emotional lives, and our internal physiology (Ornstein & Sobel 1988:11–12).

Summary

In this chapter the notion of occupational justice for older people has been considered in association with occupational therapy concepts of health. Justice, in this context, has been introduced as the enablement or empowerment of older adults to maintain or invent a lifestyle that allows them to continue to thrive. It has been argued that this is a matter of human rights and a matter of justice because occupation is intimately related with health, wellbeing, morbidity and mortality. As part of this, for individuals to reach towards their potential as part of an active ageing process, occupations must provide them with opportunity to meet unique occupational wants and needs.

In western societies in the present day, the occupational wants and needs of people beyond paid employment years are marginalised, commonly and patronisingly in the name of risk management. This encourages restrictive, externally imposed strategies that are disempowering to older people. Such strategies must not be ignored. Rather, change should be pursued rigorously and systematically as part of everyday practice because common attitudes and approaches are antithetical to occupational justice at legislative, societal and personal levels. However, it must be recognised that occupational justice has profound social and economic implications. These could be disempowering for occupational therapists seeking to implement change in the direction discussed. That means that a more proactive stance towards occupational justice needs to be taken at every level so that the idea is promulgated widely and change towards occupational justice for older people made possible.

References

Armstrong H (2000) Reflections on the difficulty of creating and sustaining equitable communicative forums. *Canadian Journal for Studies in Adult Education* 14, 67–85.

Botes A (2000) A comparison between the ethics of justice and the ethics of care. *Journal of Advanced Nursing* 32(5), 1071–1075.

Broadhead P (1985) Social status and morbidity in Australia. *Community Health Studies* IX(2), 87–98.

Clark F, Azen SP, Zemke R *et al.* (1997) Occupational therapy for independent-living older adults: a randomized controlled trial. *Journal of the American Medical Association* 278(16), 321–326.

Commission on Social Justice (1994) *Social Justice: Strategies for National Renewal.* The Report of the Commission on Social Justice. London: Vintage.

Daniels N, Kennedy BP, Kawachi I (1999) Why justice is good for our health: the social determinants of health inequalities. *Daedelus* 128(4), 215–251.

Daremberg, C. In: Ordronaux J (1870) *Regimen Sanitatis Salernitanum: Code of Health of the School of Salernum.* Philadelphia: JB Lippincott.

Department of Public Information (1982) *Yearbook of the United Nations 1982.* New York: United Nations.

Dubos R (1959) *Mirage of Health: Utopias, Progress and Biological Change.* New York: Harper and Row.

Flynn-Connors E (ed.) (1989) *Yearbook of the United Nations 1989.* The Hague: Martinus Nijhoff.

Gilbert N (1995) *Welfare Justice: Restoring Social Equity.* New Haven and London: Yale University Press.

Glass TA, de Leon CM, Marottoli RA, Berkman LF (1999) Population based study of social and productive activities as predictors of survival among elderly Americans. *British Medical Journal* 319, 478–483.

Gordon K (ed.) (1999) *Yearbook of the United Nations 1999.* New York: United Nations.

Gordon K (ed.) (2001) *Yearbook of the United Nations 2001.* New York: United Nations.

Hart JT (1982) The Black Report: a challenge to politicians. *Lancet* Jan 2, 35–36.

Kalisch D (1991) The active society. *Social Security Journal* August, 3–9.

Marshall W, Schram M (eds) (1993) *Mandate for Change.* New York: Berkley.

Martin GS (1976) *Social/Medical Aspects of Poverty in Australia.* Government Commission of Inquiry into Poverty. Canberra: Australian Government Publishing Service.

Metz T (2000) Arbitrariness, justice, and respect. *Social Theory and Practice* 26(1), 24–45.

Opit LJ (1983) Economic policy and health care: the inverse care law in Australia. *New Doctor*, 38–42.

Organisation for Economic Cooperation and Development (1988) *The Future of Social Protection*. Paris: OECD.

Organisation for Economic Cooperation and Development (1989) Editorial: The path to full employment: structural adjustment for an active society. *Employment Outlook* 7, July 1989. Paris: OECD.

Ornstein R & Sobel D (1988) *The Healing Brain: A Radical New Approach to Health Care*. London: Macmillan.

Piachaud D (1993) Social policy – parasite or powerhouse of the economy. In: Saunders P & Shaver S (eds). *Theory and Practice in Australian Social Policy: Rethinking the Fundamentals*. Proceedings of the National Social Policy Conference, Sydney, July 14–17.

Rawls J (1975) A Kantian conception of equality. *Cambridge Review* 96(2225), 94–99.

Risse GB (1993) History of western medicine from Hippocrates to germ theory. In: Kipple KF (ed.) *The Cambridge World History of Human Disease*. Cambridge: Cambridge University Press, pp. 11–19.

Starbuck R, Whitehead B, Holdsworth C *et al.* (1999) Unpublished. *Notes from Occupational Justice Workshop. Australian Occupational Therapists Conference*. Canberra: Australia.

Townsend E (1993) Muriel Driver Lecture: Occupational therapy's social vision. *Canadian Journal of Occupational Therapy* 60(4), 174–184.

Townsend E & Wilcock A (2004) Occupational justice. In: Christiansen C & Townsend E (eds). *Introduction to Occupation: The Art and Science of Living*. New Jersey: Prentice Hall, pp. 243–273.

United Nations (1982) *The Vienna International Plan of Action Ageing*. United Nations.

United Nations (2001) *Commission on Human Rights. Report on the Fifty-Seventh Session (9th–17th April)*. Economic and Social Council Official Records: United Nations.

Wilcock AA (1998) *An Occupational Perspective of Health*. Thorofare, NJ: Slack.

Wilcock A & Townsend E (2000) Occupational justice: occupational terminology interactive dialogue. *Journal of Occupational Science* 7(2), 84–86.

World Health Organisation, Health and Welfare Canada, Canadian Public Health Association (1986) *Ottawa Charter for Health Promotion*. Ottawa: Canadian Public Health Association.

World Health Organisation (2002) *Active Ageing: A Policy Framework*. Second United Nations World Assembly on Ageing, Madrid, Spain. Geneva: WHO.

Young IM (1990) *Justice and the Politics of Difference*. Princeton, NJ: Princeton University Press.

Chapter 3

THE SOCIAL CONTEXT OF OLDER PEOPLE

Frances Reynolds and Kee Hean Lim

People in their later years are as different in their skills, needs, resources and interests as younger people, yet they are often represented in both the health professional and public media as a homogeneous group. Negative stereotypes of older people are unfortunately widespread in our culture and are frequently reinforced by the negative images and information presented in the mass media. Jones (1993:58) reiterates this view when he states 'Everyone over the retirement age is seen as a strange homogenous mass, with limited abilities, few needs and few rights.' Such negative and stereotypical representations of older people appear to influence health professionals as much as other people. Thane (2000:16), in her book examining historical changes in English attitudes and policies towards older people, expresses her intention 'to help us think in less stereotyped ways about the most stereotyped of age groups.' We have a similar focus in writing this chapter and challenge our readers to explore these issues for themselves and to discover the implications that their own attitudes and perceptions may have upon their relationships and interactions with older people.

We begin this chapter by firstly addressing some of the factors that influence how older people are sometimes treated within the health and social care system. Unthinking internalisation of negative sociocultural attitudes, assumptions, and stereotypes about older people can lead not only to prejudicial thinking but also to discriminatory actions. We will examine a variety of issues relevant to ageism, prejudice and discrimination and encourage readers to reflect on personal values and wider sociocultural norms. Occupational therapists need to be aware that negative social attitudes not only affect people's own experience of the ageing process, but also shape social and health care service provision. Furthermore, it can be argued that ageism has even penetrated the rehabilitation research agenda.

As well as examining personal attitudes, we need to be sensitive to the cultural dimensions of ageing. We do not live in a homogeneous culture, so it is important for occupational therapists to be attuned to the various patterns of social support and prevalent attitudes towards ageing that are commonly found in different ethnic and cultural groups. Such cultural sensitivity enhances the therapists' capacity to form effective partnerships with older people from diverse social groups.

We will also explore the immediate social context of older people, including family, friends, pets, health professionals and local communities. We will show how older people live within a variety of social support networks, each having a char-acteristic influence over the individual's quality of life, identity/self-esteem, and strat-egies of coping with ill health. Moreover, the size and functioning of the social network may even influence physical health and longevity, and we will consider the mechanisms that may be involved. Far from presenting older people as passively dependent upon care, the chapter will explore the complex *reciprocal* relationships that form part of the majority of older people's everyday experience.

Some of the challenges inherent in residential settings will also be highlighted. Sadly, this social context may, at its worst, completely undermine the older person's wellbeing, and some of the psychosocial factors associated with neglect and abuse will be mentioned. The chapter ends by considering certain strategies that occu-pational therapists may adopt to improve partnership-working with older people, and to help older clients strengthen and extend their social networks. Such strat-egies help clients to gain better health and quality of life. Much of the chapter is based on published research, but on the basis of personal clinical experiences we offer two case studies, and a collection of quotations and recounted incidents, to illustrate the points made and to encourage personal reflection.

Ageist attitudes, values, assumptions, and stereotypes

In the prevailing culture of materialism, where those perceived not to be contributing economically are viewed as less important or significant members of society, older people are often marginalised. Their wealth of experience is overlooked. Rather than being valued as persons in their own right, older people are generally subject to negative stereotyping (Killoran *et al.* 1997; Henley & Schott 1999). Williams & Giles (1998) suggest that some stereotypes present older people as frail and useless, whereas others are equally condescending in presenting this age group as especially worthy and deserving. Both forms of stereotype neglect the individual-ity of each older person, and place older people in a special social ghetto. If older people were more often represented in the media and elsewhere as treasured assets rather than as drains upon health and social care resources, it is likely that health professionals' perceptions and attitudes towards older clients would be signific-antly different.

What shapes our personal attitudes towards older people? A variety of per-sonal/social values and norms directly impact upon how we relate and respond to others (Gross *et al.* 2000). A necessary starting point is to undertake some self-examination, as we are better able to form a non-judgemental therapeutic relationship with the older client if we are aware of our own values, and possible prejudices. We need reflective self-awareness also as health professionals so as not to impose our own values and beliefs on our clients and their carers. Gross (2001:351) defines value as a sense of what is desirable, good and worthwhile . . . 'This corresponds to the affective component of an attitude.'

What we may consider to be important will not necessarily be of importance to another person and we need to beware of our own beliefs and prejudices. The dangers of presuming that we know best what our clients would like or what is good for them, becomes all too apparent when we have clients who become non-compliant, demotivated, disgruntled or simply absent from treatment. Being able to understand what is important to each older person is crucial if we are to be able as practitioners to respond effectively to individual needs (Lilja *et al.* 2003).

So how do the assumptions that we make about others influence how we behave and relate towards them? Assumptions are defined in the Oxford Dictionary (2001) as 'the act or an instance of accepting without proof.' Assumptions are often inherent in the attitudes that we hold towards others. For example, racist attitudes may be grounded in unexamined assumptions that the target group is lazy or violent. Henley & Schott (1999:51) define attitude as 'A settled opinion or way of thinking, which is reflected in behaviour.' The authors argue that the way we think about or perceive others has an impact upon our actions and behaviour towards them. One reason for making assumptions and holding prejudicial attitudes is arguably to cope with the huge variety of social information to which we are exposed (Wetherell 1996). If instead of processing information about every person as an individual, we categorise them as members of homogeneous social groups (for example, 'old', 'black', 'body-builders', or whatever), our thinking becomes simplified. We seem to draw such stereotyped representations particularly from the mass media, which often portray members of certain groups in highly clichéd terms (Williams & Giles 1998). For example, an older woman is often presented in terms of the 'battling granny' stereotype or the 'mugging victim' rather than as an adult with many different responsibilities and skills. Unfortunately, stereotypes can act as self-fulfilling prophecies. If, for example, we treat all older clients as passive or dependent, we may precisely encourage the negative behaviour that we have anticipated. Unexamined assumptions about members of other groups may ultimately contribute to discriminatory practices as well as perpetuating myths and simplified perceptions. As health professionals it is important that their validity is challenged.

One of the key characteristics of stereotyping is that a single piece of information about an individual (such as age, gender and race) generates inferences about all other aspects of that person including personality, interests, aspirations, and so on (Levy *et al.* 1998). Stuart-Hamilton (1997) suggests that stereotypes of older people are even more deeply entrenched (and taken for granted) than misconceptions about gender differences. Ageism therefore tends to give rise to hidden oppression (Koch & Webb 1996). Given such social attitudes, it is not surprising that many people are overwhelmingly unenthusiastic about becoming old.

Ageism and discrimination

Ageism is defined by Killoran *et al.* (1997:42) as 'The unfair discrimination against older people, influenced by beliefs and assumptions.' Henley & Schott (1999:32) suggest that 'Ageism stereotypes older people's experience and knowledge as irrelevant and worthless, their intellectual powers as declining and their habits and attitudes as inflexible.' In a social context where ageism, prejudice and discrimination are widespread, older people have to be incredibly resourceful and flexible if they are to flourish.

Killoran *et al.* (1997:47) further suggest that some of the initiatives that health and social services can take to address ageism are:

- Promoting better use of services by older people.
- Professional education on attitudes to old age, special problems of ill health in old age.
- Action on age-related discrimination in provision of health care.
- Increased participation of older people in service planning.

These are important issues that need to be carefully considered if we are serious about eliminating both ageism and discrimination. It is also important to recognise that the economic and social marginalisation of older people further compounds existing health inequalities. For example, older people are confronted by the economic and social constraints of being pensioners; they may feel less entitlement to health care if they believe that they are being categorised as non-productive members of society; and they are less likely to be in position to demand or pay for care that is tailored to their needs (Young & Olson 1991; Buckwalter *et al.* 1993).

Clearly many older people play an important role in their communities, whether at the organisational level (e.g. Women's Institute, craft guilds, and religious organisations) and at the family level (e.g. caring for grandchildren). However, long-term health problems and financial constraints can jeopardise such roles. One of the recommendations from the Health and Education Authority review of the Green Paper, Our Healthier Nation (1997), further highlights the central importance of enabling older people to participate in their communities, whether defined narrowly in terms of family, or more widely through strong social networks and responsive services. The need to promote greater autonomy for the older person is essential if we are to ensure that older people have full status in the communities and societies in which they reside. Every attempt must be made at all levels to involve older people in every aspect of their treatment, and care provision, as well as in the planning of future services (Killoran *et al.* 1997; Department of Health DH 2001).

Cross cultural perspectives on ageing and older people

Differences exist in how older people are perceived within different cultures. In the west, growing old is often viewed negatively, being linked with images of disease, illness, dependence on others, loss of status and diminished autonomy. This depressing image is not found in more traditional and eastern societies, where being old is synonymous with attaining greater wisdom and knowledge. In such societies, older people are generally revered and recognised as having a great wealth of knowledge and life experience (Henley & Schott 1999; Helman 2000).

Sociocultural norms around respect for others directly influence how society treats older people. Reported cases of older people being abused or violated in their own homes or discriminated against by their own communities, illustrate the problem of limited respect for older people in western societies (Ting-Toomey 1999).

However presuming that all older people in the west are treated poorly, whilst all older people in more traditional societies are treated well is both inaccurate and naïve. What is evident is that the norms of the community and society in which we live have a significant influence in determining what attitudes and behaviours are socially and culturally legitimated.

Within 'traditional' or eastern families and communities, older people tend to have a recognised role in offering advice, guidance and sharing experiences. They also contribute actively to caring for other family members. For example, the older person may play an active and culturally valued role as grandparent, cook, and housekeeper in extended families. These roles and responsibilities promote the health, self-worth and wellbeing of older people, as they provide real purpose and opportunities to keep active, and involved (Mandel *et al.* 1999). We must, however, as health professionals be aware of culturally bound stereotypes. To immediately assume that all 'traditional' families are willing to care for their older relative, without seeking any form of help or support from statutory services, is too presumptuous. It is also important to realise that different ethnic/cultural groups and communities may have different ideas and understanding of what contributes to an individual's health and wellbeing. Whilst remaining mindful of broad cultural differences in family structures and values, we need to treat each client as an individual, with specific needs and requirements. Only in this way can we effectively provide culturally sensitive and appropriate care for each specific client (Mandel *et al.* 1999; Helman 2000; Mattingly & Garro 2000; Wells & Black 2000; Lim 2001).

The College of Occupational Therapy Code of Ethics and Professional Conduct (2000) suggest that occupational therapists shall ensure that they provide equitable manner and that they must be sensitive to the cultural and lifestyle differences. Occupational therapy **services** must reflect and value these differences. Standard 2 of the NSF for Older People (DH 2001) similarly supports the need to be person-centred (see Chapter 4).

Exploring the social networks of older people

There are two fairly widespread, somewhat contradictory, stereotypes about the social context of older people. The first is that older people are much more likely than younger people to be living alone, isolated and lonely. The second unwarranted assumption is that older people have a child-like status, passively dependent upon the care of their families, especially daughters. Research is showing that neither pattern of living is widespread and that the social networks of older people are typically rich and complex. Even older people who do live alone usually do so by choice, and retain regular contacts with a variety of relatives and friends. According to a review of four surveys carried out between 1945 and 1999, on average about 5–9% of older people regard themselves as often lonely (rising to 14% of those living alone), a pattern that shows little change over time (Victor *et al.* 2002). Similarly, Mullins & Dugan (1991) surveyed low-income older people and found that 95% were satisfied with the frequency of their social contacts and 96%

were satisfied with their quality. As reviewed by Thane (2000), surveys have revealed that large numbers of older people have contact with their adult children on at least a weekly basis. In addition, about a third of the care provided to older people is carried out by individuals who are themselves over the age of 65 years. Whilst therapists need to be aware that loneliness and isolation can have very detrimental effects on the lives of some older people, being particularly associated with **depression** (Mullins & Dugan 1991), the majority of people in their later years appear to live within networks of social relationships that they regard as acceptable (Central Office of Statistics 2001).

A social network comprises all of the interlinked relationships of a person. It can be regarded as a system of giving and receiving that can influence the social behaviour of all network members. Kahn & Antonucci (1980) propose the more dynamic concept of the social network 'convoy', comprising the numerous relationships – some stable, some changing – that accompany people over the course of their lives. As years pass, some relationships continue, some people enter the convoy (e.g. new friends, new grandchildren), and some leave the convoy, because of death, divorce, or migration to other localities.

A case study is presented in Box 3.1 to highlight and illustrate social network and cultural issues for Mr Edward Jameson.

Box 3.1

Read the case study and identify the members of Mr Jameson's social network:

Mr Edward Jameson is 81 years old. He is in fair health, but experiences chronic pain from **osteoarthritis**, particularly in his knees and back. He came to the attention of occupational therapists, after a knee replacement operation. It emerges that he cares for his wife, Dorothy, who is 78 years old. She had a **stroke** two years ago and requires considerable help with transfers and personal care, but is cognitively bright and usually cheerful. Mr Jameson does most of the housework, although his daughter, Anne, who lives nearby, brings in shopping. There is a close bond between Anne and her parents. The Jamesons see much less of their son-in-law, Paul, but they enjoy quite a positive relationship with him. Mr Jameson sometimes helps his daughter with jobs such as checking that her rather ancient car has sufficient oil, and taking it to the garage for servicing. As well as having a daughter, the Jamesons have a twelve-year old grand-daughter, Claire, whom they sometimes care for during half-term holidays. The Jamesons have a mutual friend, Emily, whom they met shortly after their wedding. They now keep in touch by letter, but they rarely see her since she moved into a residential home about 50 miles away. Mrs Jameson's closest friend died about a year ago, leaving a void in her life. Because it is difficult for her to get out of the house, she sees few other people apart from her immediate family. Mr Jameson is friendly with one of the next-door neighbours, Jim Crabtree, who is a widower, and they often chat over the garden fence. The neighbour is **diabetic** and Mr Jameson keeps a watchful eye to make sure that he is not becoming ill. The neighbour often has to attend hospital appointments, and Mr Jameson always takes him there in his car, and brings him home. Mr Jameson himself is wary of doctors and hospitals, regarding himself as 'strong' and 'uncomplaining'. Only severe pain some months ago made him attend for a medical consultation about his knee.

Mapping social networks

When exploring social networks, it can be helpful to draw a diagram of the person's relationships. Networks can be represented in many ways. For example, in Mr Jameson's case, the social network may be represented as shown in Figure 3.1.

No health professional is represented in this network, as Mr Jameson has been fiercely independent and has made minimal use of any health or social service until recently.

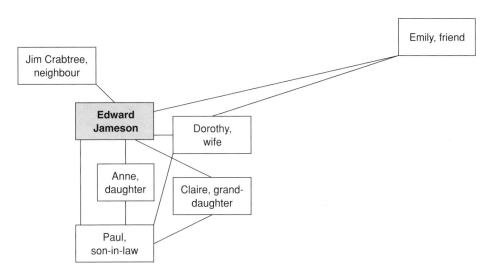

Figure 3.1   A diagram of Mr Jameson's social network.

You can be creative in the way that you represent relationships in the social network. In the example in Figure 3.1, the lengths of lines mirror emotional intimacy. As you can see from the diagram, Mr Jameson feels emotionally closer to his neighbour than to his son-in-law. You may also vary the length of lines according to

Box 3.2   Activity: mapping a social network.

If possible, carry out this activity with another person, a fellow student or trusted colleague, so that you can compare the different patterns of older people's social networks. You do not need to create a visual masterpiece – some networks will inevitably look 'messy' if there are many interconnected relationships! Consider an older person that you know well. Map out their main social relationships, with shorter lines indicating closer emotional ties. Compare the network that you have drawn with Mr Jameson's networks. Is the social network that you have mapped out more complex? Does it contain more relatives or more friends? Are health and social care professionals important or not in this network? Do pets appear?

What do you think the strengths of this social network might be, compared with those of Mr Jameson? Under what circumstances, might this network become vulnerable, or strained?

frequency of contact. Whilst intimacy and frequency of contact tend to be associated, it is possible for people to remain emotionally close (for example, with adult children or siblings) even when they are separated by great distances, and conduct most of the relationship by telephone.

Types of social support

Several large social surveys have shown that not only are most older people satisfied with their social context, but that the relationships of older people – except among the oldest or most frail – are usually characterised by reciprocity, that is, mutual support rather than one-way caring. This is shown in the case study (Box 3.1). In line with theories of friendship that propose stable relationships to be founded on an equitable basis of give-and-take, the networks of older people seem generally to both give help to the older person and to receive help from this person. What forms of help and support may be exchanged in older people's social networks?

Various studies have attempted to classify different types of social support. For example, Kahn & Antonucci (1980) suggest that support is of three main types:

- Aid/instrumental support: comprising practical assistance, including helping with tasks in the home and garden, financial aid, information.
- Emotional support: including empathy, trust, intimacy, love.
- Affirmation: including validation and acceptance, which strengthen identity and self-esteem.

Weiss (1974) offered a somewhat different perspective, arguing that social relationships could satisfy the following needs:

- Attachment (affection, security, intimate disclosure).
- Reliable alliance (lasting bonds that provide instrumental support, but not necessarily emotional intimacy).
- Enhancement of worth (recognition and affirmation of personal value).
- Social integration (companionship, access to expertise and information).
- Opportunities for nurturance (caring, giving love and support to others).

Krause & Markides (1990) have published a useful scale that measures the social support of older people, with special reference to assessing the kinds of support that are useful to help the person cope with stressful experiences. They grouped statements under four main types of social support, namely, informational support, tangible (practical) support, emotional support, and integration (which assesses ways in which the older person gives advice, practical assistance, comfort and so on to others). An example of a tangible support statement is 'provided you with some transportation'. For each statement, respondents were asked to indicate whether the form of support had been received (or given) never/once in a while/fairly often/very often, in the last year. The researchers found that 90% were satisfied with the amount of tangible support that they had received, whereas 39% wished they could have provided more support to others (making the integration scale the lowest scoring).

Close family members tend to provide most of the long-term instrumental/practical support that is available to older people, although neighbours may offer short-term help (e.g. information, or help with fairly straightforward practical tasks, such as moving a heavy dustbin). In white UK families, it appears that extended kin are rarely expected to offer practical assistance, but the norms in certain ethnic minority groups are different. Close friends tend to offer emotional support, and have a large impact on morale (Henley & Schott 1999; Litwin 2001). Friends may offer practical assistance when family members are not available for whatever reason, but there is some evidence that friendship relationships can become more quickly strained by non-reciprocal helping (Crohan & Antonucci 1989). The sense of obligation plus the presence of long-standing emotional attachments encourage close family members, especially daughters, to continue in practical caring for long periods, sometimes even at the expense of their own health and wellbeing.

The emotional support and affirmation offered by friends – as well as close family members – tend to play an important role helping the older person to maintain a familiar identity, and self-esteem, as well as offering opportunities to share stressful experiences, and perhaps to gain advice. Friends of similar ages also help to 'normalise' difficulties (such as bereavement, or disability), helping the person to feel more accepting of the challenges that later life can present (Day 1991). They may act as models of positive ageing. Siblings of the older person also tend to be key supports for similar reasons. Clearly, older people are more likely to lose their siblings and friends through death, rather than their children. Their friends and siblings, by virtue of advanced age, are also more vulnerable to cognitive impairment, or serious ill health, which may also undermine their availability and effectiveness in the social network. Loss of peers in the social network can leave the older person without confidantes, especially among those over 80 years old (Wenger & Jerrome 1999). This experience can result in emotional loneliness, and susceptibility to **depression** (Mullins & Dugan 1991). Women seem particularly likely to be devastated by loss of a confidante, even when they have a spouse (Crohan & Antonucci 1989; Wenger & Jerrome 1999). Any loss of close friends from the social network can also create strains for other family members who may attempt to plug the gaps, by for example, making more visits or inviting the older person to stay. These adaptive changes can work well for some families, but increase strain or conflict for others, for a number of reasons. Some older people do not like to feel 'indebted'; some feel awkward because they never had close emotional ties with their adult children in previous years; some family members feel overwhelmed by conflicting role obligations (to their own families, to their work and to the older person).

Although loss of peers is an inevitable part of growing older, not all social networks shrink dramatically with increasing age. Some older people – particularly women – seem able to maintain their support 'convoys', through for example, joining new organisations, doing voluntary work, remaining active within religious organisations, and making new friends (Wright 1989). Older men are particularly vulnerable to losing work-mates on retirement, and many come to depend on a few female relatives for social support, especially their spouse. Older men's social networks seem more vulnerable than women's to shrinkage. Not only do women seem on average to be better at 'relationship work', but widowhood is a more 'normal' experience for women. There are fewer widowers than widows, because of the differential longevity of men and women. This can result in greater loneliness for men who have lost their wives (who were often their sole confidantes), than for women, as it can be difficult for them to meet widowed men in a similar social situation. Older women seem to have more social organisations open to them than do men (e.g. the Women's Institute), facilitating new social contacts. Peer support appears to be as important to the wellbeing of older people living in residential settings as for those in the community (Carpenter 2002), suggesting that staff in such settings need to ensure that opportunities exist for social contact and friendship, for example by making available a wide range of sociable leisure activities (Silverstein & Parker 2002; Atwal *et al.* 2003).

Some older people extend their social networks by volunteering. The psychological importance of volunteering has been noted by Barlow & Hainsworth (2001), who found that older people with arthritis who volunteered to lead an arthritis self-help group reported less pain, and described feeling more motivated and rejuvenated once they had taken on this role. Warburton *et al.* (2001) found that older volunteers appreciated the opportunity to gain social contacts in roles recognised as useful to the community. Such experiences seem to enhance morale, and decrease the risk of **depression**. As well as enhancing personal wellbeing, research shows that older people make an enormous contribution to their families and communities, through for example volunteering, civic roles, charity work, church activities and grandparenting (Moody 1998). The findings challenge traditional stereotypes of the needy older person, who is simply in receipt of care. Even in residential homes, where possibly one might have strongest expectations that the residents are dependent upon care, a considerable exchange of social support has been observed, such as buddy systems where individuals look out for each other (Lawrence & Schigelone 2002). These supportive alliances increase feelings of solidarity and wellbeing.

Certain occupations apart from volunteering help to extend social networks – as they do for all people regardless of age. Some older people take up new activities during retirement that successfully extend their social networks. For example, a woman in her 60s who had recently had treatment for breast **cancer** described in an interview (with the first author) some of her experiences since starting a fine arts degree course. As well as enabling her to engage in a creative occupation that she had never had enough time for during her working life, the course provided her with valued, new social contacts:

'I just love being with younger people, there's a group of about thirty on the foundation course, they're just absolutely lovely to be with, I just love it, I mean they're so daring with their art-work . . . I'm really enjoying being with [other students] and I've met other people along the way as well, and so it's been a good move really. I've found it quite stimulating . . . I feel I've 'come home' in a way, I can talk about things I want to talk about.'

Box 3.3 Activity: Enquiring further into the influence of social context.

Look at the interview extract above, and interpret what the person might gain from these new social relationships. Are there any psychological benefits that have not been identified in the classifications of support outlined previously?

Clearly, the fellow students in the example above may offer an intellectual stimulus to the older person – in this case, new ideas, fresh thinking, new techniques and styles of artwork. These experiences may all contribute to the older person's process of learning and self-development, enhancing positive feelings such as curiosity, enthusiasm, and creativity and helping the person to strengthen her positive identity – in this case as an artist. However, we also need to recognise that certain social barriers can prevent older and younger people from forming positive social relationships with each other. If the younger people hold stereotyped views, or express ageist sentiments, the older person may feel ostracised or stigmatised, with potentially detrimental consequences for wellbeing. On the other hand, certain intergenerational projects have successfully challenged the stereotypes that both older and younger people sometimes hold about each other. Granville (2001) describes a project in which older people met regularly with children at school, working together as equal partners to enhance the local environment. They discovered many mutual concerns – for example about litter, vandalism, safety and poor local amenities – and gained respect for each other's skills and distinctive contribution to the project.

Types of support network

As well as documenting the size of social networks and their various supportive functions, some researchers have attempted to categorise different types of social network, exploring their relative strengths and vulnerabilities for supporting the older person. Wenger (1994) has put forward a five-fold classification, based on a longitudinal study of older people in North Wales. Firstly, let us consider aspects of the research method.

Focus on research: the social networks of older people in North Wales

The Bangor Longitudinal Study consists of a number of surveys carried out since 1978, in which a cohort of older people have been followed up every few years to document stability and change in their social support networks, in relation to factors such as illness, bereavement and migration (Wenger & Jerome 1999). In one analysis, carried out in the 1990s, the social networks of people in rural North Wales were compared with those in Liverpool (Wenger 1995). Wenger's analysis uncovered five main types of family network among older people in North Wales.

These should not be regarded as totally fixed, because changes in a person's network can occur over time, as friends, offspring and siblings die, move away, or move nearer to the older person. The birth of grandchildren can have positive effects on the network, but changes in the health of the older person can have negative effects. Also, the increasing prevalence of divorce, re-marriage and step-families complicates the social networks of older people in ways that require much greater attention from researchers. According to Wenger (1994), the five main types of network are as follows:

- **Local family dependent:** In these networks, the older person has close ties with at least some family members who live close at hand – at least within five miles. Such family members – typically one or more daughters – are in regular contact, offering assistance and emotional support. The older person tends to have few ties outside the family (e.g. with friends or neighbours). This network type is more common among widowed older people, and among those in poorer health.
- **Locally integrated:** Such networks are characterised by the presence of friends and neighbours as well as family members, living locally. The person may have close ties with church and voluntary bodies, and the social network, developed over a long period, may be large. Older people in these networks tend to be in better health.
- **Local self-contained:** These networks tend to be small, and consisting of only a few relatives, sometimes emotionally as well as geographically distant. The older person is unlikely to know many people in the local community, but may be reliant on neighbours in times of emergency.
- **Wider community-focused:** Older people in this type of network tend to have a large number of ties with the local community, including membership of local clubs, societies, charitable organisations and so on. They are often involved in helping others, and have relatively little need for assistance, at least when in good or fair health.
- **Private restricted:** These networks are tiny, and may reflect only minimal contacts with a few friends – who may in reality be more like acquaintances. Wenger argues that in many cases it represents a life-long pattern of extreme independence or indeed, aloofness.

Pets as members of the older person's social context

In recent years, there has been increasing recognition that pets may be much-loved members of the older person's social context. It is not easy to measure the effects of having a pet on the wellbeing of older people, but caring for a pet seems to satisfy the human need to nurture and care for another living being, and the pet's loyalty and affection may be perceived as a form of unconditional emotional support. Pets also provide a valued sense of continuity and identity (Cookman 1996), and may encourage better self-care and more active daily routines. Raina *et al.* (1999) noted that older people who owned a dog or cat seemed to maintain their engagement in activities of daily living over the course of a year to a greater extent than those who lacked a companion animal, even when other factors such as age had been taken into account. Having a dog may be particularly health-promoting. A small-scale study of ten older people living in a residential setting observed that those with a dog walked further than those without (Herbert & Greene 2001). As pets are important members of the social context of many older people, their death can be as distressing as the loss of a friend or relative, and yet this distress may not be socially recognised or accepted.

Health professionals as sources of social support

It is difficult to generalise about the contribution that health professionals make to the social support systems of older people. Wenger (1994) argues that the formal support provided by social and health care professionals can offer a valuable supplement to the smaller family-based social networks, in particular. However, a qualitative study by Tanner (2001) reveals that seeking and accepting professional help can be a source of discomfort and stigma, as it may be experienced as threatening the older person's view of self as independent.

Some older people do not perceive their rehabilitation specialists to be emotionally supportive or holistic, but rather to operate within the medical discourse that treats patients primarily as objects of treatment (Lund & Tamm 2001). Some older men treated for coronary artery disease saw their health care professionals as offering limited tangible or emotional support, and instead regarded their relatives as their main source of comfort (Yates 1995). Yet others regard the communications that they have with health care professionals as highly supportive and empowering. A recent review of research suggests that professionals who establish continuities in their relationships with older people, and who listen effectively and invite the older person to be a collaborative partner in decision-making are likely to achieve the most satisfactory outcomes (Stewart *et al.* 2000).

Dysfunctional social contexts

Sadly, in some cases, the social context has deleterious effects on the physical and psychological wellbeing of the older person. For example, the family can behave in disempowering and infantilising ways, even whilst intending to act in the older person's best interests. Even more worrying, Comijs *et al.* (1998) estimate that about 5% of older people live within neglectful and abusive contexts. Verbal abuse, intimidation and humiliation by caregivers demean and frighten the older person, and contribute to feelings of worthlessness and depression. Financial, physical and sexual forms of abuse may also occur, although because of their particularly hidden nature, their prevalence is difficult to estimate. Medical practitioners and other healthcare professionals have been called upon to be vigilant for instances of abuse of older people (Bradley 1996).

Which network types are most prone to neglect and abuse? Clearly, the more private networks, in which the older person is supported with minimal outside contact, are most capable of hiding abuse. Whilst some research suggests that highly neglectful or abusive family members are likely to have mental health or alcohol problems (Pillemer & Finkelhor 1989), some findings encourage us to look at the functioning of the network as a whole. Clinicians and researchers adopting the systemic perspective do not seek to condone abuse, but argue that effective intervention depends upon identifying all the factors that contribute to dysfunctional social contexts. Neglect and abuse are likely to occur when support systems are shrinking and under heavy strain (Bradley 1996; Shugarman *et al.* 2003), when care-givers have a history of conflictual relationships with the older person (who may also have been abusive as a parent), and/or when carers are experiencing prolonged stress associated with poverty or looking after other family members. Victims of mistreatment tend to be highly vulnerable, for example, suffering from **depression** or **dementia**, possibly as a result making many demands upon caregivers (Dyer *et al.* 2000). However, we must also acknowledge the influence of the social and physical environment, as well as wider social attitudes that devalue older people. Even though many people feel frustrated from time to time when caring for family members, most do not act out these feelings. Enclosure within the home, and family withdrawal from external social contacts, heighten the risk for the vulnerable older person.

The social context, health and longevity

The chapter so far has suggested that the older person's social context exerts a powerful influence over morale and wellbeing. Through emotional intimacy, affirmation, advice and practical assistance, the older person may be supported in living independently and with dignity. The social context may also offer the older person a strong sense of continuity with past identity, and self-esteem. Rather than being in passive receipt of care, the social context for most older people is a place where equitable relationships and reciprocal support occur. Such relationships affirm beliefs in one's usefulness. Social contacts can also offer stimulation, fun and challenge, and they may empower collective action. These experiences all help to reduce the individual's risk of **depression** and helplessness. As a result, the older person may be better able to cope with chronic pain and functional limitations. Such effects have been shown in a study of older people with **osteoarthritis** (Blixen & Kippes 1999). Perceived health appears to be greater among older people who belong to groups and associations which have a community-oriented purpose, perhaps because of the validation offered by others (Young & Glasgow 1998).

In addition to the psychological and perceived health benefits, some evidence exists that social support confers greater objective physical health and longevity. In a classic study, Berkman & Syme (1979) surveyed a large representative sample of the general community-dwelling population in California to establish whether those with fewer social ties were more susceptible to death over a period of nine years.

They obtained a questionnaire return rate of 86%, and a fairly complete number of death certificates, ensuring valid data. The authors reported that people aged 30–69 years old, who had a large number of social ties (including married partners, friends, family, church membership and membership of community groups) had significantly lower mortality rates over the nine-year period. The most isolated men were 2.3 times more likely to die than the men with extensive social contacts. The risk for isolated women was even greater. These findings were not confined to a single survey. House *et al.* (1988), for example, also showed that socially integrated individuals had improved longevity. This has important implications for the occupational therapist as it reinforces the importance of encouraging older people to maintain their social networks through involvement in meaningful occupations and engagement in social activities.

Box 3.4   Activity: How may social support affect physical health?

Take a few moments to reflect on the processes that may be involved.
Consider the person whose social network was represented in Box 3.2.
If certain supportive relationships were removed from this network, what effects might this have on the person's physical, as well as psychological, health?

The mechanisms linking social support to physical health are hotly debated. Some have questioned whether cause and effect are being confused in these research studies, and whether the apparent link exists simply because the healthier, more mobile person is better able to sustain social relationships (Vaillant *et al.* 1998). Alternatively, it may be questioned whether other factors such as poverty are influencing both social context and mortality. However, Berkman & Syme (1979) considered these issues carefully, and showed through their statistical analysis that the people with fewer social ties had a greater risk of premature death, even when other health jeopardising factors such as smoking status, obesity, alcohol use, and physical activity were taken into account. There may be several processes linking social context to physical health:

- Supportive friends and family in the local vicinity may alert the older person to the need to consult medical practitioners, or to take medication, in times of illness. Early action may then result in more effective treatment for health problems, and/or better adherence to treatment. The unsupported older person may neglect to act so promptly when physical symptoms of ill health appear, and may forget to take medication. Berkman & Syme (1979) showed that people with more extensive social networks tended to use preventive health services more often.
- The older person may engage in more health-promoting activities when part of a social network. For example, it has been found that having supportive friends to walk with encourages older people to take more exercise (Booth *et al.* 2000).

People living alone may get by on snacks rather than making the effort to prepare nutritious meals. Berkman & Syme (1979) showed that people with more
numerous social ties adopted healthier lifestyle behaviours, such as eating
breakfast, exercising and having sufficient sleep.

- The social context may affect health through the buffering effects of support
against stress. Older people who have less support (for example, when providing
care to a partner with chronic illness or dementia) suffer prolonged physiological stress responses. Such changes eventually lead to the down-regulation of the
immune system, leaving the body more vulnerable to infection. Chronically stressed
people who lack support also experience slower healing (e.g. of wounds). Any
long-term down-regulation of the immune system may also elevate the risk of
cancer. These links are subject to much current investigation (Evans *et al.* 2000).

Implications for occupational therapists

This chapter has shown that the social context of the older person has profound
effects on wellbeing, identity, capacity to cope with functional impairments, and
physical and psychological health. Many studies emphasise that large numbers
of older people are involved in giving care to others, and that relatively few are
passive recipients of care. Indeed, some older people are so determined to care for
others that they neglect treatment for their own health, for fear that a spouse or
disabled adult child will go into a residential setting should they be hospitalised.
Older people provide a great deal of reciprocal support within their social contexts, affirming their adult status, identity and self-esteem. Older clients may
therefore benefit psychologically and physically within the therapy process from
identifying the support that they already make to others in their social network
(whether emotional, informational, or practical), and by exploring, if they so wish,
how they can make further contributions to their communities – for example, in
volunteering, charity work and through providing emotional support to others.
Explicit recognition that older people make an enormous difference to the people
they serve may help to enhance self-esteem (Kincade *et al.* 1996; Wheeler *et al.* 1998).

Occupations that provide opportunities to forge new social contacts (e.g. through
joining adult education classes) may enhance the quality of life and self-confidence
of older people. Nevertheless, it is important for therapists to avoid an over-
romantic ideal of social support. Some older people, by reason of their upbring-
ing and personality, have always been socially quite isolated, and for some,
meeting new people is an anxiety-provoking experience. Therapists also need to
be mindful that some older people dislike age-segregated activities. Yet engagement
in meaningful occupations within a social context can help older people to develop
new relationships, and to break out of a highly family-focused network. These are
important goals as similar aged friends make a distinctive contribution to morale
(Litwin 2001). Some older people may benefit from interventions specifically
designed to help them to extend their social networks. Stevens (2001) describes
working with older people to help them analyse their social networks, and to

identify their friendship goals and strategies. This was a helpful intervention as one year later, the participants reported being less lonely and having more friends.

For relatively isolated older people, group-based therapy, or support groups, can offer empowerment and assistance. Groups that share common experiences and coping strategies, help to achieve collective action, and challenge helplessness and **depression**. Occupational therapists need to be mindful of the older person's social network type. Each type has distinct strengths and vulnerabilities. When it functions well, the smaller, more integrated network types can offer high levels of emotional and practical assistance, but they are liable to place more strain on care-givers. The wider community-focused type can provide excellent practical help, over fairly short time-scales, but may leave an older person who is in failing health with very limited emotional support. The more intense, private networks may hide abuse in a minority of cases, and health professionals need to be vigilant about this. Family structures and attitudes towards older people in different ethnic and cultural groups also differ and result in varying levels and sources of support.

Intergenerational projects may be worthwhile for enhancing social integration. As noted previously, Granville (2001) described a project involving older people working successfully on equal terms with children in a school setting to improve the local environment. Both groups found that the experience dismantled their prejudices and were surprised at finding so many shared concerns and goals. The collaborative project provided purpose and promoted self-worth. Occupational therapists can do much to assist older clients to gain quality of life through extending their social support networks, participating in health promotion and engaging in meaningful leisure pursuits (Wilcock 1999; Mayers 2000).

Occupational therapists need to work more extensively with older people in residential settings, as meaningful occupations can facilitate social contacts and friendship. Residents commonly value both social relationships and absorbing occupations, but often find that neither is facilitated. Instead, they are left to sit in large common rooms with other residents with little common purpose (Atwal *et al.* 2003). This practice continues even though there is evidence that increased participation in leisure activities makes an important contribution to quality of life, especially among people in their 80s with few relatives (Silverstein & Parker 2002). Better consultation with residents to establish their needs and preferences is a first step towards assisting them to engage in meaningful and rewarding occupations (Squire 2001).

Sensitivity is required by all therapists offering or setting in place formal supports, as some older people may regard external help as demeaning and threatening to their familiar identity (Tanner 2001). Client-centred practice, in which therapists really listen to their clients' preferences in relation to therapy and social support, is vital. Furthermore, it is crucial that occupational therapists and other health and social care professionals do not impose their own value system on others but focus on negotiating acceptable goals with each individual client. Such an imposition of an intervention on an older client is illustrated in the case of Mrs Lewis in Box 3.5.

The health and social care professionals, together with the family, all believed that they were acting in Mrs Lewis' best interest. Yet they had in fact failed to take into account her wishes. As occupational therapists we must ensure we do not make

Box 3.5 Why can't Mrs Lewis make herself heard?

When reading the case study, reflect on why the health professionals ignored Mrs Lewis' views. To what extent might ageist stereotypes – or other factors – have played a part? What ethical (and emotional) conflicts do therapists face when the older client rejects assistance that they regard as promoting safety and security?

Mrs Lewis, aged 76, was admitted to hospital following a fall. After a stay in hospital, Mrs Lewis was discharged home where she lived on her own. Social Services were requested to conduct a needs assessment and to provide her with a care package. They decided to look into adapting her bathroom which was too small to allow Mrs Lewis the required space to get in and out of her bath safely. On the assessment visit, both the occupational therapist and social worker agreed with Mrs Lewis that having a shower installed in place of her bath would allow her to manoeuvre around her bathroom more freely.

Unknown to Mrs Lewis, an additional assessment was made during the visit. This concerned the possibility of having central heating installed. Although the professional team appeared to have Mrs Lewis' best interest in mind when deciding that having central heating would be beneficial to her, they did not directly consult with her about her needs and preferences. Mrs Lewis was therefore surprised to discover on the second visit, that this additional project had been planned and agreed upon. She was also upset at the prospect of vacating her home for at least three months, whilst the additional work was carried out. Mrs Lewis objected that she had lived in the same house contently for over 50 years, with only a gas fire in her lounge and electric blankets. She did not see any need for central heating, and disliked what she called 'stuffy' environments. She was also anxious about the temporary living arrangements that the project required. Her views were, however, disregarded by her family, social services and health professionals alike. All were adamant that her quality of life and comfort would be greatly improved. This case example, taken from recent clinical practice, highlights a professional failure to consult fully with the older client and the imposition instead of personal values and judgements. Mrs Lewis' encounter with the occupational therapist and social worker was clearly disempowering and upsetting.

the error of imposing our own values and preferences on our older clients. It is important that we work in partnership with the client and their carers to arrive at a mutually acceptable solution. Nevertheless, skills are needed to resolve the ethical dilemmas that can surface when clients' values conflict with professional opinion, as research by Pursey *et al.* (1995) reveals. We also need to be involved in the process of advocating and supporting the autonomy of older people by ensuring that their views and opinions are expressed and listened to by those in authority and power. Wilcock & Townsend (2000) would go as far as challenging us to confront incidents of discrimination, and social or occupational injustice in order to redress the current imbalance and lack of opportunities for older people.

Sensitivity to the cultural and ethnic needs and preferences of our clients must also be paramount. Diversity and difference should be celebrated rather than frowned upon. Therapists need to find ways of resolving conflicts between personal and professional viewpoints and older clients' preferences. Identifying our own ageist and culturally blinkered views and stereotypes through self-examination is the first step to dismantling them. Berlin & Fowkes (1982) proposed the use of the five-stage *LEARN* Model to assist the process of understanding the client's perspective. This may be a useful guide when working in partnership with older clients from any cultural background. The five stages to the model are:

L: Listen to the client's perception and view of their problem.
E: Explain your own perception, viewpoint and understanding of why they may be experiencing that particular problem – whether it be physical, emotional or psychological.
A: Acknowledge and discuss the similarities and differences between the two perceptions of the presenting problem.
R: Recommend measures to address and resolve the presenting difficulties or problem.
N: Negotiate and get agreement on the treatment plan proposed, incorporating specific aspects of the individual's culture where appropriate in providing the treatment and care.

In conclusion, the challenge for occupational therapists working with older people is firstly to counter any ageist attitudes that may guide their thinking and practice. Secondly, they need to engage older people as equal partners in every stage of the occupational therapy process to avoid infantilising or patronising them. Thirdly, it is crucially important that occupational therapists are also involved in enhancing the quality of life of the older person through health promotion, meaningful occupation, providing autonomy and choice, and by assisting the client to enlarge their social support networks. Finally, therapists need to be mindful of the various strengths and vulnerabilities of the different network types that older people inhabit, and adapt their interventions accordingly.

References

Atwal A, Owen S, Davies R (2003) Struggling for occupational satisfaction: older people in care homes. *British Journal of Occupational Therapy* 66(3), 118–124.

Barlow J & Hainsworth J (2001) Volunteerism among older people with arthritis. *Ageing and Society* 21(2) 203–217.

Berkman L & Syme S (1979) Social networks, host resistance, and mortality: a nine-year follow-up study of Alameda County residents. *American Journal of Epidemiology* 109, 186–204.

Berlin E & Fowkes W (1982) A teaching framework for cross-cultural health care. *Western Journal of Medicine* 139(6), 938–943.

Blixen C & Kippes C (1999) Depression, social support, and quality of life in older adults with osteoarthritis. *Journal of Nursing Scholarship* 31(3), 221–226.

Booth M, Owen N, Bauman A, Clavisi O, Leslie E (2000) Social-cognitive and perceived environment influences associated with physical activity in older Australians. *Preventive Medicine* 31(1), 15–22.

Bradley M (1996) Caring for older people: elder abuse. *British Medical Journal* 313, 548–550.

Buckwalter K, Smith M, Martin M (1993) Attitude problem. *Nursing Times* 89(5), 55–58.

Carpenter B (2002) Family, peer and staff social support in nursing home patients: contributions to psychological well-being. *Journal of Applied Gerontology* 21(3), 275–293.

Central Office of Statistics (2001) *Social Trends 2001*. London: HMSO.

College of Occupational Therapists (2000) *Code of Ethics and Professional Conduct for Occupational Therapists*. London: COT.

Comijs H, Pot A, Smit J, Bouter L, Jomker C (1998) Elder abuse in community: prevalence and consequences. *Journal of the American Geriatrics Society* 46(7), 885–888.

Cookman C (1996) Older people and attachment to things, places, pets and ideas. *Image: The Journal of Nursing Scholarship* 28(3), 227–231.

Crohan S & Antonucci T (1989) Friends as a source of social support in old age. In: Adams R & Blieszner R (eds). *Older Adult Friendship: Structure and Process*. Newbury Park, CA: Sage, pp. 129–146.

Day A (1991) *Remarkable Survivors: Insights into Successful Aging Among Women*. Washington: The Urban Institute Press.

Department of Health (1997) *Health of the Nation: A Strategy for Health*. London: HMSO.

Department of Health (2001) *National Service Framework for Older People*. London: HMSO.

Dyer C, Pavlik V, Murphy K, Hyman D (2000) The high prevalence of depression and dementia in elder abuse or neglect. *Journal of the American Geriatrics Society* 48(2), 205–208.

Evans P, Hucklebridge F, Clow A (2000) *Mind, Immunity and Health: The Science of Psychoneuroimmunology*. London: Free Association Books.

Granville G (2001) Intergenerational health promotion and active citizenship. In: Chiva A & Stears D (eds). *Promoting the Health of Older People*. Buckingham: Open University Press, pp. 40–50.

Gross R (2001) *Psychology: The Science of Mind and Behaviour*, 4th edn. London: Hodder & Stoughton.

Gross R, McIlveen R, Coolican H, Clamp A, Russell J (2000) *Psychology: A New Introduction*. London: Hodder & Stoughton.

Helman CG (2000) *Culture, Difference and Healthcare*. Oxford. Butterworth Scientific.

Henley A & Schott J (1999) *Culture, Religion and Patient Care in Multi-ethnic Society*. London: Age Concern Books.

Herbert J & Greene D (2001) Effects of preference on distance walked by assisted living residents. *Physical and Occupational Therapy in Geriatrics* 19(4), 1–15.

House J, Landis K, Umberson D (1988) Social relationships and health. *Science* 241, 540–545.

Jones H (1993) Altered images. *Nursing Times* 89(5), 58–60.

Kahn R & Antonucci T (1980) Convoys over the life course: attachment, roles and social support. In: Baltes P & Brim O (eds). *Life-span Development and Behavior*, Vol 3. New York: Academic Press, pp. 253–286.

Killoran A, Howse K, Dalley G (1997) *Promoting the Health of Older People: A Compendium*. London: Health Education Authority.

Kincade J, Rabiner D, Bernard S, Woomert A (1996) Older adults as a community resource: results from the National Survey of Self-Care and Aging. *Gerontologist* 36(4), 474–482.

Koch T & Webb C (1996) The biomedical construction of ageing: implications for nursing care of older people. *Journal of Advanced Nursing* 23(5), 954–959.

Krause N & Markides K (1990) Measuring social support among older adults. *International Journal of Aging and Human Development* 30(1), 37–53.

Lawrence A & Schigelone A (2002) Reciprocity beyond dyadic relationships. *Research on Aging* 24(6), 684–704.

Levy S, Stroessner S, Dweck C (1998) Stereotype formation and endorsement: the role of implicit theories. *Journal of Personality and Social Psychology* 74, 16–34.

Lilja M, Bergh A, Johansson L, Nygard L (2003) Attitudes towards rehabilitation needs and support from assistive technology and social environment among elderly people with disability. *Occupational Therapy International* 10(1), 75–93.

Lim KH (2001) A guide to providing culturally sensitive and appropriate occupational therapy assessments and interventions. *Mental Health Occupational Therapy Magazine* 6(2), 26–29.

Litwin H (2001) Social network type and morale in old age. *Gerontologist* 41(4), 516–524.

Lund M & Tamm M (2001) How a group of disabled persons experience rehabilitation over a period of time. *Scandinavian Journal of Occupational Therapy* 8(2), 96–104.

Mandel DR, Jackson JM, Zemke R, Nelson L, Clark, FA (1999) *Lifestyle Redesign: Implementing the Well Elderly Program.* Bethesda: The American Occupational Therapy Association.

Mattingly C & Garro LC (2000) *Narratives and the Cultural Construction of Illness and Healing.* Berkeley: University of California Press.

Mayers CA (2000) The Casson Memorial Lecture 2000: Reflect on the past to shape the future. *British Journal of Occupational Therapy* 63(8), 358–366.

Moody H (1998) *Aging: Concepts and Controversies.* Beverley Hills, CA: Pine Forge Press.

Mullins L & Dugan E (1991) Elderly social relationships with adult children and close friends and depression. *Journal of Social Behaviour and Personality* 6(2), 315–328.

Oxford Dictionary (2001) Oxford: Oxford University Press.

Pillemer K & Finkelhor D (1989) Causes of elder abuse: caregiver stress versus problem relatives. *American Journal of Orthopsychiatry* 59(2), 179–187.

Pursey A & Luker K (1995) Attitudes and stereotypes: nurses' work with older people. *Journal of Advanced Nursing* 22(3), 547–555.

Raina P, Waltner-Toews D, Bonnett B, Woodward C, Abernathy T (1999) Influence of companion animals on the physical and psychological health of older people: an analysis of a one-year longitudinal study. *Journal of the American Geriatrics Society* 47(3), 323–329.

Shugarman L, Fries B, Wolf R, Morris J (2003) Identifying older people at risk of abuse during routine screening practices. *Journal of the American Geriatrics Society* 51(1), 24–31.

Silverstein M & Parker M (2002) Leisure activities and quality of life among the oldest old in Sweden. *Research on Aging* 24(5), 528–547.

Squire A (2001) Health-promoting residential settings. In: Chiva A & Stears D (eds). *Promoting the Health of Older People.* Buckingham: Open University Press, pp. 120–131.

Stevens N (2001) Combating loneliness: a friendship enrichment programme for older women. *Ageing and Society* 21(2), 183–202.

Stewart M, Meredith L, Brown J, Galajda J (2000) The influence of older patient–physician communication on health and health-related outcomes. *Clinics in Geriatric Medicine* 16(1), 25–36.

Stuart-Hamilton I (1997) Adjusting to later life. *Psychology Review* 4(2), 20–23.

Tanner D (2001) Sustaining the self in later life: Supporting older people in the community. *Ageing and Society* 21(3), 255–278.

Thane P (2000) *Old Age in English History: Past Experiences, Present Issues.* Oxford: Oxford University Press.

Ting-Toomey S (1999) *Communicating Across Cultures.* New York: Guilford Press.

Vaillant G, Meyer S, Mukamai K, Soldz S (1998) Are social supports in late mid-life a cause or result of successful ageing? *Psychological Medicine* 28(5), 1159–1168.

Victor C, Scambler S, Shah S *et al.* (2002) Has loneliness amongst older people increased? An investigation into variations between cohorts. *Ageing and Society* 22(5), 585–597.

Warburton J, Terry D, Rosenman L, Shapiro M (2001) Differences between older volunteers and nonvolunteers: attitudinal, normative and control beliefs. *Research on Aging* 23(5), 586–605.

Weiss R (1974) The provisions of social relationships. In: Rubin Z (ed.) *Doing Unto Others*. Englewood Cliffs, NJ: Prentice Hall.

Wells SA & Black RM (2000) *Cultural Competency for Health Professionals*. Bethesda: The American Occupational Therapy Association.

Wenger GC (1994) *Support Networks of Older People: A Guide for Practitioners*. Bangor: Centre for Social Policy Research and Development, University of Wales.

Wenger GC (1995) A comparison of urban with rural support networks: Liverpool and North Wales. *Ageing and Society* 15(1), 59–82.

Wenger GC & Jerrome D (1999) Change and stability in confidante relationships: findings from the Bangor Longitudinal Study of Ageing. *Journal of Aging Studies* 13(3), 269–294.

Wetherell M (1996) Group conflict and the social psychology of racism. In: Wetherell M (ed.) *Identities, Groups and Social Issues*. London: Sage, pp. 175–238.

Wheeler J, Gorey K, Greenblatt B (1998) The beneficial effects of volunteering for older volunteers and the people they serve: a meta-analysis. *International Journal of Aging and Human Development* 47(1), 69–79.

Wilcock AA (1999) Reflections on doing, being and becoming. *Australian Occupational Therapy Journal* 46(1), 1–11.

Wilcock AA & Townsend E (2000) Occupational justice: occupation terminology, interactive dialogue. *Journal of Occupational Science* 7, 84–86.

Williams A & Giles H (1998) Communication of ageism. In: Hecht M (ed.) *Communicating Prejudice*. Thousand Oaks, CA: Sage, pp. 136–160.

Wright P (1989) Gender differences in adults' same and cross-gender friendships. In: Adams R & Blieszner R (eds). *Older Adult Friendship: Structure and Process*. Newbury Park, CA: Sage, pp. 197–221.

Yates B (1995) The relation among social support and short- and long-term recovery outcomes in men with coronary heart disease. *Research in Nursing and Health* 18(3), 193–203.

Young RF & Olson EA (1991) *Health, Illness and Disability in Later Life: Practical Issues and Interventions*. London: Sage.

Young RF & Glasgow N (1998) Voluntary social participation and health. *Research on Aging* 20(3), 339–362.

Chapter 4

SYSTEMS, SERVICES AND POLICIES

Anita Atwal

In the United Kingdom current **health care policy** has transformed the way in which services will be delivered to older people. These policies regulate not only the health and social care system but also the way in which occupational therapy services will be organised and structured. **Systems, services and policies** other than those of health and social care such as housing, education, employment and transportation also determine the functioning and well being of older people and these are expanding areas for the occupational therapy profession. Policies on ageing need to promote the well being of older people and ensure that they promote economic independence, equity, independence and the right of self-determination.

Whilst occupational therapists strongly support the notion of client-centred practice, they have been criticised for not fully participating and or understanding the importance of participating in political and social policy making (Cameron & Masterson 1998; Wilcock 1998). In order to influence the policy making process and professional issues, occupational therapists could become members of professional special interest groups, write in professional journals, vote in a general election or become an active member of a political party or community action group such as Age Concern or Help the Aged.

Countries have different approaches to the types of services that they provide to older people. For example, support services such as meals on wheels are well established in the United Kingdom, Netherlands and Denmark but are less established in countries where the family provides care for example Greece, Spain and Portugal. In Germany and Japan public long-term insurance predominates whereas in Australia long-term care is provided predominantly by the private sector (profit and non-profit organisations). For this reason, making comparisons with the United Kingdom and other countries is tenuous. Devolution in the United Kingdom in the late 1990s also means that there are differing priorities, systems, services and policies in England, Scotland, Wales and Northern Ireland. This chapter considers mainly English systems, services and policies and the reader is referred to pages 224–8 for United Kingdom, European and international government websites. Whilst there are no universal health objectives for older people, in 1984 the World Health Organisation's (WHO) European Region Health for All programme adopted 38 regional targets (WHO 1985). However since 1984 these targets gave been modified (WHO 1993, 1994, 1998) and there are currently three targets on life transitions and health (focusing on infants and pre-school children, young people and older people). Attempts have also been made to share knowledge across countries.

Table 4.1 Core values of occupational therapy (College of Occupational Therapists 2000) compared with the Human Rights Act (United Kingdom Parliament 1998a) and the National Health Service from the NHS Plan England (DH 2000).

Human Rights Act	Occupational therapy (OT) core values	National Health Service (NHS) core principles
Article 3: No-one shall be subjected to torture or to inhuman or degrading treatment.	OTs reflect on their practice and strive to improve it. Each OT has a responsibility to ensure that he or she provides a high quality service which meet the client's needs and does no harm. OT is part of the total care of the client and the OT is a member of the multidisciplinary team.	The NHS will help keep people healthy and work to reduce health inequalities. The NHS will provide a universal service for all based on clinical need, not ability to pay. The NHS will provide a comprehensive range of services. The NHS will work continuously to improve quality services to minimise errors. The NHS will support and value its staff. Public funds for health care will be devoted solely to NHS patients. The NHS will work together with others to ensure a seamless services.
Article 8: Everyone has the right to respect his/her private life, his/her home and his/her correspondence.	OT practice is culturally sensitive and culturally relevant. The clients' goals take precedence in the treatment programme. OTs promote personal identity by giving information and choices to their clients.	The NHS will respond to the different needs of different populations. The NHS will respect the confidentiality of individual patients and provide open access to information about services, treatment and performance.
Article 9: Everyone has the right to freedom of thought, conscience and religion. Article 10: Everyone has the right to freedom of expression.	OTs listen to their clients in order to make informed choices about their care.	The NHS will shape its services around the needs and preferences of individual patients, their families and carers.

In the UK there is still no specific legislation to outlaw age discrimination, although anti-discriminatory practice is a fundamental element of occupational therapy practice (see Table 4.1). Legislation does exist to protect older people against sex, race and disability discrimination (Sex Discrimination Act 1975; Race Relations Act of 1976; Disability Discrimination Act 1995). However on a positive note, in the United Kingdom older people in care homes have recently been given the same rights as older people living at home, with the Royal Commission (1999) recommending that older people in care homes should receive free nursing care. The current government is planning to implement a European Directive to introduce age discrimination legislation by 2006.

The aim of this chapter is not to focus on the historical perspective of social policy but rather to examine and debate how current and past systems, services and policies can impact upon how older people live. This chapter will use the narratives of the Mrs Lewis and Mr Jameson from Chapter 3.

The development of services for older people

Policies for older people have advanced for many different reasons, such as trade unions, media and political pressure, and lobbying from charities representing the rights of older adults. Even in 1947 newspapers such as the *Evening Standard* and the *Daily Mail* drew the public's attention to the difficulties that older people faced. Indeed the meals on wheels service developed as a result of these concerns. Significant reports and commissions that have impacted upon older people are shown in Table 4.3 (p. 52). If we examine the core principles of the National Service Framework for Older People (DH 2001) (Table 4.2) with relevant reports and commissions it is evident that most of its key recommendations are not new (Table 4.3). What is new is the way in which these ideas will be implemented and put into practice, for example the need for interprofessional collaboration through the single assessment process.

Table 4.2 The eight standards of the National Service Framework for Older People (DH 2001).

Standard 1 – Rooting out age discrimination
NHS services will be provided, regardless of age, on the basis of clinical need alone. Social care services will not use age in their eligibility criteria or policies, to restrict access to available services.

Standard 2 – Person-centred care
NHS and social care services treat older people as individuals and enable them to make choices about their own care. This is achieved through the single assessment process, integrated commissioning arrangements and integrated provision of services, including community equipment and continence services.

Standard 3 – Intermediate care
Older people will have access to a new range of intermediate care services at home or in designated care settings, to promote their independence by providing enhanced services from the NHS and councils to prevent unnecessary hospital admission and effective rehabilitation services to enable early discharge from hospital and to prevent premature or unnecessary admission to long-term residential care.

Standard 4 – General hospital care
Older people's care in hospital is delivered through appropriate specialist care and by hospital staff who have the right set of skills to meet their needs.

Standard 5 – Stroke
The NHS will take action to prevent strokes, working in partnership with other agencies where appropriate. People who are thought to have had a **stroke** have access to diagnostic services, are treated appropriately by a specialist stroke service, and subsequently, with their carers, participate in a multidisciplinary programme of secondary prevention and rehabilitation.

Table 4.2 (cont'd)

Standard 6 – Falls
The NHS, working in partnership with councils, takes action to prevent **falls** and reduce resultant **fractures** or other injuries in their populations of older people. Older people who have fallen receive effective treatment and rehabilitation and, with their carers, receive advice on prevention, through a specialist falls service.

Standard 7 – Mental health in older people
Older people who have mental health problems have access to integrated mental health services, provided by the NHS and councils to ensure effective diagnosis, treatment, and support, for them and for their carers.

Standard 8 – The promotion of health and active life in older age
The health and wellbeing of older people are promoted through a coordinated programme of action led by the NHS with support from councils.

Table 4.3 Analysis of the key standards of the National Service Framework.

Standard 1
The Carnegie Inquiry into the Third Age (1993) found age barriers in the recruitment and use of volunteers and recommended that decisions should be taken on the individual capability and not age.

Standards 2 and 3
Guillebaud Report (Ministry of Health 1956) and the Royal Commission on Doctors' and Dentists' Remuneration (1960). Discussed the costs of health care. Both reports suggested that health and welfare departments could be combined.

Joint Care Planning health and local authorities Circular 4C(77) 17/LAC(77) 10 (Department of Health and Social Security [DHSS] 1977). Local authorities were recommended to set up joint planning committees with health to plan and co-ordinate services for older people.

Gillie Report (Standing Medical Advisory Committee Report 1963): Emphasised the need for improved teamwork between doctors and primary care workers.

A Happier Old Age (DHSS 1978). A discussion document that looked at services for older people. The report highlighted the contribution of the voluntary and private sector.

Consultation document Priorities for Health and Personal Social Services in England (Department of Health and Social Security 1976) proposed an expansion in community services.

Care in Action (DHSS 1981). A handbook outlining national guidelines for health and social services. Older people were considered a priority group. Four objectives were given: to strengthen community and voluntary services, to promote independence in older people and enable them to return home, maintain capacity in the acute sector to treat older people, to maintain provision for older people requiring long-term support in came homes or long-term care.

Wagner Report (National Institute for Social Work 1988) on residential care listed a number of rights that older persons should have who reside in institutions.

Minister of Housing and Local Government (1961) called for greater co-operation between housing, local health and welfare authorities and voluntary organisations.

Standard 4
Wagner report (National Institute for Social Work 1988) emphasised the importance of training in a report on residential care.

A joint report from Royal College of Physicians and Royal College of Psychiatrists (Royal College of Physicians 1989) stressed the importance of training for doctors working with older people.

Standards 5, 6, 7, 8
Choosing Health: making healthier choices easier (DH 2004b); a document published in order to develop a health promotion strategy and to focus on the promotion of good health and well being as well as providing information and practical support.

Finance and employment

The average age for retirement and the way in which pensions are funded and organised varies across countries. Despite these variations a report by the Organisation for Economic Co-operation and Development (OECD) (2001) concluded that real wellbeing in older people in a range of European and North American Countries was remarkably similar. In all nine countries studied (Canada, Finland, United States, Sweden, the Netherlands, Italy, Japan, UK and Germany) older people had on their retirement 70 to 80% of the income of comparable groups during later working lives.

Table 4.4 Significant Acts relating to pensions.

1946: National Insurance Act (Ministry of National Insurance and National Insurance Advisory Committee 1946). A compulsory system of insurance that guarantees people financial assistance during periods of sickness unemployment and retirement.

1957: The National Insurance Act (National Insurance Advisory Committee 1957) Enabled retirement and widowed pensioners under the age of 70 (65 for women) to delay their retirement and to earn additions to their retirement which would be paid when they stopped working.

1961: Graduated Pensions Scheme (Ministry of Pensions and National Insurance 1962). Higher pensions were to be payable in return for higher contributions related to higher earnings.

1980: Social Security Act which amended the 1975 Social Security Act (Department of Health and Social Security 1980). All benefit increases were to be related to the movement of prices.

1986: Social Security Act (DHSS 1986) This saw the introduction of means-tested benefits. One of the main aims was to harmonise rules for calculating entitlement to benefits and housing benefit (this Act replaced supplementary benefit with income support and introduced the concept of the social fund).

Since 1945, a succession of Acts has been introduced to extend pensions to nearly all old people in the UK (Table 4.4). However despite these Acts, two million older people still live in poverty in the United Kingdom and over 25% live below the Government's official poverty line (Department of Work and Pensions 2002). Furthermore around 70% of the world's population live in developing countries (WHO 2002). An analysis of inequality in the UK places nearly two-thirds of those over 70 among the poorest 40% of the population, and are only half as likely as the average of other age groups to be among the richest 40% of the population (Goodman *et al.* 1997). If we consider Mr Jameson and Mrs Lewis, it is likely that they have made very different provisions for their retirement. Strategies to prevent poverty in older age have included changes to the pension system. An initiative aimed at enhancing quality of life for older people include the introduction of Minimum Income Guarantee (MIG) and Pension Credit. It is important to note that external factors such as a volatile stock market can impact upon older person's finances.

In the UK it has been suggested that in order to support an ageing population the State Pension age for men and women should rise to 72 or even 75 (O'Connell 2002). This could have personal and professional implications for occupational therapists. There are still barriers to overcome if this policy is to be implemented, namely that of discrimination in the work place. In 1999 the Government published the Code of Practice on Age Diversity in Employment that set the standard for non-ageist approaches to recruitment, training, and development, promotion, redundancy and retirement.

Driving and transportation

The use of public and private transport services are closely linked with older people's feelings of independence and enhanced quality of life (Gilhooly *et al.* 2003). However Gilhooly *et al.* (2003) identified that transport operators tend to focus on the needs of disabled passengers (particularly wheelchair users) in response to the Disability Discrimination Act (DDA) (1995) rather than the older passenger or those with cognitive or sensory impairment. In the UK even though many buses are now provided with level or ramped access these are not always operated, with the bus moving away before the older person is seated in an attempt not to waste time (Department for Transport [DfT] 2000; Gilhooly *et al.* 2003). Alternative schemes run by local authorities such as Dial-a-Ride, though successful, can also have barriers that prevent older people from using these schemes, such as the need to book ahead for usage (DfT 2002).

Access to transport is important for maintaining social relationships and independence (Gilhooly *et al.* 2003). Focus groups conducted by the Department of the Environment, Transport and Regions (DETR) in 1999 found that travel was very important for entertainment, participation independence and social interaction; however only 50% of older people in the UK actually take up the travel concessions to which they are entitled (Burnett 2004). The trend of building out-of-town shopping centres, the placing of retirement and residential homes on the outskirts of towns, alongside privatisation and deregulation of public transport services can also deprive older people access to these necessary amenities (DfT 2000; Gilhooly *et al.* 2003).

The barriers that older people perceive to using public transport are:

- Personal security – especially at night.
- Risk of falls on moving transport.
- Carrying of heavy loads (e.g. shopping).
- Unreliable services.
- Isolated stops with a long distance between them.
- Poor lighting in waiting areas.
- Cost of travel.
- Difficulty boarding and alighting from vehicles.
- Confusion over use and access to information.

In order to overcome some of the **environmental barriers** preventing older people from using public transport, Section 46 of The DDA (1995) gave the Secretary of State the power to ensure that all new trains, trams and other track-based systems are accessible to disabled people. Consequently the Rail Vehicle Accessibility Regulations 1998b (RVAR) came into force in November 1998, with the Public Services Vehicles Accessibility Regulations (2000: PSVAR) affecting all new bus and coach vehicles, from December 2000. The DDA (1995) also requires service providers such as hotels, tour operators to make 'reasonable adjustments' so that disabled people can use their facilities. However for disabled air travellers only a voluntary code of practice is currently in existence (Access to Air Travel for Disabled People Code, available from www.dft.gov.uk).

The National Travel Survey (Department of Environment, Transport and the Regions [DETR] 1998) found that the single factor most affecting travel by older people is access to a car (both as a driver and as a passenger). Possible reasons for this can be attributed to limited finances and or disability (Office for National Statistics [ONS] 1999). An ageing population will mean an even greater number of people wanting to continue driving (Automobile Association 2000).

There is little consensus about what constitutes fitness to drive (Karagiannidou & Foot 2003). In the UK the driving licence is valid until 70 years when fitness to drive is determined every 3 years by the completion of a health declaration, with the onus on the driver to complete this accurately and honestly. (More information can be obtained from the Driving and Vehicle Licensing Agency Medical Rules www.dvla.gov.uk/drivers/dmed1.htm.) Many older people feel that fitness to drive should be determined by a medical examination or assessment (Gilhooly *et al.* 2003), with evidence that self-report is unreliable as many older people lack insight and awareness of their driving ability (Karagiannidou & Foot 2003).

Occupational therapists therefore have an important role in enabling older people to use transportation. This may include giving advice on safe driving methods, assisting reapplication for driving licenses, transport training and education. An occupational therapist could assess and advise Mr Jameson on manual handling issues when assisting his wife Dorothy who has had a **stroke** to get in and out of the car as well as advice on car seating because of his **osteoarthritis**.

Older people can be facilitated in maintaining safe driving by:

- Regularly driving to maintain skills.
- Preparing routes in advance.
- Choosing the most appropriate time for travel.
- Avoiding fatigue by sharing driving or taking frequent rests.
- Avoiding distractions.
- Avoiding adverse weather conditions.
- An awareness of the side effects of medications.

Other opportunities to encourage safer driving are:

- Advice on buying a car with power-assisted steering.
- Clear (not tinted) windows.

- Good all-round visibility.
- Wide-angled door mirrors.
- Front and side impact air bags.
- Being supported to recognise their decline in abilities.
- Being encouraged to make appropriate lifestyle and transport changes without a car.

Housing and adaptations

Housing is a pre-requisite for independent living and for the well being of older people. A range of housing options is available to older people and in the United Kingdom housing is commonly classified according to tenure. The main tenures are owner-occupation, local authority housing, private rented housing and Housing Associations. An influential report by Townsend in 1964, concluded that many older people were placed in care homes because they lacked adequate income and housing.

Occupational therapists in partnership with other professionals need to ensure that older people's housing needs are considered in relationship to positive lifestyle choice. For example, Mrs Lewis is not consulted about the provision of central heating in her home. Consequently this can have a negative impact upon her well-being. Older people need to be supported through the decision-making process to make the best decision for them. When assisting older people to make informed choices it is important to consider certain factors that include their current need for health and social care services and their anticipated future needs. Consideration should also be given to the income and capital circumstances of the potential house-mover such as the running costs of the new accommodation (food, heating, and taxes), the tenure of the old and new accommodation, and the location of the property in relation to Post Offices, doctors' surgeries, shops, or places of worship.

Occupational therapists have an important role in the removal of environmental barriers that constrain the way people wish to live, and hinder independence. Indeed, a principal role of many occupational therapists is to ensure that older adults can perform occupations in accessible environments. Hence, occupational therapists might consult with those designing and building new nursing homes, hospitals, hotels, museums, restaurants and other public spaces, as well as providing educational services to architects, planners and developers (CAOT 2002).

Box 4.1

The Elderly Accommodation Counsel has implemented a project which focused on the piloting of choice-based lettings for sheltered housing by listing sheltered housing vacancies on its website www.housingcare.org

Box 4.2

> **Refer back to Mrs Lewis' story from Chapter 3:**
> Is central heating an essential item for health and wellbeing?
> How would Barbara have funded the provision of central heating and the bathroom modification?

It has been acknowledged that financial barriers can impact upon adaptations and modifications being made to the home. Consequently the Regulatory Reform Act (2001a) has given local authorities wide discretionary powers to provide financial assistance for repairs, improvements and adaptations of living accommodation. The power is also available to help with the cost of moving and adapting or improving another property where this is thought to be the more cost-effective option.

Health and social care

Table 4.5 Influential Acts impacting on older people.

1968: Health Service and Public Health Act gave local authorities a general responsibility to promote the welfare of older people and made the provision of home-help a mandatory service.

1962: Amendment Act (Ministry of Health 1962). The National Assistance Act (Ministry of Health 1948) was amended so local authorities could directly provide meals on wheels service.

1970a: Local Authority Service Act: Restructuring of **social services** based on the Seebohm Report. Saw the establishments of new departments to meet the social needs of individuals, families and communities. Residential homes for older people, equipment and adaptations, home help service, meals on wheels were all included in this new department.

1970b: The Chronically Sick and Disabled Persons Act. This required local authorities to provide practical assistance in the home, provision of, or assistance in obtaining radio, television, library or similar recreational facilities, lectures, games, outings if other recreational facilities outside of the home, or assistance in taking advantage of educational facilities available, facilities for, assistance in, travelling to and from home for various purposes, assistance in arranging adaptation to the home, or the provision of additional facilities designed to secure greater safety, comfort or convenience, facilitation the taking of holidays, meals, whether at home or elsewhere.

Provision, or assistance in obtaining a telephone and any special equipment needed to enable the disabled person to use it.

1990: Community Care Act (1989b). Main changes were:
Separation of responsibility for commissioning and providing services (purchaser–provider split).

Introduction of competition into health and social care (internal market, fund holding general practitioners).

The expectation that services are to be provided by the local authority and the introduction of the independent sector.

Table 4.5 *(cont'd)*

The introduction of care management.

Social Services departments became responsible for the assessment and financial arrangements for people needing admission to a care home.

1997: White Paper NHS Modern and Dependable (DH 1997) Main changes were to replace competitiveness with co-operation by removing the internal market, the purchaser/provider split and fund holding general practitioners.

Primary care groups (PCGs), instead of health authorities would be responsible for the commissioning of services.

1999: Royal Commission on the problems of funding long-term care for older people (Royal Commission 1999). The commission recommended that 'hands-on care' should be free, irrespective of income for older people living at home or in care homes.

There is evidence that a considerable proportion of the health and social care budget is spent on people aged 65 and over. In 1998–99, nearly two-fifths of hospital and community health service expenditure in England was spent on people aged 65 and over. How the NHS should be funded has long been an area of considerable debate and controversy. The National Health Service Act (1956) enabled a health service to be set up that is free at the point of need and financed by general taxation. Alternative funding arrangements have been debated in order to ensure that the health service can deliver effective care. Suggestions have included adopting individual charges for social insurance and private insurance. General taxation is still thought to be the best system to deliver a free NHS service that is based upon need and not on the ability to pay.

Quality in health and social care

Whilst services for older persons have improved, there is still evidence that variation in the treatment and management for older people exists between hospital trusts. Furthermore there is evidence that a shortage of professionals and of skilled personnel directly impact upon standards of care. The setting and implementation of national standards is an attempt to reduce unacceptable variations in standards of care and treatment that have been reported within the United Kingdom. Occupational therapists need to be aware of government performance measures and ensure that their input contributes to achieving these goals. However, there has been considerable criticism over the use of performance indicators as a means of demonstrating quality. For example it can mean that some health trusts are so concerned with meeting targets that they ignore other aspects of patient care. Furthermore some of the targets have been regarded as unrealistic and unachievable.

In order to monitor quality, key agencies have been given a specific role (Table 4.6). The performance of NHS trusts will be assessed under the five domains of the NHS Performance Framework (Table 4.7). The performance of social services is con-

Table 4.6 Key roles of agencies to promote quality in health and social care.

The National Care Standards Commission	Responsible for the registration and inspection of health and social care services in England. It is a non-departmental public body, established by the Government under the Care Standards Act 2000(a).
Commission for Social Care Inspection	Established in April 2004 under the Health and Social Care (Community Health and Standards) Act 2003. It is the single, independent inspectorate for all social care services in England. It promotes improvements in social care and has both a national and local role. Its national role is to draw together all the information about the quality of social care provision in a local area in order to form a national picture of the state of social care in England. Its local role is to ensure that social care in each council area is of high quality, and ensures this by regularly inspecting and reviewing all care services.
Commission for Healthcare Audit and Inspection	Formed by the Health and Social Care (Community Health and Standards) Act 2003 and launched in April 2004. Its role is to promote improvement in quality of health care in England and Wales. In England only, this includes regulation of the independent health care sector. The Healthcare Commission has a wide range of functions that includes independently assessing the performance of the health services from patients' perspectives, discovering how effectively public funds are used within health care, investigating serious failures in healthcare services, and publishing ratings of NHS hospitals and trusts, and an annual report on health care in England and Wales.

Table 4.7 Health Improvement Framework.

Fair access

Effectiveness delivery of appropriate care

Efficiency

Patient/carer experience

Health outcomes of NHS care

sidered within the equivalent PSSS Performance Assessment Framework (PAF) whose five domains are the same as those used by all the local governments.

Patient/carer experience

Traditionally older people have been seen as passive consumers of services. For example whilst the Chronically Sick and Disabled Persons Act (1970) places a duty on local authorities to identify the number of disabled people and to publish information on the type of services that they offer (under Section 2 of the Act), it says little about the quality of services that older people can expect to receive. Hence older people will often complain that they have to comply with the daily routines of their home help, such as being assisted to bed at 6.00 p.m. instead of their later chosen time.

However, systems need to be in place that protects patients' rights. Although we have no Bill of Rights, **legislation** that has enhanced the power of patients includes the Mental Health Act (1983) and the 1990 National Health Service and Community Care Act. Recent legislation has strengthened the involvement of older people in the decision-making process (Health and Social Care Act 2001b).

In the UK, choice and involvement was facilitated by the 1990 National Health Service and Community Care Act, that recommended that people were given a copy of their care plan. In addition, the Data Protection Act (1998c) strengthened patients' rights to access their own health care records. Hence, good practice in occupational therapy means that older adults are given a copy of all relevant documentation. This in turn will ensure that the patient and the therapist are striving for the same goal. In order to meet this standard it is suggested that occupational therapists will need to provide information to carers and older persons, explaining the results of assessments and or any decisions that have been made regarding their care.

One of the major changes and possibly the most controversial change to occur in the organisation of health and social care is the policy of devolution. The development of foundation hospitals will impact upon the role of occupational therapist. Foundation hospitals will treat NHS patients according to NHS principles and NHS standards, but they will be controlled and run locally, not nationally.

Occupational therapists need to be sensitive to the needs of carers of older people, as these have not always been safeguarded. There are about 5.7 million people providing some type of informal care (Office for National Statistics 1998), most of whom will be caring for older people (see Table 4.8).

More women than men provide informal care and people aged between 45 and 64 comprise the single largest group of unpaid carers. Research from London Economics for Carers National Association (1998) found that unemployed people were less likely to provide unpaid care, and that carers not living with an older person were more likely to provide care if they were better off. The Royal

Table 4.8 Characteristics of people providing informal care (Office for National Statistics 1998) based on General Household Survey 1995.

		All carers (%)
Carers:	Men	40
	Women	60
Aged:	16–24	32
	45–64	48
	65+	20
Dependant's relationship to care:	Spouse	19
	Parent/parent in-law	43
	Child (any age)	9
	Other relative or friend	28
	TOTAL	100

Commission (1999) suggests that it is important to consider whether there will be a reduction in the supply of unpaid care in the future. It is important to consider the effects on the supply of unpaid care because of changes in family structure brought about by falls in birth rates, higher divorce rates, re-marriage, greater family mobility and less living together of families across generations.

Under the Carers (Recognition and Services) Act (1995), occupational therapists had a duty to assess the needs of a carer only if the person they are caring for is being assessed. However new legislation (The Carers and Disabled Children Bill 1999a) gives carers the right to have their own needs assessed in cases where the person they are caring for has refused an assessment. A conflict of interest may occur if both the carer and the client have different opinions and needs. Perhaps the solution is to make appropriate use of patient advocates, which have been introduced as part of the NHS Plan (DH 2000). The Practical Guide for Disabled People or Carers is a useful guide which tells people where to find information, services and equipment for older people and or support (DH 2003).

When working with older people and their carers, occupational therapists need to be aware of health and safety **legislation** in order to ensure their own safety but also that of clients, colleagues and carers. In particular it is estimated that over 50% of all injuries in the health and social care sector are due to manual handling (Health Service Executive 1998). The Health and Safety Act (1974c) and the Management of Health and Safety at Work Regulation (1992a) cover some of the most important aspects of health and safety legislation. In particular, occupational therapists need to be aware of the Manual Handling Operations Regulations (MHORs) (Health Service Executive 1992a,b) and the need to carry out risk assessment. Further guidance can be obtained from Health and Safety Executive (http://www.hse.gov.uk/).

Such legislation has been interpreted locally and occupational therapists need to be aware of their local policy on MHORs as well as other local policies affecting the health and safety of clients and themselves, such as the Control of Substances Hazardous to Health (COSHH) and Control of Infection. A local control of infection policy will advise occupational therapists working with older people with infectious diseases such as methicillin-resistant *Staphylococcus aureus* (MRSA), tuberculosis, and hepatitis B and C, ensuring safe practice and minimising the risk to clients and practitioners (COT 2004).

Efficiency

Integrated working and partnership is at the centre of current health care policy (DH 2000). The need for integration is highlighted by the fact that care is often uncoordinated; there is weak communication between professional and different agencies; assessments are often duplicated; and physical, social, psychological problems can be missed or go unreported. The National Service Framework for Older People and the NHS Plan (DH 2000 and 2001) have emphasised the need for an integrated health and social care system to eradicate the problems cited above.

Specific changes in practice also include the introduction of intermediate care and integrated health and social care. As a response to this policy shift the College of Occupational Therapists has published the document 'From Interface to Integration' (COT 2002) which outlines proposals for an integrated occupational therapy service.

Effective delivery of appropriate care

Occupational therapists have a professional duty to provide good quality care (COT 2000). In the UK ways of enhancing quality have been brought under the umbrella term of clinical governance, which aims to safeguard quality and effectiveness of **services** (DH 1998). It aims to achieve this by implementing quality improvement, good practice, and detecting and minimising adverse events, addressing poor performance and thorough professional development. For occupational therapists working with older people this means that they have a duty to ensure that they are addressing and implementing quality activities which may include evidence-based practice, clinical audit, setting standards, involving users, and through lifelong learning. The National Service Framework for Older People (DH 2001) has placed a specific emphasis on competence, and occupational therapists will need to ensure that they are able to demonstrate that they have specific training that enables them to work with older people. Thus there is the need for continued professional development through lifelong learning.

The need for effective assessment and treatment will be reinforced by the Community Care Discharge Act (DH 2004a). If older people remain in hospital because social services have not fulfilled their responsibility, then the costs will be passed onto the social services department. For occupational therapists this may bring increased interprofessional and intraprofessional tension. Furthermore it may hinder the ethos of partnership-working as discharge planning is a process that is dependent on interprofessional collaboration between health and welfare professionals. Consequently, occupational therapists will need to ensure that they continue to support the principles of collaborative working.

Health outcomes of NHS care

Occupational therapists need to be aware of the milestone for each standard in the NSF so that appropriate changes in practice can occur and that progress can be made within local health and social care systems. For example, the rise in the number of older people living at home will result in more occupational therapists working with older people in the community. Some milestones from the Department of Health – Public Service Agreement (2002) are:

- To improve the quality of life and independence of older people so that they can live at home wherever possible, by increasing by March 2006 the number

of those supported intensively to live at home to 30% of the total being supported by social services at home or in residential care.

- To reduce the maximum wait for an outpatient appointment to 3 months, and
the maximum wait for inpatient treatment to 6 months by the end of 2005, and
achieve progressive further cuts with the aim of reducing the maximum inpatient and day case waiting time to 3 months by 2008.

In order to measure the quality of services from the consumers' opinions the
NHS Plan requires all NHS and Primary Care trusts to carry out local surveys.
Occupational therapists need to ensure that they have the skills and the expertise
to capture the opinions of users (see Chapter 1).

Box 4.3

Download a patient survey from:

www.dh.gov.uk/PublicationsAndStatistics/PublishedSurvey/NationalSurveyOfNHSPatients/fs/en

Is it the best tool for ascertaining older people's opinions?

Summary

Occupational therapists need to have an excellent understanding of many different current **policies** in order to ensure that older people receive equitable care to
facilitate their health, functioning and wellbeing. Occupational therapists need to
become more aware of the challenges facing health and special care and ensure
that the profession has suitably trained therapists with both the skills and the
motivation to promote active ageing.

References

Automobile Association [AA] (2000) *Helping the Older Driver*. London: AA.
Burnett A (2004). *Forum Brief. Bus Passes*. Accessed 14.05.2004.
  http://www.epolitix.com/EN/ForumBriefs/200212/F7662DCC-9C04-4D8E-B1D4-
  BFB84493AD17.htm
Cameron A & Masterson A (1998) The changing policy context of occupational therapy
  British Journal of Occupational Therapy 61(12), 556–560.
Canadian Association of Occupational Therapists (2002) *Report of the Professional Issue
  Forum on Universal Design for Growing Through Occupation*. http://www.caot.ca/p59
Carnegie Inquiry into the third age (1993) *Life, Work and Livelihood in the Third Age*.
  Dunfermline, Scotland: Carnegie UK Trust.
College of Occupational Therapists (2000) *Code of Ethics and Professional Conduct for
  Occupational Therapists*. London: College of Occupational Therapists.

College of Occupational Therapists (2002) *From Interface to Integration. A Strategy for Modernising Occupational Therapy Services in Local Health and Social Care Communities*. A Consultation Document. London: College of Occupational Therapists.

College of Occupational Therapists (2004) *Providing a Safe Service to People with Infectious Diseases*. COT/BAOT Briefing. London: College of Occupational Therapists.

Department of the Environment, Transport and the Regions (1998) *National Travel Survey, 1996–1998*. London: HMSO.

Department of Environment, Transport and the Regions (1999) *Road Accidents in Great Britain 1998: The Casualty Report*. London: HMSO.

Department of Health (1997) *The New NHS Modern and Dependable*. London: HMSO.

Department of Health (1998) *A First Class Service. Quality in the New NHS*. London: HMSO.

Department of Health (2000) *The NHS Plan*. London: HMSO.

Department of Health (2001) *The National Service Framework for Older People*. London: HMSO.

Department of Health (2002) *Public Service Agreement*. Accessed 14.05.2004. http://www.hmtreasury.gov.uk/Spending_Review/spend_sr02/psa/spend_sr02_psaindex.cfm

Department of Health (2003) *A Practical Guide for Disabled People or Carers Where to Find Information, Services and Equipment*. London: HMSO.

Department of Health (2004a) *The Community Care (Delayed Discharges etc) Act*. London: HMSO.

Department of Health (2004b) *Choosing Health: making healthier choices easier*. London: HMSO.

Department of Health and Social Security (1976) *Priorities for Health and Personal Social Services in England*. Consultative document. London: DHSS.

Department of Health and Social Security (1977) *Joint Care Planning Health and Local*. (Circular 4C(77) 17/LAC(77) 10). London: HMSO.

Department of Health and Social Security (1978) *A Happier Old Age: A Discussion Document*. London: HMSO.

Department of Health and Social Security (1980) *Social Security Act*. London: HMSO.

Department of Health and Social Security (1981) *Care in Action*. London: HMSO.

Department of Health and Social Security (1986) *Social Security Act*. London: HMSO.

Department for Transport (DfT) (2000) *Understanding People's Needs: Older People: Their Transport Needs and Requirements – Summary Report*. London: DfT.

Department for Transport (2002) *Inclusive Mobility; A Guide to Best Practice on Access to Pedestrian and Transport Infrastructure*. London: DfT.

Department for Work and Pensions (2002) *Pensioners' Guide – England and Wales*. The Pension Service. London: HMSO.

Gilhooly M, Hamilton K, O'Neill P, Gow J, Webster N, Pike F (2003) *Transport and Ageing. Extending Quality of Life via Public and Private Transport*. Economic Social Research Council Growing Older Programme. Accessed 29.05.2004. http://www.shef.ac.uk/uni/projects/gop/MaryGilhoolyTransp.htm

Goodman A, Johnson P, Webb S (1997) *Inequality in the UK*. Oxford: University Press.

Health Service Executive (1992a) *Management of Health and Safety at Work Regulations 1992*. London: Health and Safety Commission.

Health Service Executive (1992b) *Manual Handling Operations Regulations 1992*. London: Health and Safety Executive.

Health Service Executive (1998) *Manual Handling Operations Regulations 1992*. Guidance on regulations. Sudbury: HSE Books.

Karagiannidou E & Foot H (2003) *The Impact of Keeping a Diary on Older Drivers*. Royal Society for the Prevention of Accidents Road Safety Congress, Blackpool.

London Economics (1998) *The Economics of Informal Care*. A report by London Economics to the Carers National Association. London: Economics/Carers National Association.

Ministry of National Insurance and National Insurance Advisory Committee (1946) *National Insurance Act, 1946*. London: HMSO.

Ministry of Health (1948) *National Assistance Act*. Circular 87/48. London: HMSO.

Ministry of Health (1956) *Report of the Committee of Enquiry into the Cost of the National Health Service (The Guillebaud Committee)*. London: HMSO.

Minister of Housing and Local Government (1961) *Services for Older People Report*. London: HMSO.

Ministry of Health (1962) *National Assistance Act 1948 (Amendment) Act*. Circular 7/62. London: HMSO.

Ministry of Pensions and National Insurance (1962) *Ministry of Pensions and National Insurance: Report for the Year 1961*. London: HMSO.

National Institute for Social Work (1988) *A Positive Choice*. The Wagner Report, Vol. 1: Report of the Independent Review of Residential Care. London: National Institute for Social Work.

National Insurance Advisory Committee (1957) *Report in Accordance with Section 41 (3) of the National Insurance Act, 1946 on Part-time Employment*. London: HMSO.

O'Connell A (2002) *Raising State Pension Age. Are We Ready?* A discussion paper. London: Pensions Policy Institute.

Office for National Statistics (1998) *Informal Carers: Results of an independent study carried out on behalf of the Department of Social Security as part of the 1995 General Household Survey*. London: HMSO.

Office for National Statistics (1999) *The Family Expenditure Survey 1996/97*. London: HMSO.

Organisation for Economic Co-operation and Development (2001) *Ageing and Income: Financial Resources and Retirement in Nine OECD Countries*. Paris: OECD.

Royal College of Physicians (1989) *Care of Older People with Mental Illness*. Report of a Joint Working Party of the Royal College of Physicians and The Royal College of Psychiatrists. London: Royal College of Physicians.

Royal Commission (1960) *Royal Commission on Doctors' and Dentists' Remuneration, 1957–1960*. Report. London: HMSO.

Royal Commission (1999) *Royal Commission on the Funding of Long Term Care with Respect to Old Age: Long Term Care – Rights and Responsibilities*. London: HMSO.

Standing Medical Advisory Committee Report (1963) *The Field of Work of the Family Doctor (The Gillie Report)*. London: HMSO.

Townsend P (1964) *The Last Refuge*. London: Routledge and Kegan Paul.

United Kingdom Parliament (1956) *The National Health Service Act 1956*. London: HMSO.

United Kingdom Parliament (1968) *Health Service and Public Health Act 1968*. London: HMSO.

United Kingdom Parliament (1970a) *Local Authority Service Act 1970*. London: HMSO.

United Kingdom Parliament (1970b) *The Chronically Sick and Disabled Persons Act 1970*. London: HMSO.

United Kingdom Parliament (1974a) *The Housing Act*. London: HMSO.

United Kingdom Parliament (1974b) *The 1974 Rent Act*. London: HMSO.

United Kingdom Parliament (1974c) *Health and Safety at Work Act 1974*. London: HMSO.

United Kingdom Parliament (1975) *Sex Discrimination Act 1975*. London: HMSO.

United Kingdom Parliament (1976) *Race Relations Act of 1976*. London: HMSO.

United Kingdom Parliament (1980) *Housing Act 1980*. London: HMSO.

United Kingdom Parliament (1983) *The Mental Health Act 1983*. London: HMSO.

United Kingdom Parliament (1984) *Housing Act 1984*. London: HMSO.

United Kingdom Parliament (1988) *Housing Act 1988*. London: HMSO.

United Kingdom Parliament (1989a) *Local Government and Housing Act 1989*. London: HMSO.

United Kingdom Parliament (1989b) *National Health Service and Community Care Act 1990*. London: HMSO.

United Kingdom Parliament (1995) *The Disability Discrimination Act 1995*. London: HMSO.

United Kingdom Parliament (1995) *Carers (Recognition and Services) Act 1995*. London: HMSO.

United Kingdom Parliament (1998a) *Human Rights Act* (Chapter 42), which incorporates the European Convention on Human Rights into English Law. London: HMSO.

United Kingdom Parliament (1998b) *The Rail Vehicle Accessibility Regulations (RSVAR) 1998*. London: HMSO.

United Kingdom Parliament (1998c) *Data Protection Act 1998*. London: HMSO.

United Kingdom Parliament (1999a) *Carers and Disabled Children Bill 1999*. London: HMSO.

United Kingdom Parliament (1999b) *Health Act 1999*. London: HMSO.

United Kingdom Parliament (2000a) *The Care Standards Act 2000*. London: HMSO.

United Kingdom Parliament (2000b) *The Public Services Vehicles Accessibility Regulations 2000*. London: HMSO.

United Kingdom Parliament (2001a) *The Regulatory Reform Act 2001*. London: HMSO.

United Kingdom Parliament (2001b) *Health and Social Care Act 2001*. London: HMSO.

United Kingdom Parliament (2002) *National Health Service Reform and Health Care Professions Act 2002*. London: HMSO.

United Kingdom Parliament (2003) *Health and Social Care (Community Health and Standards) Act 2003*. London: HMSO.

Wilcock AA (1998) *An Occupational Perspective of Health*. Thorofare, USA: Slack.

World Health Organisation/Europe (1985) *Targets for Health for All*. European Health for All Series, No 1. Copenhagen: WHO Regional Office for Europe.

World Health Organisation/Europe (1993) *Health for All Targets. The Health Policy for Europe*. Copenhagen: WHO Regional Office for Europe.

World Health Organisation/Europe (1994) *Health in Europe: The 1993/1994 Health for All Monitoring Report*. Copenhagen: WHO Regional Office for Europe.

World Health Organisation/Europe (1998) *Health 21 – The Health for all Policy for the WHO European Region: 21 Targets for the 21st Century*. Copenhagen: WHO Regional Office for Europe.

World Health Organisation (2002) *Active Ageing. A Policy*. Geneva: World Health Organisation.

Chapter 5
PATHOLOGIES OF OLD AGE

Introduction

Older people differ from younger people in the way they respond to illness and disability. Consequently, it is essential that older people have access to appropriate specialists who are skilled in and who have relevant expertise in working with and for older people. Working with older people is particularly stimulating as they often present with multiple pathology. For this reason occupational therapists need to be able be able to assess and evaluate how each pathology as well as social, psychological, spiritual and cultural factors impact upon an older person's health and wellbeing.

The United Kingdom (UK) government's National Service Frameworks (NSFs) have highlighted key services, targets and assessments which will influence the delivery of occupational therapy services and therefore these have been used to provide a structure for this chapter. The most obvious of these, the NSF for Older People (DH 2001a) has far reaching implications for services and has already been discussed in Chapter 4. The pathologies discussed in this chapter are presented in alphabetical order and are chosen because of recent concern surrounding best practice. The pathologies can be seen in Box 5.1 and have been illustrated by the use of case studies. Outcome measures enable therapists to demonstrate with confidence that a change in a client's wellbeing be attributed to their intervention. The data generated by such assessments can be used not only by practitioners, but also by managers to monitor quality assurance and to develop health and social care policy and research. However, occupational therapists need to try to find an outcome measure that is right for their client group and organisation and there is increasing evidence that therapists are finding this a difficult and challenging task (Stubbs *et al.* 2004). In this chapter, many of the outcome measures are not pathology specific such as the Canadian Occupational Therapy Performance Measure (COPM) (Law *et al.* 1998), or occupational therapy specific, and can be used by different team members. It is also important that occupational therapists consider using quality of life measures to ascertain the older person's perspectives on their health and wellbeing (Liddle & McKenna 2000). A useful resource is an information pack for occupational therapists on outcomes measures published by the College of Occupational Therapists (Clarke *et al.* 2001).

Box 5.1

- Cancer
- Dementia
- Depression
- Diabetes
- Falls
- Fractures
- Heart failure
- Learning disability
- Musculoskeletal problems
- Respiratory problems
- Stroke (cerebrovascular accident)

CANCER

Helen Barrett and Anna Kittel

Box 5.2

Mrs Mullin is a 70-year-old woman with breast cancer, which was diagnosed 5 years ago. At the time she had a mastectomy of her right breast and subsequently received chemotherapy and radiotherapy treatment. She has developed lymphoedema in her right arm. She has a husband who is a retired builder and two grown-up daughters who are married with families. Mrs Mullin has recently developed lung metastases and has had a pleural effusion drained. However, she has noticed that she still becomes breathless when doing the housework or walking upstairs, and becomes anxious when this happens. She enjoys seeing her three grandchildren but finds she gets very fatigued.

Over 70% of all newly diagnosed cancers occur in people aged 60 or over. For men the most common type of cancer is lung cancer (19%), prostate cancer (17%), large bowel cancer (14%) and bladder cancer (7%). In contrast, for women the most common type of cancer is breast cancer (29%) (like Mrs Mullin in Box 5.2), large bowel cancer (12%), lung cancer (11%), and cancer of the ovary (5%) (Cancer Bacup 2002).

Cancer is one of a group of many related diseases that commence at cellular level. Normally cells grow and divide when required by the body. However if cells keep dividing when new cells are not needed they can form a mass of tissue, called a growth, tumour or neoplasm, which can be benign or malignant. Benign tumours are not cancerous, but like malignant tumours, can impinge upon the function of surrounding organs. Cells from malignant tumours can break away and spread to other locations within the body, known as a metastasis.

A number of factors that increase a person's chance of developing cancer have been identified. These include tobacco, diet, alcohol, ultraviolet radiation, ionizing radiation, chemicals and other substances, hormone replacement therapy (HRT), diethylstilbestrol (DES), and having close relatives with certain types of cancer. Consequently as some risk factors can be avoided, occupational therapists have an important health promotion role both within primary, secondary and tertiary health promotion (National Cancer Institute 2002).

Age discrimination has taken place within cancer care for older people in relation to preventive screening and treatment (Turner *et al.* 1999). Furthermore, there is evidence that doctors fail to inform older patients of their diagnosis despite research that suggests the contrary (Ajaj *et al.* 2001). In order to ensure that cancer patients receive a first class service, the National Health Service Cancer Plan (DH 2000a) has presented a radical reorganisation of cancer services in order to promote survival and wellbeing.

A diagnosis of cancer and the treatment itself can cause consider psychological problems to cancer patients and their families (Bottomley & Jones 1997). Indeed one of the most common psychological symptoms is anxiety and patients may experience different levels of anxiety dependent upon the disease type, the stage of the disease and doctor preference treatment (Bottomley 1997). Depression is also common with a cancer diagnosis (Bottomley *et al.* 1996). Indeed Mrs Mullin's anxiety could be exacerbating her ability to perform her daily occupations. Consequently, occupational therapists require excellent communication skills and strategies to manage psychological issues and to deliver client-focused services. The NHS Cancer Plan (DH 2000a) has outlined the importance not only of good communication skills but has highlighted the importance of making high quality information available to cancer patients.

Whilst some cancers are responsive to treatment, others are not. The term 'palliative care' is used to define 'the active care of patients and their families by a multiprofessional team when the patient's disease is no longer responsive to curative treatment' (WHO Expert Committee 1990:1). Occupational therapists are often members of the multiprofessional team, which should also include specialist medical and nursing staff, social workers, and physiotherapists and should work closely with dietetics and chaplaincy (DH 1995).

Consequently, the primary role of occupational therapy is to enhance wellbeing and quality of life through engagement in meaningful occupation (Penfold 1996). Indeed, in Mrs Mullin's case, an occupational therapist would need to consider interventions that would enable Mrs Mullin to manage her fatigue, anxiety and breathlessness so she can continue to visit her grandchildren and participate in occupations which she values. A survey by Anderson *et al.* (2001) identified that most frequent problems for palliative care patients were pain (49%), loss of independence (30%), and difficulty walking (27%). Consequently specific interventions used by occupational therapists need to address these identified problems. A survey by Meek & Atwal (2004) into the role of the occupational therapist in palliative care found that the most frequently used interventions by occupational therapists were daily living assessments, team working and collaboration with other agencies, home visits and rehabilitation. Furthermore, the same survey found that a key role of the occupational therapist within palliative care is within discharge planning.

Table 5.1 Assessment and outcome tools used by occupational therapists in oncology and palliative care.

Canadian Occupation Performance Measure (COPM). A client-centred outcome measure, which can be used to detect change over time of a person's self-perception of occupational performance (Law *et al.* 1998).

Westcotes Measure (Eames *et al.* 1999). Uses goal-setting to measure outcomes. The scoring system is designed so that it is able to identify statistically significant change (Eva 2000).

Goal Setting. Involves identifying, SMART (specific, measurable, achievable, realistic, timely) goals in collaboration with clients, relating to an occupational performance. A baseline measure of performance is made from which change can be measured following intervention (Eva 2000).

World Health Organisation Quality of Life Scales (WHOQOL-100 and WHOQOL-BREF). Suitable for all areas of practice and assesses physical health, psychological state, personal beliefs, social relationships and relationship with the environment (University of Bath 2004).

Whilst the role of the occupational therapist within palliative care is emerging, it is hindered by the absence of robust research to demonstrate the effectiveness of occupational therapy. It is essential that occupational therapists use outcome measures to evaluate their interventions and occupational therapists need to consider using quality of life measures. Possible outcome measures that could be used with older people with cancer have been suggested in Table 5.1.

DEMENTIA

Alison Warren

Box 5.3

> Mrs Davies is an 80-year-old lady who has been referred to a community mental health team. George, her husband had become worried as she has become repetitive, tearful, forgetful (losing objects) and disorientated in her local community. Mrs Davies now requires assistance with cooking and shopping. Until recently Mrs Davies attended church regularly where she sings in the choir. Mr Davies is too worried to let Mrs Davies walk to the shops and does not like leaving her alone. This means that Mr Davies has now stopped attending the Bowls club and they spend all of their time together.

Mrs Davies' narrative (Box 5.3) describes some of the early signs that could possibly lead to a diagnosis of dementia. Dementia is an umbrella term, a syndrome that describes the signs and symptoms of several diseases that are linked to the degeneration or death of brain cells. The WHO (1992) ICD-10 diagnostic guidelines define dementia as a decline in memory and thinking. This in turn impacts on activities of daily living and is progressive in nature. Dementia mainly affects older people although its onset can be under the age of 65 years (Harvey *et al.* 1998).

According to the Alzheimer's Society (2003) there are over 100 different types of dementia with Alzheimer's disease, vascular dementia and Lewy body being the most common. Depending on the area of the brain affected by the degenerative process, the disease will present differently.

There are many changes for the individual and family when a person has dementia. By looking at Mrs Davies' narrative, there is evidence of cognitive, behavioural, emotional, physical and occupational performance difficulties.

The role of occupational therapy in dementia care is diverse, challenging and exciting. It provides us with an opportunity to be truly holistic using our unique focus on the therapeutic use of occupation for people with dementia and their carers.

Historically, occupational therapists have struggled to practice effectively in dementia care (Perrin & May 2000). The deteriorating nature of dementia has often made it a challenge for occupational therapists and other professionals who have attempted to use rehabilitation models. Occupational therapy is not only concerned with promoting independence but also promoting wellbeing through the use of occupation with both the person with dementia and their carers.

Occupational therapists can provide a valuable contribution within a multidisciplinary team. This includes working in memory clinics, community teams, day services and inpatient facilities as well as networking with other agencies. There are various models adopted by multidisciplinary teams, with professionals being viewed as specialists or generic workers.

Members of the multidisciplinary team each have a role to play in the assessment of people with dementia. This often includes using a variety of screening tools to assist with diagnosis and problem identification (Naidoo & Bullock 2001). The assessment tools will vary depending on whether they are diagnostic in nature or designed for planning intervention (see Table 5.2). Occupational therapists assess individuals with dementia in order to ascertain their functional ability/occupational performance needs and abilities. The occupational therapists will assess in the

Table 5.2 Key assessment tools used by occupational therapists in dementia care.

Large Allen's Cognitive Level Screen (LACLS). One of several assessment tools designed to be used in conjunction with the Cognitive Disabilities Model (Allen *et al.* 1992). The client is given a rectangular piece of leather with holes around the edge and instructed to complete three different types of stitch and to correct certain errors. This screening tool identifies a client's cognitive level, which should always be backed up by a practical assessment and by talking to carers. The client's intervention can then be planned in order to maintain or maximise the client's functional performance.

Assessment of Motor and Process Skills (AMPS). An observational functional assessment tool that examines both the motor and process elements of the activity. Training via a specific AMPS course (Fisher 1995).

Canadian Occupational Performance Measure (COPM) (Law *et al.* 1998).

Pool Activity Level Instrument (PAL). Developed to engage people with dementia in meaningful occupation. Comprises of a checklist completed by both formal and informal carers to recognise the activity level of an individual and provide appropriate activities to promote wellbeing (Pool 2002).

areas of self-care, productivity and leisure as well as performance components (Canadian Association of Occupational Therapists [CAOT] 2002). Performance components include affect, cognition and physical ability and are also assessed by other disciplines. It is important to carry out assessments in the home environment to increase the accuracy of information gained (Naidoo & Bullock 2001).

Within dementia there tends to be a focus on the assessment of **impairment** particularly cognition for example the **Mini Mental State Examination** (Folstein *et al.* 1975) or the **Middlesex Elderly Assessment of Mental State** (Golding 1989). It is important that the areas of **activity limitation** and **participation restriction** are not overlooked. It is important that a multidisciplinary approach is acknowledged with risk assessment when identifying risk and accepting that people are allowed to take risks (Bullock 2002).

Traditionally in dementia care the interventions of reality orientation (Holden 1988) validation therapy (Feil 1993) and reminiscence therapy (Coleman 1986) have been used which have changed in popularity. Over recent years there has been the introduction of sensory work with people in the late stage of the disease (Pinkney 1997), and also assistive technology with people at the early stage, to enable them to remain living in their home environment (Doughty & Burton 2002).

The interventions offered by the multidisciplinary team are varied and involve both the person with dementia and their carers. Interventions offered should be shaped around individual need, and appropriate for the stage of the disease. The intervention may be on an individual or group basis.

Occupational therapists in dementia care make use of their holistic and problem-solving approach. The range of interventions can include providing equipment to assist with bathing, providing visual cues in order to maintain skills and safety in the kitchen, or advising on an environment that provides stimulation with the aim of enhancing wellbeing.

Evaluating outcomes can be difficult when working with people who have dementia, as there is not an expectation that there will be functional improvement because of the nature of the disease (Clarke *et al.* 2001).

There are many outcome measures available to occupational therapists and other members of a multidisciplinary team. In the area of dementia care, it would be most appropriate to use outcome measures that are not only charting the progression of the disease but those which examine quality of life, wellbeing and meaningful goals for the individual and their carer. Therefore to provide continuity for the client and carer and to assist in the collection of outcome information, it can be useful for professionals to work across service areas.

DEPRESSION

Alice Mackenzie

Present studies show that the prevalence of depression is the most common mental health problem in older adults (Beekman *et al.* 1999). These studies suggest

Box 5.4

Mr Jones is 75 years old and lives in a one-bedroom flat in the city. He has been referred to the community mental health team for older people for assessment and treatment. His wife died 1 year ago after 47 years of marriage. Mr Jones has a daughter who lives about 50 miles away and a son who lives overseas. Nine months ago Mr Jones was diagnosed with angina and prescribed medication. Two months ago Mr Jones's daughter suggested he saw his GP because he seemed to be more anxious than normal; worrying about things going wrong in his flat that would not have worried him before and also being preoccupied with his physical health. He had been neglecting his shopping and cooking, and did not want to socialise with his friends at the pub or work on his allotment. He has become increasingly bad tempered and irritable with his daughter. He complains of being forgetful, sleeping poorly and expresses feelings of hopelessness with regard to the future.

that the number is between 10% and 16%, rising to 20% in the over 80s (Audit Commission 2000). These figures can be doubled for these older people with physical health problems (Banerjee *et al.* 1996). In this case study (Box 5.4) Mr Jones has been diagnosed with angina and seems to be more anxious than normal. He is also complaining of being forgetful, sleeping poorly and expresses feelings of hopelessness with regard to the future. Depression has been shown to be greater in patients with **heart disease** and **diabetes mellitus** than in controls (Katon & Ciechanoweki 2003).

There is evidence that clinical depression among older people can often go undiagnosed and untreated (Crawford *et al.* 1998). Suggested explanation for this is related to poor detection, and the fact that older people often present with physical conditions or have complex social problems that lead professionals to discount symptoms as 'understandable' or just a symptom of old age (Bagley *et al.* 2000). Older people are more likely to present with somatic complaints rather than feelings associated with depression (Mayall *et al.* 2004). This is rather disturbing since depression is the risk factor most often associated with suicide (Zweige & Hinrichsen 1993).

The most common form of intervention with older people is pharmacological. One study found that only 5% of older people received counselling or supportive therapy, despite evidence that older people have a lower drop-out rate than younger people when using psychological therapies (Blanchard *et al.* 1999). Other effective forms of treatment include exercise to improve depressive symptoms among older people who are not responsive to medication (Mather *et al.* 2002).

It is important to differentiate between low mood or sadness that everyone can experience from time to time, and the symptoms of clinical depression. Depression is classified as a mood disorder (WHO 1992). Key symptoms which guide the diagnosis and degree of severity of a clinical depression are:

- Loss of concentration and attention.
- Loss of energy, psychomotor retardation.
- Sleep disturbance.

- Feelings of guilt.
- Feelings of sadness and hopelessness.
- Suicidal thoughts or impulses.
- Psychosomatic symptoms.
- Memory problems.

When the depression is severe the person may present with paranoid delusions and ideation. Ballard & Eastwood (1999) report an overlap of symptoms between severe depression and dementia. Not only does depression occur in **dementia**, but dementia can also be caused by **depression** (pseudodementia).

Evidence of physical illness (**angina**) and stressful life events, especially those associated with loss (such as with Mr Jones); causing a person to develop clinical depression is ambiguous. But there are a number of contextual factors (Beekman *et al.* 1999; Tijhuis *et al.* 1999) associated with clinical depression, for example:

- A previous history of depression.
- Family history of depression.
- Poverty.
- Social isolation.
- Poor physical health and/or developing a life threatening illness.
- Moving into residential care.
- Bereavement of spouse or a child, or close family/friends.
- Retirement.
- Lack of satisfaction with life.

It should be emphasised that clinical depression is not an automatic response to deficits or excesses of these factors (Minardi & Blanchard 2004).

Occupational therapists and multidisciplinary teams have an important role in the early detection and management of depression in older people both in the community, care homes and physical and mental health setting. The primary aim of intervention is to enable older persons to engage with everyday roles and daily occupations. In the case of Mr Jones, the occupational therapist will need to ensure that the participation restrictions affecting his ability to perform his chosen occupations are identified.

A number of assessments and outcome measures could be used with Mr Jones. However occupational therapists must ensure that the tools have reliability and validity for use in older persons (Table 5.3).

Occupational therapists work with both individuals and groups using a diverse range of **activities**. The intervention will be dependent on priorities and goals identified from the assessment by the client and the occupational therapist. However interventions are aimed at helping people retain a sense of purpose and self-worth (College of Occupational Therapists 2001). These can be broken down to short-term goals as the client's motivation may be affected by their mood. Therefore it would be appropriate to set short-term goals initially that the client feels they are able to meet. Since attending his allotment is an important occupation for Mr Jones this can be a central focus of occupational therapy intervention.

Table 5.3 Assessment and outcome measures for older people with depression.

Geriatric Depression Scale (GDS). A self-report inventory with simple yes/no format. For 30-item scale, scores of 0–10 are indicative of non-depression; 11–20 of mild depression and 21+ of severe depression. Probably the most widely used instrument in older persons' psychiatry. Several versions exist: 30-item; 15-item and 4-item (Yesavage *et al.* 1982–83).

Brief Assessment Schedule Depression Cards (BASDEC). Consists of a 19-item deck of cards, to elicit a response of 'true', 'false' or 'I do not know'. Two items are weighted to give two points, with a maximum score of 21. A score of seven or above suggests a 'case' of depression, i.e. depressive symptoms of sufficient severity to warrant intervention. BASDEC is user-friendly and can be administered by non-medical staff at the bedside (Adshead *et al.* 1992).

The Assessment of Occupational Functioning – Collaborative Version (AOF-CV). A semi-structured, self-report instrument designed to yield qualitative and quantitative information about how a person is functioning relative to key components of the Model of Human Occupation. It is appropriate for use with older people in inpatient settings Version (AOF-CV 2003).

Canadian Occupational Performance Measure (Law *et al.* 1998).

As a client's improvement may in part be due to positive effects of medication; lifting the client's mood and increasing their motivation or spontaneous recovery from the depression it is important to keep clear records of **occupational performance** when reviewing (multidisciplinary) outcomes.

DIABETES

Lindy van den Berghe

Box 5.5

> Mr Crabtree is 85 and was diagnosed with type II diabetes 20 years ago. Mr Crabtree's wife and family returned to the Caribbean island of St Lucia 45 years ago and he has had little contact with them. He has lived alone ever since but enjoys the company of his neighbour, Mr Jameson. He has never been keen on cooking and tends to eat ready meals or take-aways from the local shops. Mr Crabtree has been advised about what he should eat as a diabetic several times when he attends the diabetic clinic both at the hospital and also at the GP surgery but 'can't be bothered with all that fuss'. He takes his diabetic medication and checks his blood sugars when he remembers. He has regular ophthalmology check-ups and has had deteriorating eyesight for several years. Mr Crabtree is now seeing the district nurse on a regular basis because he has recently developed an ulcer on his big toe after an ingrowing toenail became septic – he had not realised this because he has had poor sensation in both feet for many years. His main complaint is that he now can't get to the pub to play dominoes with his friends.

Mr Crabtree's situation is not uncommon (Box 5.5). In the United States 18.3 percent of all people age 60 and over have diabetes (National Diabetes Information

Clearing House 2004). It is vital these people are managed carefully and properly by the multidisciplinary healthcare team from the time of diagnosis to minimise and avoid the long-term complications. It is also important to diagnose diabetes in older people before it causes complications.

The exact causes of type II diabetes are not known and probably vary for different individuals. Environmental factors, including obesity, inactivity, and diets with a high saturated fat content appear to be factors in its development because its incidence is rapidly increasing. Other factors known to be associated with a higher risk for developing type II diabetes are age between 40 and 75, a family history of diabetes, and Asian or African-Caribbean genes.

Whatever the cause of type II diabetes, defects in insulin secretion and insulin action (either of which may be the main feature) and liver glucose production result in the high blood glucose (Stratton *et al.* 2000; Ousman & Sharma 2001).

This involves frequent monitoring of blood glucose and appropriate treatment with a diet (restricting glucose intake), oral hypoglycaemic drugs (to stimulate insulin production or sensitivity to insulin), or insulin.

Over many years, diabetes causes a variety of effects on different parts of the body associated with damage to blood vessel walls. These are thought to result from biochemical and other mechanisms associated with high blood glucose. In particular damage to small blood vessels affects:

- The retina of the eye (diabetic retinopathy), resulting in deteriorating vision and eventually blindness.
- The kidney (diabetic nephropathy), resulting in poor kidney function and eventually kidney failure, which is fatal without dialysis or a kidney transplant.
- The nerves (diabetic neuropathies), causing a variety of syndromes associated with loss of and abnormal sensation.

Damage to large blood vessels affects:

- The heart, causing angina and heart attacks.
- The brain, causing **strokes**.
- The legs, resulting in intermittent claudication (exercise-limiting pain in the calves on walking), ulcers, and gangrene.

Treatment needs to be sensibly balanced against other factors such as life expectancy and coexisting disease. Guidelines for treatment have been produced for the National Institute for Clinical Excellence (UK Prospective Diabetes Study [UKPDS] 1998b; Hutchinson *et al.* 2002).

Mr Crabtree has diabetic peripheral neuropathy, as demonstrated by the loss of sensation in his feet. He was therefore unaware that his ingrowing toenail was cutting into his toe. The subsequent injury to Mr Crabtree's toe became infected by contamination from his toenail and because Mr Crabtree's poorly controlled diabetes increases his susceptibility to infection. Diabetic foot ulcers are the most common cause of lower limb amputations in the UK, and in one study 25% of patients admitted to a university hospital with a diabetic foot ulcer ended up having an amputation. Consequently the podiatrist is an essential member of the multi-disciplinary team (Apelqvist & Agardh 1992).

Mr Crabtree, like many other older diabetics, has deteriorating eyesight. Although this is commonly caused by cataracts and macular degeneration in older people, people like Mr Crabtree probably have diabetic retinopathy as well. Regular ophthalmological follow-up and treatment are essential to maximise vision and avoid preventable blindness. There is a strong correlation between long-term poor control of the blood glucose level and the development of diabetic eye disease (The Diabetes Control and Complications Trial [DCCT] 1993; UK Prospective Diabetes Study [UKPDS] Group 1998a).

Diabetes is a neglected area of occupational therapist practice since there is lack of evidence demonstrating the effectiveness of the occupational therapist's role. An occupational therapist may be involved in the assessment and rehabilitation of an older person who has an amputation as a consequence of their diabetes, where diabetes is secondary to the amputation. Consequently occupational therapists must ensure that they understand how the primary and secondary diagnosis impacts upon their quality of life and wellbeing. For this reason the assessment tools and outcome measures will vary; however therapists could use many of the tools listed in this chapter. Occupational therapists tend to be involved with enabling older people engage in daily occupations and in **health promotion** for those clients with complications of their diabetes, such as visual impairment and amputation.

Occupational therapists have an important role in enabling the older client to compensate for vision loss with regard to their daily occupations. Cate *et al.* (1995) offer useful advice for guidelines for the treatment and management of occupational therapy and the person with diabetes and vision impairment. Important areas are domestic tasks such as self-care, monitoring glucose and drawing insulin, domestic tasks, using public transport, hobbies and leisure. Occupational therapists can introduce the client to alternative techniques and strategies to carry out difficult tasks and should consider appropriate **products and technology** that will enable older people to maintain and or enhance quality of life.

Assessment of sensory loss also needs to incorporate the extent of this **impairment** within the older person's occupations. As demonstrated by this case study, loss of sensation can eventually lead to amputation. Since diabetes rather than trauma is the primary cause of amputations, occupational therapists have an important role in educating the older persons about management of post-operative pain, rehabilitation goals and strategies. Furthermore older people need support to adapt to the loss of the limb and the resulting change in **body function** and image. Grieving should be regarded as a normal response to an amputation. However therapists need to be aware of symptoms of **depression**. Some older people may experience phantom pain or sensation. Phantom sensation, the feeling that all or part of a missing limb is still intact, is common among people with limb loss. Treatment of phantom pain includes measures to make the residual limb less sensitive, transcutaneous electrical nerve stimulation, biofeedback and guided imagery.

Pre- and post-operative rehabilitation is an important part of the occupational therapist's role. This will include a graded programme to enhance daily occupations and in particular strengthening activities. Other aspects will include modifications of the home **environment**, wheelchair mobility, management of the wound, pressure care and skin care and the management of the prosthesis.

Within activities of daily living occupational therapists have an important **health promotion** role and should address this when carrying out assessment of **activities** of daily living. For example when carrying out a self-care assessment, occupational therapists can emphasise the need for older people to pay particular attention to their feet and of the need for suitable footwear. The therapist could refer to the podiatrist for further advice and could recommend that the client receive assistance with foot care if they are unable to carry out this **activity**. When carrying out domestic assessments, the therapist can reiterate the need for a healthy diet and may work closely with the dietician. The occupational therapist could also be part of a team that runs specific healthy lifestyle courses which reiterate the importance of diet, exercise and education about diabetes.

FALLS

Anne McIntyre

Box 5.6

> Mr Partick Duffy is 91, lives alone in a council flat since the death of his sister 5 years ago. He is rather a loner and only sees his niece once a week when she takes him to Sunday mass. A few Saturdays ago Mr Duffy fell for the first time in the bathroom and couldn't get up. He lay on the floor of the bathroom for nearly 24 hours before his niece discovered him. He was admitted to hospital and was found to be malnourished and dehydrated. The nurses told Mr Duffy and his niece that he was very lucky that it was summer time otherwise he would have got hypothermia. Mr Duffy lost his confidence when transferring, standing and walking and even though he is frightened of returning home alone and of falling again he is adamant that he does not want to go into residential care.

Mr Duffy's story is not unusual (Box 5.6), and even though a fall is not a disease in itself, falls in older people have dramatic consequences, with the incidence of a fall often being an indicator of underlying pathologies. A fall is defined as unintentionally coming to rest on the ground or a lower level – not as a result of an intrinsic event such as **syncope** or **stroke** or because of an extrinsic **environmental hazard** (Tinetti *et al.* 1988).

Falls are the leading cause of death in the over-75 age group in the UK with 300 000 older people being seriously injured enough to require hospital treatment (Department of Trade and Industry [DTI] 2001). Tinetti *et al.* (1988) estimated that 30% of adults over 65 years and 50% of adults over 80 years fall at least once a year and people with dementia are said to have rates double that of the cognitively normal population. However, as falls are commonly under-reported, it is likely that these are conservative estimates (Campbell *et al.* 1990). It also has to be said that older people do not fall more than younger people do, but the consequences are usually more severe.

Falls cost the UK approximately £100 million and the US $1000 million each year (Rowe 2000; Scuffham *et al.* 2003). Falls in older people are a major factor in premature admission to permanent residential care (Audit Commission 1995) and also result in an early reduction in everyday activity and increase in support services (McIntyre 1999). However, fall rates and fracture risks increase in people in institutional settings with approximately 10% of older people who fall having a resultant fracture (Rowe 2000). People with dementia are more likely to have a 'bad fracture', with poorer recovery and three times higher mortality rates than cognitively normal older people (Baker *et al.* 1978). Common consequences of falls are:

- Minor injury.
- Hypothermia.
- Bronchopneumonia.
- Pressure sores.
- Reduced mobility.
- Reduced independence.
- Fear of falling.
- Social isolation and loneliness.
- Loss of self-efficacy.

There is much research on management and risk identification of falls in cognitively normal older people, with older people with cognitive impairment and dementia commonly excluded from research (Bartlett & Martin 2000). Gillespie *et al.* (2002) identified that falls research in older people is still in its infancy, with methodological issues in current research needing resolution. However, the UK National Institute for Clinical Excellence (NICE) in 2004 has produced clinical practice guidelines for the assessment and treatment of falls based on the best available current evidence.

Research has identified intrinsic and extrinsic risk factors associated with falls, with the following being the most common:

Intrinsic factors:
- Age >80 years.
- Falls history.
- Muscle weakness.
- Mobility and gait impairment.
- Balance impairment.
- Fear of falling.
- Limitations in everyday activity.
- Visual impairment.

- Cognitive impairment.
- Depression.
- Musculoskeletal problems.
- Urinary incontinence.

Extrinsic factors:
- Environmental hazards.
- Incorrect use of equipment.
- Polypharmacy.
- Psychotrophic and cardiovascular medications.
- Poorly fitting clothing and footwear.

(American Geriatrics Society [AGS] 2001; NICE 2004).

Occupational therapists and physiotherapists are recommended to use assessment and outcome measures that consider activity (see Table 5.4), and these measures should include at least one of the following domains:

- Falls.
- Physical function.
- Activities of daily living.
- Gait or balance.

(Chartered Society of Physiotherapy [CSP];
College of Occupational Therapy [COT] 2002).

The evidence for unidimensional interventions (including environmental modifications) is currently weak. However significant evidence exists for multifactorial, interdisciplinary, person-centred and individually tailored programmes (Gillespie *et al.* 2002). Mr Duffy was offered a programme that addressed occupational performance, modification of environmental hazards, strength and balance retraining, vision assessment, medication review and education of falls prevention (including regular exercise).

Table 5.4 Assessments and outcome measures commonly used with older people who fall.

Falls Efficacy Scale (FES) – a 10-point scale measuring confidence in everyday activities without falling. Has test–retest reliability. Based on interviews with clients and professionals, but administered by professional. Easy to administer and score. (Tinnetti *et al.* 1990).

Westmead Home Safety Assessment – identifies 72 potential extrinsic fall hazards in the home environment such as trafficways, bedroom layout, seating, footwear and medication. Devised for older people, therapist administered. No training or equipment required, clear to administer and easy to score (Clemson 1997).

Get Up and Go Test – valid and reliable test of functional balance for use with older adults. The subject is observed and scored in their ability to stand unaided from a chair, turn around, then sit themselves down again (Mathias *et al.* 1986).

Occupational therapists are commonly involved in primary, secondary and tertiary health promotion in falls management, offering advice about environmental adaptation, self-care and productivity within rehabilitation programmes, falls prevention and enhancement of self-efficacy to both the 'well' older client group as well as those who have already fallen.

FRACTURES AND OSTEOPOROSIS

Jill Lloyd

Box 5.7

> Mrs Burns is an 85-year-old widow who lives alone in a two-bedroomed house. She has a bathroom on the ground floor level, but sleeps upstairs. Mrs Burns has two daughters, one of whom lives locally and works as a teacher, and she and her husband are very supportive of Mrs Burns. She was found by her home carer on the floor 3 weeks ago having fallen whilst going to the bathroom at around 7 a.m. Mrs Burns was subsequently admitted to the local district general hospital, where an examination revealed a fractured neck of femur which was confirmed on X-ray. Management of her hip problem included a hemi-arthroplasty which was inserted under epidural anaesthesia. Her post-operative recovery was uneventful following the local integrated care pathway of early mobilisation and planned discharge at 10 days post-surgery.

The most common fractures in older people are those involving the hip, wrist, vertebrae and shoulder (proximal humerus) with osteoporosis being linked to 90% of hip fractures and 75% of wrist fractures (Tugwell *et al.* 2004).

Osteoporosis is accelerated bone loss above that of the usual ageing process (see Chapter 7) with 1 in 3 women and 1 in 5 men aged over 50 having osteoporosis. Risk factors for osteoporosis are:

- Age 70 plus.
- Female gender.
- Caucasian or Asian race.
- A decline in oestrogen following the menopause or early hysterectomy.
- Amenorrhea as a result of excessive dieting or over-exercising.
- Low levels of testosterone in men.
- Long-term use of corticosteroids.
- Malabsorption syndromes.
- Family history of osteoporosis.
- Previous fracture.
- Low body weight.
- Inactivity and lack of weight-bearing exercise.
- Smoking.

- Alcohol abuse.
- Malnutrition.
- Lack of dietary calcium.
- Lack of sunlight exposure.

(National Osteoporosis Society 2003; Woolf & Åkesson 2003).

The rising incidence of fractures is not only linked with osteoporosis but also with an increasing tendency to fall (see previous section) and deterioration in protective reflex mechanisms with ageing. Fractures at the wrist and shoulder tend to lead to a temporary reduction in activity and participation, with vertebral fractures being, in the main, asymptomatic. However, 1 in 5 people die after a hip fracture and 1 in 4 older people are less independent as a result (Gillespie 2001). In the UK, hip fractures cost the public sector £1.7 billion annually and the cost to individuals' independence and quality of life cannot be measured in monetary terms. A study by Salkeld et al. (2000) identified that many older women feared a deteriorating quality of life and said that they would prefer death than loss of independence and admission to residential care following a bad hip fracture.

The majority of those experiencing hip fractures (87%) are like Mrs Burns (see Box 5.7), over 65; and like many older people her hip fracture occurred as a result of a fall. Internal fixation of non-displaced and joint replacement of displaced fractures are the interventions of choice with older people as both allow early weight-bearing through the affected hip and therefore return to independent living and mobility. Mrs Burns had a total hip replacement (THR), because her fracture was displaced and she had evidence of osteoporosis. She was admitted to a geriatric orthopaedic rehabilitation unit (GORU), which had an early supported discharge (ESD) programme. Even though GORUs are not considered cost-effective, ESDs and geriatric hip fracture programmes (GHFP) are considered to be effective for the more active older person (such as Mrs Burns), significantly facilitating return home with previous levels of activity and participation (Cameron et al. 2000). Members of the ESD team not only include occupational therapists but also physiotherapy, medical, nursing and social work colleagues, with many teams having a discharge liaison co-ordinator.

Client-centred interventions should be prepared as soon as Mrs Burns has recovered from the acute episode and aim to stimulate musculoskeletal, postural, sensory, cognitive and psychosocial components to enhance independence (Stinnett 1996). Mrs Burns' ESD programme involved balance and mobility exercises with the physiotherapist and education in the use of walking products (see Chapters 8 and 10), both on level surfaces and stairs. Mrs Burns' occupational therapist concentrated on working with her on a return to full participation in daily occupations. It has been found that all people benefit from occupational therapy intervention following hip fracture. An American study compared the use of the occupational adaptation model with the biomechanical–rehabilitation model and found that the occupational adaptation method was associated with a better outcome and preferred by the patients (Jackson & Schkade 2001). There are no specific occupational therapy measures for this client group; however some of the outcomes measures already discussed in this chapter are relevant.

Both Mrs Burns' physiotherapist and occupational therapist followed and incorporated local total hip replacement precautions and guidelines into their programmes, ensuring that Mrs Burns was able to incorporate and generalise these into everyday life. Such precautions are taken to reduce the risk of dislocation of the replaced joint in the early weeks of recovery; however there are no universal guidelines as yet for THRs and these may alter within localities (depending on the decision by the orthopaedic surgical team), as well as between them.

Pre-discharge home assessments are commonly carried out with this client group to promote independence, prevent joint dislocation or further injury. Mrs Burns would have been provided with appropriate modifications and assistive technology for either the short or longer term.

Once discharged, continuation of mobility practice, monitoring by the discharge liaison co-ordinator, re-assessment of occupational needs and demands, provision of appropriate community services and valuable support from her family as Mrs Burns progressed, enabled her to be independent in all self-care activities and most domestic activities 6 months post-fracture. Continuing support of her family also encouraged her to resume most of her leisure interests after this time; however the return of Mrs Burns to her former functional level is unfortunately not typical of older people with fractures around the hip.

In order to prevent Mrs Burns having any further fractures the following strategies are likely to have been implemented:

- Calcium and vitamin D supplementation and/or bisophosphonates to decrease bone resorption thus increasing bone mass.
- Reduction in the incidence in falls through admission to a falls management programme (see this chapter).
- Reduction in injuries associated with falls through the use of hip protectors or home modification. However there is no current evidence to support either of these for not living in residential care (Lyons *et al.* 2004; Parker *et al.* 2004).
- Encouragement of a healthy lifestyle through maintenance of physical activity and good nutrition for example (see Chapter 8).

Prevention of osteoporosis in older age has also been part of many health promotion strategies, however it seems that few older people with fractures have limited knowledge of osteoporosis and its strong association with fractures, with what little information they have acquired being given by the media rather than by a health professional (Pal 1999). A 'bone-friendly' lifestyle throughout the lifespan can maximise peak bone mass to withstand bone loss through the normal ageing process through a calcium-rich diet with adequate protein, weight-bearing exercise, cessation of smoking and moderate alcohol consumption (National Osteoporosis Society 2003). It is therefore useful for occupational therapists to remember these primary health promotion strategies when working with clients of any age.

HEART FAILURE

Kirsty Tattersall

Box 5.8

> Mrs Rose Smith is a 79-year-old lady who has been referred to the occupational therapist whilst she is in hospital. Mrs Smith has a history of coronary artery disease and frequent hospital admissions, having recently been diagnosed with heart failure. Her husband and daughter are concerned about her shortness of breath on activity, and her extreme tiredness. They now assist with most of the housework and cooking. Mrs Smith finds it difficult to walk around the supermarket and has stopped going to her bridge club because of the flight of stairs to get there. She is spending much of her time at home and reports feeling quite low.

Heart failure is a common chronic condition, the prevalence of which increases markedly with age. It is the only major cardiovascular disease with increasing prevalence, incidence and mortality. This is particularly due to better overall treatment of coronary heart disease among younger people and an ageing population. Heart failure accounts for about 5% of all medical admissions to hospital and readmission rates are the highest for any common condition in the UK (DH 2000b).

Heart failure occurs when the heart muscle is unable to maintain an effective pumping action to meet the body's needs. The heart does not function with maximum efficiency. By looking at Mrs Smith's narrative (Box 5.8), she is displaying some of the main symptoms of heart failure, that of fatigue and breathlessness. Loss of energy is a common problem, making it difficult to carry out normal everyday activities. Failure of the left side of the heart to pump blood into the arteries results in 'back pressure' in the circulation. This can cause fluid to accumulate in the air spaces of the lungs resulting in breathlessness (British Heart Foundation [BHF] 2002).

The impact of heart failure on a person's life may be related as much to psychological adaptation to the disease as to impairment in physical functioning. In people with heart failure functional disability has been found to be a strong predictor of poor quality of life (Grady *et al.* 1995). Symptoms such as breathlessness can severely limit activity and cause avoidance of situations that might precipitate it. This can lead to further problems such as disuse atrophy and social isolation, both of which are evident for Mrs Smith (Fitzgerald 2000). Psychosocial function is also commonly affected; with depression being found to occur in approximately 33% of people with heart failure and frequently goes untreated (BHF 2001). For Mrs Smith the negative impact of heart failure on her ability to carry out her roles of homemaker and caregiver may be having a profound effect on her feelings of self-worth and quality of life.

Occupational therapists have an important role to play in the assessment and treatment of people with heart failure due to their holistic approach and ability to analyse activity, with a major occupational therapy aim being to assist them in

Table 5.5 New York Heart Association classifications.

Class I: No symptoms.

Class II: Symptoms of fatigue, palpitation, dyspnoea or angina pain on ordinary physical activity.

Class III: Symptoms in less than ordinary activity. Comfortable at rest.

Class IV: Symptoms at rest and unable to carry on physical activity without discomfort.

making a positive adjustment to their condition. An older person has to adjust to living with new limitations and the knowledge that life expectancy may be shortened.

'Heart failure care should be delivered by a multidisciplinary team with an integrated approach across the health-care community' (NICE 2003). The occupational therapist is an integral member of the multidisciplinary team working closely with the specialist heart failure nurses to ensure that the person and their carers fully understand the disease and are able to monitor and manage it themselves, which will help reduce hospital readmission (Stewart *et al.* 1999).

Assessments will be undertaken by the multidisciplinary team, assessing both the symptoms of the disease and the effects they are having on the person. People with heart failure are routinely categorised by the cardiologist on discussion of symptoms according to the New York Heart Association (NYHA) classifications (Bowling 1995) (see Table 5.5).

Occupational therapists can add to the quality of information about the person's functional ability in the areas of self-care, productivity and leisure through the use of observations and standardised assessment and outcome measures (Table 5.6). It is important to also assess the person's view of their quality of life and mood as these are known to be poor in people with heart failure.

Table 5.6 Key assessment and outcome measures used by occupational therapists in heart failure care.

Assessment of Motor and Process Skills (Fisher 1995).

Canadian Occupational Performance Measure (Law *et al.* 1998).

MOS 36-Item Short-Form Health Survey (SF-36) (Ware & Sherbourne 1992). Thirty-six questions which focus on eight health concepts. It is suitable for self-administration or administration by (and has been successfully used with) older people (Clarke *et al.* 2001; Ware 2002).

Hospital Anxiety and Depression Scale (HAD) (Zigmund & Snaith 1994). An easy-to-use self-report questionnaire measuring anxiety and depression in and outside hospital and community settings. Originally constructed for use with adults, additional validation has enabled its use with older people (Snaith 2003).

Occupational therapy interventions target the symptoms of fatigue and breathlessness that affect occupational performance. Dyspnoea on exertion and fatigue are expected symptoms of heart failure and for Mrs Smith and her family knowing this can alleviate some of the anxiety when performing activities.

Teaching energy conservation techniques through the use of pacing, time management and cycles of rest and activity can lead to a marked reduction in breathlessness and fatigue. This will help Mrs Smith regain some of her roles within the house and feel a valued member of her family. Assistive products and technology may be used to achieve energy conservation, but also increase independence and maintain safety.

Anxiety can trigger dyspnoea and tax cardiopulmonary function. The teaching of breathing control techniques such as diaphragmatic breathing and promotion of a relaxed and gentle breathing pattern should be considered along with other types of relaxation techniques. These are effective for the relief of anxiety and help in slowing breathing patterns (Keable 1997).

Exercise can improve exercise tolerance and symptoms for people with heart failure (Coats *et al.* 1990) and referral to a cardiac rehabilitation programme may be appropriate. A multidisciplinary approach to cardiac rehabilitation will provide exercise, education and support.

Reassessment of psychological status should be undertaken once treatment for the symptoms has been carried out to determine if any depression was precipitated by the symptoms. This will assist the multidisciplinary team to plan future treatment if needed.

Current treatment for heart failure does not arrest progression of the disease. A palliative care approach may need to be considered for end-stage heart failure. The teams approach should be one of aiming at maintaining quality of life and good symptom control (BHF 2001).

LEARNING DISABILITIES

Zoe Harvey-Lee

Box 5.9

Miss Jean Carter has difficulty understanding and remembering certain things and can be impulsive, while others often find it difficult to understand what she is doing or trying to say. Recently, her already unsteady walking and poor eyesight have worsened and Miss Carter has fallen, breaking her arm badly. This situation causes her confusion; she has become more frail and has problems with things like eating and dressing. Miss Carter has great difficulty understanding how to cope in these unfamiliar circumstances and that unless she takes particular care she may exacerbate her condition or worse still fall again.

Today older people like Miss Carter (Box 5.9), who also experience a learning disability, have equal rights to health care (DH 2001b). Many such individuals suffered years of inequitable health provision, social prejudice and marginalisation.

They lived much of their life in long-stay hospitals which lacked opportunities otherwise afforded to the general population.

However since the 1970s there has been a substantial shift in **social attitudes and policy**, and today's older person with a learning disability usually lives in the community either with family or in a care setting, where they are encouraged to engage within broader society.

Currently there are no precise estimates as to the number of people over 65 with a learning disability. However it is accepted that as a percentage of the rising older population their numbers are expanding disproportionately (Holland 2000), thanks largely to improvements in the quality and access to medical care and better **social support**.

For these older people their learning disability has been a lifelong condition, acquired before, during, or soon after birth. It has had an enduring effect on their development, causing a reduction in their ability to learn or to understand new or complex information, and will have affected to some degree their adaptive and social functioning.

Many factors can lead to a person's learning disability. It may have been due to some genetic abnormality, as for those with Down's syndrome, or due to an environmental factor such as maternal malnutrition. Whatever its cause, the nature and severity of the learning disability will vary from person to person and is commonly accompanied by conditions such as autism, epilepsy, sensory or neurological deficits, or other physical or mental health problems.

For some people their intellect, health and general functioning may only be mildly influenced by their learning disability, in which case they may be virtually independent. Alternatively someone may be profoundly affected by multiple disabilities, and have experienced a lifelong dependency on others. However independence levels and abilities will always be influenced by the opportunities afforded in earlier life. Those from institutional backgrounds are often disadvantaged in this respect, having never learnt to optimise their potential for independence.

For older people with a learning disability, as with the general population, the implications of ageing depend on a range of individual factors. Those with more profound physical disabilities still tend to die younger, while those who are more able can experience some degree of acceleration in the ageing process (Ward 1998).

Typical problems of ageing are a decline in mobility, hearing and sight. Cardiovascular, respiratory and neurological complications are also common (Beange 2002). In Miss Carter's case, it would be necessary to ascertain why she fell and to minimise risks. Although these parallel ageing in the general population, such complaints in a learning disabled person, often compound an already compromised physical and mental state, leading to more significant functional losses in later life. In particular people with Down's syndrome are susceptible to developing early onset, and often aggressively active, **dementia** conditions (Dodds *et al.* 2002). In Miss Carter's situation, it would be necessary to ascertain and assess whether her ability to remember and understand events has deteriorated over a period of time. Such conditions are often difficult to detect due to already established cognitive impairments; however it is a growing focus of research given the increasing older population.

There is very little research that delineates occupational therapy specific to older people with a learning disability, despite the growing need for clarification. However just as with other older clients, occupational therapy for this group aims to optimise independence in self-care, productivity and leisure, so that individuals can fulfil meaningful roles in self-determined **social contexts**.

Increasingly medical and therapeutic interventions for common physical complaints are delivered through mainstream services. However there is still much work to be done in this area and in mental health services, before truly equitable access to the most appropriate medical and social care is achieved.

Clients are currently referred to the Community Team for People with Learning Disabilities (CTPLD), particularly if they have more complex and challenging problems. Team members work in a multidisciplinary way and in partnership with care managers, social services, private and charitable organisations.

Currently there seems no agreed definition of the specialist community occupational therapist's role. Consequently therapists develop their practice contingent on their professional areas of interest, expertise and team demands. The important thing to remember, however, is that such specialist occupational therapists complement the profession's overall understanding of the client group, and have a future role both supporting colleagues working in mainstream services, and pioneering practice innovations.

Assessment of older people with a learning disability may be undertaken as with any other older person, in the context of mainstream acute and community services. Clients may present with any manner or mix of physical, sensory or mental health problems. There may be social concerns around risk and vulnerability, or a need to evaluate social and accommodation or equipment needs. When the client is only mildly affected by their learning disability then it may be relatively easy to gain consent to occupational therapy, and for them to fully participate in a demonstration of function or undertake a home visit. Standardised assessments are, however, difficult to administer in these situations, given that they have not been developed for use with learning disabled clients.

More complex cases may be assessed by members of the CTPLD, where problems of multiple disability, impaired communication, comprehension or challenging behaviour can be managed by those skilled to do so. The occupational therapist will assess different aspects of functional performance viewed from a holistic perspective, and by determining the extent to which a person's learning disability, social history and any other associated conditions influence their abilities; they identify the areas that will respond to intervention. Such assessments may take considerable time and be achieved through a process of close working between team members, carers and outside agencies.

Intervention requires that information and client training is offered in ways that are sympathetic to the intellectual, sensory and communication level of the individual. Occupational therapists often involve carers with implementing input strategies, in order to help reinforce intervention outside the therapy sessions (Herge & Campbell 1998).

The occupational therapist may work directly with clients to maintain or develop skills, individually or in small groups. They may give advice on assistive products that enhance or enable function and access to valued activities. Commonly, input focuses on quality of life issues for the older client and carer, rather than on independence.

Because of the frequent dependence of older people on services and carers, therapists often work with these in a consultative role, looking at ways to modify types of support and the **environment**, so as to enhance client autonomy and reduce any perceived risks.

If not so commonly found in the mainstream, occupational therapy within the CTPLD is integrated into the generally held service principles of promoting participation, respect, inclusion and choice for people with a learning disability. These together with current approaches to client-centred planning, client advocacy and user-empowerment fit well within occupational therapy's holistic models of practice (Platt 1993) and afford interesting avenues for future research.

Currently there is a lack of consensus as to the most successful outcome measure for use with older people with a learning disability. As with assessments there are problems of achieving rigour using standardised instruments when individuals have essential problems understanding and participating fully in the evaluation process. Difficulties of client self-report make reference to carer perceptions an important dimension of the final outcome measurement. Occupational therapists must judge the extent to which the presenting difficulty has been resolved. However this can be difficult when problems lie in conditions such as dementia, where functional decline is an inevitable outcome.

MUSCULOSKELETAL PROBLEMS/ARTHRITIS

Mary Grant

Box 5.10

> Mr Drake is 81, and lives with his wife Dorothy. Mr Drake used to be a long-distance lorry driver until he retired 16 years ago. He had been a keen footballer in his youth, playing professional football in his early 20s. Mr Drake has osteoarthritis, and has been in chronic pain for sometime – especially in his knees and back. Mr Drake now finds he cannot walk outdoors and has difficulty getting out of his chair where he spends most of his day watching football on the television. Mr Drake has just been referred to the community therapy team.

Mr Drake's narrative (Box 5.10) describes the impact of back pain and osteoarthritis on his life. Back pain is the most frequent and yet strangely neglected musculoskeletal complaint in older people (Pitkala *et al.* 2002), with the second most common musculoskeletal condition in older people being osteoarthritis. Until recently this condition was seen as a degenerative disease and was the natural consequence of ageing and trauma, but it is now viewed as a metabolic, fundamentally reparative process (Buckwalter & Mankin 1998). Rheumatoid arthritis can present as a new onset disease in old age, but often it is seen as a sequel to earlier onset disease. Pain and functional limitation are found to decrease quality of life for older people with rheumatoid arthritis and osteoarthritis alike (Jakobsson & Hallberg 2002).

Occupational therapists work as part of the multidisciplinary team providing intervention for older people with musculoskeletal disease, which has shown to be effective in maintaining functional ability (Hakala *et al.* 1994). People with rheumatoid arthritis are likely to be managed by a secondary care hospital rheumatology service. They will be seen by the consultant rheumatologist or clinical specialists (who may be nurses, occupational therapists or physiotherapists) in order to monitor disease activity, response to drug therapy and for referral to other members of the team. People with osteoarthritis, like Robert, tend to be managed by primary care services, including community therapy services (Peat *et al.* 2001). However, if joint replacement surgery is necessary then people with joint disease will be admitted to orthopaedic wards and receive a multidisciplinary rehabilitation service. Intermediate care teams may also be involved to continue this process in the community in more complex cases.

It is likely that Mr Drake, with musculoskeletal problems, will see a physiotherapist for pain relieving modalities, exercise and hydrotherapy (Chard & Dieppe 2001). Podiatrists and dieticians are increasingly involved in providing specialised rheumatology services (Royal College of Nursing 2003). The role of complementary therapies, such as acupuncture, has also grown (Hicks 2000).

Self-management is becoming an increasingly popular concept and the voluntary sector are involved in providing self-management programmes (e.g. Challenging Arthritis run by Arthritis Care), based on a self-management programme devised by Lorig *et al.* (2000). An evaluation by Barlow *et al.* (2000) in the UK has shown positive outcomes including a reduction in visits to a physician, an improvement in self-efficacy and a more active lifestyle. It has also proved to be cost effective (Groessl *et al.* 2003). Numerous outcome measures can be used (see Table 5.7 for examples).

The occupational therapy aims for Mr Drake were to:

- Prevent loss or further loss of use of the joints.
- Restore, maintain and enhance meaningful occupations.

Table 5.7 Key assessment and outcome measures used by occupational therapists with older people in musculoskeletal care.

Canadian Occupational Performance Measure (Law *et al.* 1998).

Health Assessment Questionnaire (HAQ). A well-researched and evaluated self-report functional status measure rather than process measures (Stanford University Medical Centre (2003)).

Arthritis Impact Measurement (AIM). A self-administered questionnaire pilot tested in a mixed arthritis population. Containing nearly 80 items in a 13-page questionnaire. Most questions ask about the person's health and functioning over the previous month (Meenan *et al.* 1992).

- Maintain health and wellbeing through health promotion strategies and lifestyle management.
- Pain management strategies.

The provision of **assistive products** for Mr Drake (such as a chair raise) make daily occupations more manageable and less stressful for the joints and muscles. However, a Cochrane review concluded there was not enough information to say whether advice about using **assistive products** is helpful, but that there is strong evidence for the effectiveness of instruction on joint protection (Steultjens *et al.* 2004).

Joint Protection is often used by occupational therapist to reduce the stress on joints affected by arthritis while participating in daily occupations. The principles of joint protection include:

- Awareness and respect for pain.
- Distributing the load over several joints.
- Using stronger and larger joints.
- Using joints in their most stable and functional positions.
- Avoiding positions of deformity.

Occupational therapists need to ensure that older people like Mr Drake maintain occupational balance within their daily lives. Energy conservation and work simplification techniques are important strategies taught by occupational therapists that enable older people to carry out meaningful occupations. Other interventions that are effective as a form of pain management include relaxation therapy in reducing pain, joint inflammation and improving psychosocial functioning (Kessler 2001). Stress management techniques can be used to facilitate the use of positive coping strategies and reduces pain (Parker *et al.* 1995). The assessment and provision of orthoses is also a common occupational therapy role, with evidence of reduction of pain and also improved grip strength with their use (Weiss *et al.* 2000; Steultjens *et al.* 2004).

Occupational therapists have an important health promotion role with other team members, incorporating education about musculoskeletal conditions and ways of preventing further deterioration of joints whilst at the same time having balanced and fulfilled occupations. However it has been suggested that there is no evidence that patient education interventions on health status have long-term benefits in adults with rheumatoid arthritis (Riemsma *et al.* 2004).

RESPIRATORY DISEASE

Wendy Gregson

Respiratory conditions are prevalent within primary and secondary health-care settings, with recent figures from the British Thoracic Society (BTS) reported that respiratory disease amounted to some 38 million GP consultations and 78 000 inpatient admissions in 2000 (BTS 2001:44).

Box 5.11

> Mr John King is a 74-year-old gentleman who has been referred to the inpatient occupational therapy team. Mr King reports that he has become increasingly breathless whilst climbing the stairs to his flat. He has found that he needs to plan ahead as he finds he is becoming increasingly tired. Mr King has now sought assistance from his daughter for his shopping, as he feels anxious when going outdoors alone. Until he went to his GP, Mr King put the gradual physical and psychological changes down to his 'old age' and because he is a bit of a 'worrier'.

Respiratory disease encompasses a wide variety of conditions for example, chronic obstructive pulmonary disease (COPD); asthma; tuberculosis (TB) and pulmonary fibrosis. Discussion here will centre on occupational therapy intervention with people with COPD (such as Mr King). COPD can be defined as a chronic, slowly progressive and debilitating disease of the lungs (Bourke & Brewis 1998:112; Hansel & Barnes 2004:3) with the primary cause being smoking (The National Institute for Clinical Excellence [NICE] 2004; Hansel & Barnes 2004). Statistics from 1999 identified that 630 000 people over 65 have COPD (NICE 2003).

Recent guidelines on the management of COPD in primary and secondary care settings pay particular attention to the multidisciplinary management of this condition (NICE 2004). Owing to the high prevalence of respiratory conditions, occupational therapy services can be found in many different health settings, including palliative and hospice care.

Occupational therapists seek to enable older people to better adapt to the debilitating effects of their respiratory condition and continue participation in their life activities. Assessment seeks to identify how the individual's symptoms (such as breathlessness), may limit their **activity and participation,** as well as considering other intrinsic psychological, cognitive, **environmental** and psychosocial factors. In Mr King's case it is essential to assess the environment and how this impacts on his daily occupations. See Table 5.8 for assessment tools and outcome measures.

Persons with COPD frequently experience symptoms other than shortness of breath, such as decreased endurance and strength, rising fatigue levels as well as general malaise, poor appetite, weight loss, low mood and anxiety. Although primarily a disorder of the respiratory system, more recent evidence suggests that COPD has many secondary, systemic effects including metabolic and musculoskeletal conditions (Calverley 2000).

The nature of any respiratory condition demands continual psychosocial adjustment by the patient in terms of their lifestyle. In Mr King's case the occupational therapist would need to spend time discussing strategies and techniques with Mr King and his family to enable him to participate fully with his chosen daily occupations. Aside from managing the day-to-day practicalities of life with respiratory disease, the person must also try to maintain effective and fulfilling relationships with family and friends as life defining roles, routines and habits (Williams 1993). A high prevalence of **anxiety** and **depression** in patients with COPD has been noted (Gore *et al.* 2000).

Table 5.8 Examples of key assessment tools and outcome measures used by occupational therapists in respiratory care.

Canadian Occupation Performance Measure (COPM) (Law *et al.* 1998).

Sickness Impact Profile (SIP). A self-report or interviewer-administered tool to provide a descriptive profile of changes in a person's behaviour due to sickness. Containing 136 items grouped into 12 dimensions of daily activity; sleep and rest, emotional behaviour, body care and movement, home management, mobility, social interaction, ambulation, alertness, behaviour communication, work, recreation and pastimes, and eating (Bergner *et al.* 1981).

Medical Research Council UK Scale (MRC dyspnoea scale). Used for grading the effect of breathlessness on daily activities and allows the patients to indicate the extent to which their breathlessness affects their mobility (Fletcher 1960).

BORG Rating of perceived exertion (Borg 1982). A grading rating of perceived exertion. A score of zero indicates no breathlessness at all and a score of 10 being maximal breathlessness.

St George's Respiratory Questionnaire (SGRQ). Completed by self, face-to-face or telephone interview. Has three domains and categories: **Symptoms** (frequency and severity); **Activity** (activities that cause or are limited by breathlessness); **Impacts** (social functioning, psychological disturbances resulting from airways disease (Jones *et al.* 1991).

Hospital Anxiety and Depression Scale (HAD) (Zigmond & Snaith 1994).

As disease advances, individuals will require regular monitoring, evaluation and education throughout each stage of their disease. Successful management of the palliative and end stages of chronic disease requires a timely multidisciplinary approach to the rapidly changing physical and psychological needs of the older person and their carers.

Occupational therapy interventions could include:

- Use of activities to address specific physical, cognitive and psychosocial dysfunctions.
- Education on energy conservation and work simplification. These techniques are not only applied and integrated into the person's daily life but also to enhance self-management, in accordance with their specific medical regime.
- Anxiety management and relaxation techniques.
- Management of breathlessness – positioning, breathing and relaxation techniques, advice regarding available resources for smoking cessation.
- Fatigue management.
- Pulmonary rehabilitation aiming for reduction in disability and increase quality of life for people with lung disease, while diminishing the health care burden (British Thoracic Society Standards of Care Subcommittee on Pulmonary Rehabilitation 2001).
- Prescription and installation of assistive products and technology, in conjunction with energy conservation principles.
- Provision of education and support to carers.
- Education in self-management of the disease, which may include strategies to assist the individual in adjusting to their condition.

STROKE (CEREBROVASCULAR ACCIDENT)

Anne McIntyre

Box 5.12

> Mrs Rena Gopal is 78 and had a left-sided stroke (cerebrovascular accident [CVA]) 2 years ago. She is a small lady, and has always been overweight. She can only walk short distances indoors; she no longer climbs the stairs and has difficulty standing up from her chair or toilet. She has hemiparesis of her right side, with her right upper limb being worse than her right lower limb. Consequently her daughter-in-law helps her with all transfers, washing and dressing. Even though Mrs Gopal has no cognitive problems she does have expressive dysphasia as a result of her stroke; this is most noticeable with yes/no responses, which she finds highly frustrating. She is also unable to hold a pen and write with her right (dominant) hand. Eating food is a problem for Mrs Gopal as she has difficulties manipulating her right hand.
>
> Mrs Gpoal is less independent now than she was on discharge from hospital 2 years ago.

Stroke is a 'clinical syndrome characterised by rapidly developing clinical signs of focal (or global) disturbance lasting 24 hours or longer or leading to death with no apparent cause other than of vascular origin. The definition of stroke incorporates haemorrhagic and ischaemic lesions, with additional subtypes in both categories' (Liebeskind 2003:1085). Stroke is the second commonest cause of death in the world after ischaemic heart disease (WHO 2003), a major cause of disability in older people alongside **hip fractures** and **dementia**, and is closely associated with the onset of **dementia** (Zhu *et al.* 1998). People over the age of 70 are more likely to have a dominant (left) hemisphere infarct involving the middle cerebral artery, which supplies the frontal, temporal and parietal cortices, as well as the basal ganglia and internal capsule (Pohjasvaara *et al.* 1997).

It is important that stroke care addresses both the immediate acute medical consequences and the longer term problems of a stroke. These problems can be demonstrated in terms of the framework of the ICF (WHO 2001), using Mrs Gopal's story (Box 5.12) in Table 5.9.

In the UK, both the British Geriatric Society (BGS) (2003) and the Royal College of Physicians (RCP) (2002) have produced guidelines for stroke care, alongside those written in conjunction with the National Association for Neurological Occupational Therapists (NANOT) in 2000. These guidelines recommend that each locality should have a specialised stroke service with an occupational therapist specialised in stroke care as a key member of a rehabilitation team (RCP 2002) with care encompassing:

- Prevention of stroke (both primary and secondary health promotion principles).
- Acute care (including rapid assessment and management).
- Rehabilitation.
- Long-term support.

Table 5.9 Mrs Gopal's difficulties with functioning since her stroke.

Body function/structures	Emotional lability
	Low mood
	Difficulties expressing spoken language
	Poor proprioception and sense of touch
	Poor exercise tolerance
	Alterations in muscle tone in right side of body
	Limited voluntary movements in right side of body
Activity limitations	Difficulty with eating
	Difficulties with conversation, verbal and written communication
	Self-care – problems with washing, dressing
	Movement – changing position, walking indoors and out, climbing stairs
	Difficulty reaching, manipulating and grasping objects in right hand and use of left hand unacceptable
	Unable to perform most household tasks
Participation restriction	Difficulty following religious practice
	Loss of role within household

These guidelines were followed by joint occupational therapy standards for Stroke care in terms of service structure and process of care mainly for inpatients (COT and RCP 2002). However, where and how occupational therapy should be offered, is still debated. There is evidence for better survival, independence and return home from inpatient specialist stroke teams (Stroke Unit Triallists' Collaboration [SUTC] 2001). The long-term evidence for dedicated community services is less clear (Gilbertson *et al.* 1999; Lincoln *et al.* 2004). It is recommended that assessments should be client-centred and **activity** focused rather than **impairment** focused (as should interventions) (RCP 2002).

Occupational therapy assessment of stroke considers how the impact on an older person's physical, cognitive, perceptual and psychosocial abilities for **activity** or **participation** in their chosen physical and cultural **environment** (see Table 5.10). For Mrs Gopal, the inability to use her left hand in activities, to compensate for poor manual dexterity of the right hand was addressed sensitively by the occupational therapist.

Long-term intervention with stroke has tended to concentrate on medical management and prevention, rather than recovery of independence and quality of life both for the older person and informal carers, with many individuals (like Mrs Gopal) not retaining earlier independence (Hoffmann *et al.* 2003; Kalra *et al.* 2004).

The treatment of movement disorders after stroke is common to both occupational therapists and physiotherapists, with the use of activity analysis crucial to effective application. The most popular techniques in the UK are Bobath (Bobath 1991), motor relearning programme (Carr & Shepherd 2002) and of increasing

Table 5.10   Key assessment tools used by occupational therapists in stroke care.

Structured Observation Test of Function (SOTOF). Evaluation of everyday performance in self-care tasks, as well as body functions. Good reliability, face validity. Used as a diagnostic tool and outcome measure (Laver & Powell 1995).

Rivermead Behavioural Inattention Test (BIT). Considers everyday performance as well as 'laboratory' type tests. A diagnostic and outcome tool (Wilson *et al.* 1987).

Rivermead Perceptual assessment Battery (RPAB). For adults following CVA or TBI, has normative data for older people. Reliable and valid outcome and diagnostic tool (Whiting *et al.* 1985; Lincoln & Edmans 1990).

Rivermead Behavioural Memory Test (RBMT). This has ecological validity, assessing skills for everyday functioning. Can be used both as a diagnostic tool and as an outcome measure (Wilson *et al.* 1985).

Assessment of Motor and Process Skills (Fisher 1995).

interest, constraint-induced movement therapy (CIMT) (Taub *et al.* 1998) – however this technique would not be acceptable to Mrs Gopal. Current evidence does not favour one technique over another for long-term recovery (Langhammer & Stanghelle 2003; Sieghert *et al.* 2004). This lack of evidence is also reflected in cognitive and perceptual retraining where both transfer of training and the function approach as described by Zoltan (1996) are commonly used (Edmans *et al.* 2000).

Summary

The pathologies discussed in this chapter are complex diseases, which can have a great impact on an older person, their family and friends. **Services** provided should be client-centred, needs driven and appropriate to the nature and stage of the illness. This chapter does not provide an exhaustive list, as older people with Parkinson's disease, sensory impairment, and those who enter old age already with disability have not been addressed here. Occupational therapists need to be sensitive to the impact imposed by long-term disability and life-threatening illness. They have to be flexible to the variations in the disease trajectory: from diagnosis through to death. Occupational therapists enable the individual to maximise their quality of life regardless of life expectancy. The challenge for occupational therapist is to ensure that all interventions are based on best evidence, this means that research must become a priority within occupational therapy practice. This chapter has highlighted the need to use both functional outcome measures and quality of life measures.

The role of the occupational therapist in **health promotion** has been discussed in Chapter 1 and has been highlighted in this chapter, but further research is needed to demonstrate the effectiveness of the occupational therapist role in this area. Furthermore this chapter has emphasised the need for interprofessional and partnership working. For an effective team can enhance wellbeing, quality of life, independence, and functioning.

References

Allen CK, Earhart CA, Blue T (1992) *Occupational Therapy Treatment Goals for the Physically and Cognitively Disabled*. USA: The American Occupational Therapy Association.

Adshead F, Cody D, Pitt B (1992) BASDEC: a novel screening instrument for depression in elderly medical inpatients. *British Medical Journal* 305, 397.

Ajaj A, Singh MP, Abdulla AJ (2001) Should elderly patients be told they have cancer? Questionnaire survey of older people. *British Medical Journal* 323, 1160.

Alzheimer's Society (2003) *Facts about Dementia*. Accessed 12.05. 2004. http://www.alzheimers.org.uk/Facts_about_dementia/index.htm

American Geriatrics Society, British Geriatrics Society, American Academy of Orthopaedic Surgeons Panel on Falls Prevention (2001) Guideline for the prevention of falls in older persons. *Journal of the American Geriatrics Society* 49(5), 664–672.

Anderson H, Ward C, Gomm SA *et al.* (2001) The concerns of patients under palliative care and a heart failure clinic are not being met. *Palliative Medicine* 15(4), 279–286.

Apelqvist A & Agardh CD (1992) The association between clinical risk factors ·and outcome of diabetic foot ulcers. *Diabetes Research and Clinical Practice* 18, 43–45.

Audit Commission (1995) *United they Stand*. London: Audit Commission.

Audit Commission (2000) *Forget Me Not. Mental Health Services for Older People*. London: Audit Commission Publications.

Bagley H, Cordingley L, Burne A *et al.* (2000) Recognition of depression by staff in nursing and residential homes. *Journal of Clinical Nursing* 9(3), 445–450.

Baker BR, Duckworth T, Wilkes E (1978) Mental state and other prognostic factors in femoral fractures of the elderly. *Journal of the Royal College of General Practitioners* 28(194), 557–559.

Ballard C & Eastwood R (1999) Psychiatric assessment. In: Wilcock GK, Bucks RS, Rockwood K (eds). *Diagnosis and Management of Dementia*. Oxford: Oxford Medical Publication, pp. 62–77.

Banerjee S, Sharmash K, Macdonald AJD, Mann AH (1996) Randomised controlled trial of effect of intervention by psychogeriatric depression in frail elderly people at home. *British Medical Journal* 313, 1058–1061.

Barlow JH, Turner AP, Wright CC (2000) A randomised controlled study of the arthritis self management programme in the UK. *Health Education and Research. Theory and Practice*. 15(6), 665–680.

Bartlett H & Martin W (2000) A balancing act: dementia research runs the risk of an ethical controversy. *Guardian* September 6. Accessed 12.05.2004. http://www.guardian.co.uk/print/0,3858,4059739-103772,00.html

Beange H (2002) Epidemiological issues. In: Pasher V & Janicki M (eds). *Physical Health and Adults with Intellectual Disability*. Oxford: Blackwell Publishing.

Beekman ATF, Copeland JRM, Prince MJ (1999) Review of community prevalence of depression in later life. *British Journal of Psychiatry* 174, 307–311.

Bergner M, Bobbitt RA, Carter WB, Gilson BS (1981) The Sickness Impact Profile: development and final revision of a health status measure. *Medical Care* 19(8), 787–805.

Blanchard MR, Waterreus A, Mann AH (1999) Can a brief intervention have a longer-term benefit? The case of the research nurse and depressed older people in the community. *International Journal of Geriatric Psychiatry* 14(9), 733–738.

Bobath B (1991) *Adult Hemiplegia: Evaluation and Treatment*, 3rd edn. London: Butterworth Heinemann.

Borg GA (1982) Psychophysical bases of perceived exertion. *Medicine and Science in Sport and Exercise* 14(5), 377–381.

Bottomley A, Hunton S, Roberts G (1996) Social support and cognitive behavioural therapy with cancer patients. A pilot study of group interventions. *Journal of Psychological Oncology* 14(1), 65–83.

Bottomley A & Jones L (1997) Women with breast cancer. Their experiences. *European Journal of Cancer Care* 6(2), 124–132.

Bottomley A (1997) Psychosocial problems in cancer care: a brief review of common problems. *Journal of Psychiatric and Mental Health Nursing* 4(5), 323–333.

Bourke S & Brewis R (1998) *Lecture Notes on Respiratory Medicine*. Oxford: Blackwell Science.

Bowling A (1995) Cardiovascular diseases. *Measuring Disease*. Philadelphia: Open University Press.

British Geriatric Society (2003) *Standards of Medical Care for Older People*. Accessed 05.05. 2004 http://www.bgs.org.uk/compendium/compa3.htm

British Heart Foundation (BHF) (2001) *Palliative Care of Heart Failure*. Accessed 25.04.2004. Http://www.bhf.org.uk

British Heart Foundation (BHF) (2002) *Living with Heart Failure*. Series No. 8. Accessed 26.04.2004. Http://www.bhf.org.uk

British Thoracic Society Standards of Care Subcommittee on Pulmonary Rehabilitation (2001) Pulmonary rehabilitation. *Thorax* 56(11), 827–834.

Buckwalter JA & Mankin HJ (1998) Articular cartilage: degeneration and osteoarthritis, repair, regeneration and transplantation. *Instructional Course Lectures* 47, 487–504.

Bullock R (2002) *Building a Modern Dementia Service*. Edgeware: Altman.

Calverley P (2000) COPD. In: *British Lung Foundation (2000) Lung Report II. Lung Disease: A Shadow Over the Nation's Health*. London: British Lung Foundation.

Cameron I, Crotty M, Currie C *et al.* (2000) Geriatric rehabilitation following fractures in older people: a systematic review. *Health Technology Assessment* 4(2), 1–111.

Campbell AJ, Borrie MJ, Spears GF, Jackson SL, Brown JS, Fitzgerald JL (1990) Circumstances and consequences of falls experienced by a community population 70 years and over during a prospective study. *Age and Ageing* 19(5), 136–141.

Canadian Association of Occupational Therapists (2002) *Enabling Occupation: An Occupational Therapy Perspective*, revised edn. Ottawa: CAOT Publications.

Cancer Bacup (2002) *Cancer Type*. Accessed 29.08.2004. http://www.cancerbacup.org.uk/Home

Carr JH & Shepherd RB (2002) *Stroke Rehabilitation: Guidelines for Exercise and Training to Optimize Motor Skill*. London: Butterworth Heinemann.

Cate Y, Baker SS, Gilbert MP (1995) Occupational therapy and the person with diabetes and vision impairment. *American Journal of Occupational Therapy* 49(9), 905–911.

Chartered Society of Physiotherapy and College of Occupational Therapists (2002) *Falls Audit Pack: Guidelines for the Collaborative, Rehabilitative Management of Elderly People who have Fallen*. London: COT and CSP.

Chard J & Dieppe P (2001) The case for nonpharmacologic therapy of osteoarthritis. *Current Rheumatology Reports* 3(3), 251–257.

Clarke C, Lapes-Sealey C, Kotsch L (2001) *Outcome Measures. Information Pack for Occupational Therapists*. London: College of Occupational Therapists.

Clemson L (1997) *Home Fall Hazards and the Westmead Home Safety Assessment*. West Brunswick, Australia: Coordinates Publications.

Coats AJS, Adamopoulos S, Meyer TE, Conway J, Sleight P (1990) Effects of physical training in chronic heart failure. *Lancet* 355, 63–66.

Coleman PG (1986) *Ageing and Reminiscence Processes: Social and Clinical Implications.* Chichester: Wiley.

College of Occupational Therapists (2001) *Submission of Evidence on Management of Depression.* Accessed 24.04.2004. http://www.cot.co.uk/public/publications/nice/mental_health/intro.html

College of Occupational Therapists and Royal College of Physicians (2002) *Occupational Therapy Standards for Stroke Care.* London: NANOT, COT.

Crawford M, Prince M, Menzes P, Mann A (1998) The recognition and treatment of depression in older people in primary care. *International Journal of Geriatric Psychiatry* 13(3), 172–176.

Department of Health (1995) *A Policy Document for Commissioning Cancer Services.* London: HMSO.

Department of Health (2000a) *The NHS Cancer Plan.* London: Department of Health.

Department of Health (2000b) *National Service Framework for Coronary Heart Disease.* London: HMSO.

Department of Health (2001a) *National Service Framework for Older People.* London: HMSO.

Department of Health (2001b) *Valuing People: A New Strategy for Learning Disability for the 21st Century.* London: HMSO.

Department of Trade and Industry (2001) *International Review of Interventions in Falls Among Older People.* London: DTI.

Dodds K, Turk V, Christmas M (2002) *Down's Syndrome and Dementia: Resource Pack for Carers and Support Staff.* Kidderminster: BILD.

Doughty K & Burton L (2002) *Assistive Technology to Assess and Support Dementia Sufferers in the Community.* Paper Presentation at Occupational Therapy Conference for Older People Dementia: Clinical Forum Conference, University of Warwick.

Eames J, Ward G, Siddons L (1999) Clinical audit of the outcome of individualised occupational therapy goals. *British Journal of Occupational Therapy* 62(6), 257–260.

Edmans J, Webster J, Lincoln NB (2000) A comparison of two approaches in the treatment of perceptual problems after stroke. *Clinical Rehabilitation* 14(3), 230–243.

Eva G (2000) *Guidelines of Measuring Occupational Therapy Outcomes in HIV/AIDS, Oncology and Palliative Care.* London: College of Occupational Therapists.

Feil N (1993) *The Validation Breakthrough: Simple Techniques for Communicating with People with 'Alzheimer's-Type Dementia'.* London: Health Professions Press.

Fisher AG (1995) *Assessment of Motor Process Skills.* Fort Collins, CO: Three Star Press.

Fletcher CM (Chairman) (1960) Standardised questionnaire on respiratory symptoms: a statement prepared and approved by the MRC Committee on the aetiology of chronic bronchitis (MRC breathlessness score). *British Medical Journal* 2, 1665.

Folstein MG, Folstein SE, McHugh PR (1975) Mini-mental state: a practical method for grading the cognitive state of patients for the clinician. *Journal of Psychiatric Research* 12(3), 189–198.

Gilbertson L, Langhorne P, Walker A, Allen A, Murray GD (1999) Domiciliary occupational therapy for patients with stroke discharged from hospital: randomised controlled trial. *British Medical Journal* 320, 603–606.

Gillespie WJ (2001) Hip fracture. *British Medical Journal* 322, 968–975.

Gillespie LD, Gillespie WJ, Robertson MC, Lamb SE, Cumming RG, Rowe BH (2002) Interventions for preventing falls in elderly people. *The Cochrane Database of Systematic Reviews* (4) CD000340.

Golding E (1989) *The Middlesex Elderly Assessment of Mental State (MEAMS)*. Bury St Edmunds: Thames Valley Test Company.

Gore JM, Brophy CJ, Greenstone MA (2000) How well do we care for patients with end stage chronic obstructive pulmonary disease (COPD)? A comparison of palliative care and quality of life in COPD and lung cancer. *Thorax* 55(12), 1000–1006.

Grady KL, Jolowiec A, White-Williams C *et al.* (1995) Predictors of quality of life in patients with advanced heart failure awaiting transplantation. *Journal of Heart and Lung Transplantation* 14(1), 2–10.

Groessl EJ, Kaplan RM, Cronan TA (2003) Quality of wellbeing in older people with arthritis. *Arthritis and Rheumatism* 49(1), 23–28.

Hakala M, Nieminen P, Kolvist O (1994) More evidence from a community based series of better outcome in rheumatoid arthritis. Data on the effect of multidisciplinary care on the retention of functional ability. *Journal of Rheumatology* 21(8), 1432–1437.

Hansel T & Barnes P (2004) *An Atlas of Chronic Obstructive Pulmonary Disease*. London: Parthenon Publishing Group.

Harvey RJ, Rossor MN, Skelton-Robinson M, Garralda E (1998) *Young Onset Dementia: Epidemiology, Clinical Symptoms, Family Burden, Support and Outcome*. London: Imperial College.

Herge E & Campbell J (1998) The role of the occupational and physical therapist in the rehabilitation of the older adult with mental retardation. *Topics in Geriatric Rehabilitation* 13(4), 12–21.

Hicks JE (2000) Rehabilitation strategies for patients with rheumatoid arthritis. Part 2: Modalities, orthoses and assistive devices. *Journal of Musculoskeletal Medicine* 17(7), 385–387.

Hoffmann T, McKenna K, Cooke D, Tooth L (2003) Outcomes after stroke: basic and instrumental activities of daily living, community reintegration, and generic health status. *Australian Occupational Therapy Journal* 50(4), 225–233.

Holden UP (1988) *Reality Orientation: Psychological Approaches to the 'Confused' Elderly*, 2nd edn. Edinburgh: Churchill Livingstone.

Holland A (2000) Ageing and learning disabilities. *British Journal of Psychiatry* 176(1), 26–31.

Hutchinson A, McIntosh A, Griffiths CJ *et al.* (2002) *Clinical Guidelines and Evidence Review for Type 2 Diabetes: Blood Pressure Management*. Sheffield: ScHARR, University of Sheffield.

Jackson JP & Schkade JK (2001) Occupational adaptation model versus biomechanical-rehabilitation model in treatment of patients with hip fractures. *American Journal of Occupational Therapy* 55(5), 531–537.

Jakobsson U & Hallberg IR (2002) Pain and quality of life among older people with rheumatoid arthritis and/or osteoarthritis: a literature review. *Journal of Clinical Nursing* 11(4), 430–443.

Jones PW, Quirk FH, Baveystock CM (1991) The St George's Respiratory Questionnaire. *Respiratory Medicine* 85(suppl), 25–31.

Kalra L, Evans A, Perez I *et al.* (2004) Training care givers of stroke patients: randomised controlled trial. *British Medical Journal* 328, 1099–1101.

Katon W & Ciechanoweki P (2003) Impact of major depression on chronic illness. *Journal of Psychosomatic Research* 55(4), 859–863.

Keable D (1997) *The Management of Anxiety. A Guide for Therapists*, 2nd edn. London: Churchill Livingstone.

Kessler R (2001) CBT added to medical management improved clinical outcomes in rheumatoid arthritis. *Evidence-Based Mental Health* 4(3), 89.

Langhammer B & Stanghelle JK (2003) Bobath or motor relearning programme? A follow-up one and four years post stroke. *Clinical Rehabilitation* 17(7), 731–734.

Laver AJ & Powell GE (1995) *The Structured Observation Test of Function*. Windsor: NFER-Nelson Publishing.

Law M, Baptiste S, Carswell-Opzoomer A, McColl M, Polatajko H, Pollock N (1998) *Canadian Occupational Therapy Performance Measure Manual*. Canadian Association of Occupational Therapists Publications. Toronto, ON: ACE.

Liebeskind DS (2003) Case fatality rates after hospital admission for stroke. Definition of stroke defines stroke mortality. *British Medical Journal* 326, 1085–1086.

Liddle J & McKenna K (2000) Quality of life: an overview of issues for use in occupational therapy outcome measurement. *Australian Occupational Therapy Journal* 47(2), 77–85.

Lincoln NB & Edmans J (1990) A revalidation of the Rivermead Perceptual Assessment Battery for elderly patients with stroke. *Age and Ageing* 19(1), 19–24.

Lincoln NB, Walker MF, Dixon A, Knights P (2004) Evaluation of a multiprofessional community stroke team: a randomised controlled trial. *Clinical Rehabilitation* 18(1), 40–47.

Lorig K, Fries JF, Gecht MR, Minor M, Laurent DD, Gonzalez VM (2000) *The Arthritis Handbook: A Tested Self Management Program For Coping with Arthritis*, 5th edn. Cambridge, MA: Perseus Books.

Lyons RA, Sander LV, Weightman AL *et al.* (2004) *Modification of the Home Environment for the Reduction of Injuries* (Cochrane Review). The Cochrane Library, Issue 3. Chichester: John Wiley.

Mather A, Rodriguez C, Moyra F, Guthrie MF, McHarg AM, Reid IC (2002) Effects of exercise on depressive symptoms in older adults with poorly responsive depressive disorder *British Journal of Psychiatry* 180, 411–415.

Mathias S, Nayak US, Isaacs B (1986) Balance in elderly patients: the 'get-up and go' test. *Archives of Physical Medicine and Rehabilitation* 67, 387–389.

Mayall E, Oathamshaw S, Lovell K (2004) Developing and piloting of a multidisciplinary training course for detecting and managing depression in older people. *Journal of Psychiatric and Mental Health Nursing* 11(2), 165–171.

McIntyre A (1999) Elderly fallers: a baseline audit of admissions to a day hospital for elderly people. *British Journal of Occupational Therapy* 62(6), 244–248.

Meek S & Atwal A (2004) *Occupational Therapy in Palliative Care: A Role Evaluation*. Unpublished Paper. London: Brunel University.

Meenan RF, Mason JH, Anderson JJ, Guccione AA, Kazis LE (1992) AIMS2: the content and properties of a revised and expanded Arthritis Impact Measurement Scales Health Status Questionnaire. *Arthritis and Rheumatism* 35(1), 1–10.

Minardi HA & Blanchard M (2004) Older people with depression: pilot study. *Journal of Advanced Nursing* 46(1), 23–32.

Naidoo M & Bullock R (2001) *An Integrated Care Pathway for Dementia*. London: Mosby.

National Association for Neurological Occupational Therapists (2000) *National Clinical Guidelines for Stroke: Impact on Occupational Therapy Practice*. London: National Association for Neurological Occupational Therapists, Royal College of Physicians.

National Cancer Institute (2002) *Common Cancer Types*. Accessed 29.08.2004. http://www.nci.nih.gov/

National Diabetes Information Clearinghouse (2004) *Introduction to Diabetes*. Accessed 14.05.2004. http://diabetes.niddk.nih.gov/index.htm

National Institute for Clinical Excellence (NICE) (2003) *Chronic Heart Failure: Management of Chronic Heart Failure in Adults in Primary and Secondary Care*. Accessed 24.04.2004. http://www.nice.org.uk

National Institute for Clinical Effectiveness (NICE) (2004) *The Assessment and Prevention of Falls in Older People: NICE Guideline*. London: NICE.

National Institute for Clinical Excellence (2004) *Guidelines for the Management of Chronic Obstructive Pulmonary Disease in Primary and Secondary Care*. London: NICE.

National Osteoporosis Society (2003) *Osteoporosis: Are You at Risk?* Bath: National Osteoporosis Society.

Ousman Y & Sharma M (2001) The irrefutable importance of glycaemic control. *Clinical Diabetes* 19, 71–72.

Pal B (1999) Questionnaire survey of advice given to patients with fractures. *British Medical Journal* 318, 500–501.

Parker JC, Smarr KL, Buckelew SP *et al.* (1995) Effects of stress management on clinical outcomes in rheumatoid arthritis. *Arthritis and Rheumatism* 38(12), 1807–1818.

Parker MJ, Gillespie LD, Gillespie WJ (2004) *Hip Protectors for Preventing Hip Fractures in the Elderly* (Cochrane Review). The Cochrane Library, Issue 3. Chichester: John Wiley.

Peat G, McCarney R, Croft P (2001) Knee pain and osteoarthritis in older adults: a review of community burden and current use of primary health care. *Annals of the Rheumatic Diseases* 60(2), 91–97.

Penfold SL (1996) The role of the occupational therapist in oncology. *Cancer Treatment Reviews* 22(1), 75–81.

Perrin T. & May H. (2000) *Wellbeing in Dementia: An Occupational Approach for Therapists and Carers*. London: Churchill Livingstone.

Pinkney L (1997) A comparison of the snoezelen environment and a music relaxation group on the mood and behaviour of patients with senile dementia. *British Journal of Occupational Therapy* 60(5), 209–218.

Pitkala KH, Strandberg TE, Tilvis RS (2002) Management of non-malignant pain in home-dwelling older people: a population based survey. *Journal of the American Geriatrics Society* 50(11), 1861–1865.

Platt L (1993) Social role valorisation and the Model of Human Occupation: a comparative analysis for work with people with a learning disability in the community. *British Journal of Occupational Therapy* 56(8), 278–282.

Pohjasvaara T, Erkinjuntti T, Vataja R, Kaste M (1997) Comparison of stroke features and disability in daily life in patients with ischaemic stroke aged 55 to 70 and 71 to 85 years. *Stroke* 28(4), 729–735.

Pool J (2002) *The Pool Activity Level (PAL) Instrument for Occupational Profiling: A Practical Resource for Carers of People with Cognitive Impairment*. London: Jessica Kingsley.

Pound P, Gompertz P, Ebrahim S (1998) A patient-centred study of the consequences of stroke. *Clinical Rehabilitation* 12(4), 255–264.

Riemsma RP, Kirwan JR, Taal E, Rasker JJ (2004) *Patient Education for Adults with Rheumatoid Arthritis* (Cochrane Review). The Cochrane Library, Issue 2. Chichester: John Wiley.

Rowe J (2000) The management of falls in older people: from research to practice. *Reviews in Clinical Gerontology* 10(4), 397–406.

Royal College of Nursing (2003) Psoriatric arthritis. *Nursing Standard* 15(18), 47–52.

Royal College of Physicians (2002) *National Clinical Guidelines for Stroke: Update 2002*. London: Royal College of Physicians.

Salkeld G, Cameron ID, Cumming RG *et al.* (2000) Quality of life related to fear of falling and hip fracture in older women: a time trade off study. *British Medical Journal* 320, 341–345.

Scuffham P, Chaplin S, Legood R (2003) Incidence and cost of unintentional falls in older people in the United Kingdom. *Journal of Epidemiology and Community Health* 57(9), 740–744.

Siegert RJ, Lord S, Porter K (2004) Constraint-induced movement therapy: time for a little restraint. *Clinical Rehabilitation* 18(1), 110–114.

Snaith RP (2003) The Hospital Anxiety and Depression Scale. *Health and Quality of Life Outcomes* 1(1), 29.

Stanford University Medical Centre (2003) *Health Assessment Questionnaire (HAQ).* Accessed 12.05.2004. http://www.hqlo.com/content/1/1/20

Steultjens EMJ, Dekker J, Bouter LM, van Schaardenburg D, van Kuyk MAH, van den Ende CHM (2004) *Occupational Therapy for Rheumatoid Arthritis* (Cochrane Review). The Cochrane Library, Issue 2. Chichester: John Wiley.

Stewart S, Vandenbroek AJ, Pearson S, Horowitz JD (1999) Prolonged beneficial effects of a home based intervention on unplanned readmissions among patients with congestive heart failure. *Archives of Internal Medicine* 159(3), 257–261.

Stinnett KA (1996) Occupational therapy intervention for the geriatric client receiving acute and subacute services following total hip replacement and femoral fracture repair. *Topics in Geriatric Rehabilitation* 12(1), 23–31.

Stratton IM, Adler AI, Neil HAW *et al.* (2000) Association of glycaemia with macro-vascular and microvascular complications of type 2 diabetes (UKPDS 35): prospective observational study. *British Medical Journal* 321, 405–412.

Stroke Unit Trialists' Collaboration (2001) *Organised Inpatient (Stroke Unit) Care for Stroke* (Cochrane Review). The Cochrane Library, Issue 2, 2004. Chichester: John Wiley.

Stubbs R, Atwal A, McKay K (2004) Searching for the Holy Grail. *International Journal of Therapy and Rehabilitation* 11(6), 281–286.

The Assessment of Occupational Functioning – Collaborative Version (AOF–CV) (2003) Accessed 11.05.2004. http://www.sahp.vcu.edu/occu/html/assessment.htm

The Diabetes Control and Complications Trial (DCCT) (1993) The effect of intensive treatment of diabetes on the development and progression of long-term complications in insulin-dependent diabetes mellitus. *New England Journal of Medicine* 329(14), 977–986.

Taub E, Crago JE, Uswatte G (1998) Constraint-induced movement therapy: a new approach to treatment in physical rehabilitation. *Scandinavian Journal of Medicine and Science in Sports* 8(5 pt 1), 152–170.

Tijhuis MAR, De Jong-Gierveld J, Feskens EJM, Kromhout D (1999) Changes in factors relating to loneliness in older men. The Zutphen Elderly Study. *Age and Ageing* 28(5), 491–495.

Tinnetti ME, Speechley M, Ginter SF (1988) Risk factors for falls among elderly persons living in the community. *New England Journal of Medicine* 319(26), 1701–1707.

Tinnetti ME, Richman D, Powell L (1990) Falls efficacy as a measure of falling. *Journal of Gerontology* 45(6), 239–243.

Tugwell P, Wells G, Shea B *et al.* (2004) *Hormone Replacement Therapy for Osteoporosis in Postmenopausal Women* (Protocol for a Cochrane Review). The Cochrane Library, Issue 3. Chichester: John Wiley.

Turner NJ, Haward RA, Mulley GP, Selby PJ (1999) Cancer in old age – is it inadequately investigated and treated? *British Medical Journal* 319, 309–312.

UK Prospective Diabetes Study (UKPDS) (1998a) Group intensive blood-glucose control with sulphonylureas or insulin compared with conventional treatment and risk of complications in patients with type 2 diabetes (UKPDS 35). *Lancet* 352, 837–53.

UK Prospective Diabetes Study (UKPDS) Group (1998b) Tight blood pressure control and risk of microvascular and macrovascular complications in type 2 diabetes (UKPDS 38). *British Medical Journal* 317, 703–713.

University of Bath (2004) *WHO Field Centre for the Study of Quality of Life*. Accessed 29.08.2004. http://www.bath.ac.uk/whoqol/

Vrkljan B & Miller-Polgar J (2001) Meaning of occupational engagement in life-threatening illness: a qualitative pilot project. *Canadian Journal of Occupational Therapy* 68(4), 237–246.

Ward C (1998) *Preparing for a Positive Future*. Derbyshire: ARC Publications.

Ware JE & Sherbourne CD (1992) The MOS 36-Item Short-Form Health Survey (SF-36) *Medical Care* 30(6), 473–481.

Ware JE (2002) *SF-36® Health Survey Update*. Accessed 30.04.2004. http://www.sf-36.org

Weiss S, LaStayo P, Mills A, Bramlet D (2000) Prospective analysis of splinting the first carpometacarpal joint: an objective, subjective and radiographic assessment. *Journal of Hand Therapy* 13(3), 218–226.

Whiting S, Lincoln NB, Bhavnani G, Cockburn J (1985) *The Rivermead Perceptual Assessment Battery*. Windsor: NFER-Nelson Publishing.

Wilson BA, Cockburn J, Baddeley AD (1985) *Rivermead Behavioural Memory Test*. Bury St Edmunds: Thames Valley Test Co.

Wilson BA, Cockburn J, Halligan P (1987) *Behavioural Inattention Test*. Bury St Edmunds: Thames Valley Test Co.

Williams S (1993) *Chronic Respiratory Illness*. London: Routledge.

Wilson BA, Cockburn J, Baddeley A (1985) *The Rivermead Behavioural Memory Test*. Bury St Edmunds: Thames Valley Test Co.

Woolf AD & Åkesson K (2003) Preventing fractures in elderly people. *British Medical Journal* 327, 89–95.

World Health Organisation Expert Committee (1990) *Cancer Pain Relief and Palliative Care*. Technical Report Series 804. Geneva: World Health Organisation.

World Health Organisation (1992) *The ICD-10 Classification of Mental and Behavioural Disorders: Clinical Descriptions and Diagnostic Guidelines*, 10th edn. Geneva: World Health Organisation.

World Health Organisation (2001) *The International Classification of Functioning Disability and Health*. Geneva: World Health Organisation.

World Health Organisation (2003) *The WHO Stroke Surveillance System*. Accessed 05.05.2004. http://www.who.int/ncd_surveillance/steps/stroke/en/flyerStroke2.pdf

Yesavage JA, Brink TL, Rose TL *et al.* (1982–83) Development and validation of a geriatric depression screening scale: a preliminary report. *Journal of Psychiatric Research* 17(1), 37–49.

Zhu L, Fratiglioni L, Guo Z, Aguero-Torres H, Winbalb B, Viitanen M (1998) Association of stroke with dementia, cognitive impairment and functional disability in the very old: a population-based study. *Stroke* 29(10), 2094–2099.

Zigmond AS & Snaith RP (1994) *The Hospital Anxiety and Depression Scale*. Windsor: NFER-Nelson.

Zoltan B (1996) *Vision, Perception and Cognition: A Manual for the Evaluation and Treatment of the Neurologically Impaired Adult*, 3rd edn. New Jersey: Slack.

Zweig R & Hinrichsen G (1993) Factors associated with suicide attempts by depressed older adults: a prospective study. *American Journal of Psychiatry* 150(11), 1687–1692.

Chapter 6

BODY STRUCTURES AND BODY FUNCTIONS: PART 1

Stephen Ashford, Anne McIntyre and Trudi Minns

Introduction

In previous chapters an older person's ability to engage in meaningful occupation has been discussed in terms of their **societal** and **cultural context** – not only considering the applicable **services, legislation and policies** but also the **attitudes** of those around them. In this chapter and also in Chapter 7, the focus will be on those intrinsic or body factors that impact on an individual's ability to perform **activities** and **participate** in meaningful occupations. The WHO (2001) classifies these as **body functions** and **structures** within the ICF and these are defined as follows:

> *'Body functions are the physiological functions of body systems, including psychological functions.*
>
> *Body structures are anatomical parts of the body such as organs, limbs and their components.'*

(WHO 2001:10).

In occupational therapy it could be said that occupation and therefore activity is our core business and not impairment of body function or structure. However in many instances it is necessary for us to consider an impairment of body function or structure and the impact it has on **activity** or **participation** (and therefore **occupational performance**).

Deconstruction of an activity (activity analysis) should identify not only the demands of the activity (what, where, how often, how quickly and with what), the **context** of the activity, but also the body functions and structure required to successfully carry the activity out. These are also referred to as client factors (American Association of Occupational Therapists 2002) and performance components (Law & Baum 2001) within the occupational therapy literature.

Impairments of body structure and function may arise from pathological processes (as indeed occurs at any other age), with such changes superimposed upon normal age-related changes to body structure and function. Health professionals working with older people therefore have a responsibility to possess knowledge of these normal changes and their relationship to functional performance, whilst also understanding the additional impact of pathologies (often multiple) in this age group.

Ageing has its basis in cellular and subcellular change. Physiological theories of ageing discussed in Chapter 1 help us understand what may happen to body structures. Some cells, notably skeletal muscle fibres, cardiac fibres and neurones do not replicate at all and so these cell populations decline with age and cells are not replaced if tissue damage occurs. Also with ageing, the spontaneous binding of glucose to proteins both inside and outside cells occurs, forming irreversible links between molecules, and contributing to stiffening and loss of elasticity of tissues. An accumulation over time of oxidative damage – the action of free radicals in 'stealing' electrons from other, stable atoms to render them unstable – can lead to toxicity and chemical imbalances, cell membrane disruption and eventual cell death. It is important to remember that many individual factors impact upon the rate and extent of age-related changes – at all levels of structure and function. Heredity, gender, fitness, nutrition, rest–activity balance, habits such as smoking and drinking, these and more can affect the ageing process in one or more systems.

From the cellular level of organisation, cells become organised and grow to form tissues, which then become organised into organs (identifiable structures composed of two or more tissues). Organs are organised into systems culminating in a complex multisystem organism capable of coordinated functions that sustain life and all its features. Ultimately, changes at the cellular level culminate in the variety of age-related changes manifest in the organism, observable by others and experienced by the individual.

The ICF has been used as a classification to discuss those body functions and structures that are impacted upon in old age and also by health conditions more common in older people, including those discussed in Chapter 5. The body functions and structures considered in this chapter are listed in Box 6.1 (p. 107), and other body functions and structures will be discussed in Chapter 7.

The central nervous system

The control of human movement is a complex task and requires the interaction of a number of systems. Key to the production and control of movement is the structure and function of the nervous system. Likewise sensory perception is required to perceive the **environment** and allow movement to be meaningfully controlled producing useful behaviours to the individual.

The nervous system comprises the central nervous system (CNS) and the peripheral nervous system (PNS). The CNS has two main component parts, the brain and spinal cord. The PNS consists of peripheral nerves, which connect the CNS to the muscles or sensory receptors. Nerves linking the CNS to muscles are termed motor nerves and those linking sensory receptors to the CNS are termed sensory nerves. Many of the nerves in both the CNS and PNS are surrounded by myelin an insulating material, which improves the speed of nerve conduction.

Before reading further it would be useful for you to review the general structure and function of the nervous system. In particular it would be useful to be aware of the general anatomy and principal functions of the following:

Box 6.1

- **Structures of the nervous system**
  - Central nervous system
  - Peripheral nervous system
- **Structures and functions of voice and speech**
- **Mental functions**
  - Global mental functions
    + Consciousness and sleep
    + Orientation
    + Intellect
    + Energy and motivation
    + Personality and temperament.
  - Specific mental functions
    + Attention
    + Memory
    + Executive functions
    + Psychomotor performance
    + Emotion
    + Perception
    + Language
- **Structures and functions of the sensory system**
    + Touch
    + Pain
    + Eye
    + Ear
    + Balance

The brain's four principle regions:

(1) Cerebral hemispheres.
(2) Diencephalon (thalamus, hypothalamus and epithalamus).
(3) Brain stem (mid-brain, pons and medulla).
(4) Cerebellum.

The spinal cord:

(1) Principle regions.
(2) Motor and sensory connections to peripheral nervous system.

Apoptosis is a normal process by which cells are allowed to die. It is not a pathological process, but necessary to ensure appropriate development of connections between neurones (Joaquin & Gollapudi 2001). Apoptosis is important to consider related to normal ageing because evidence suggests that changes occur in this process, causing increased numbers of cells to die as people get older (Volloch *et al.* 1998; Savory *et al.* 1999; Fillenbaum *et al.* 2001).

Other factors are also thought to contribute to normal ageing at a neural cell level. Some processes may also contribute to certain pathological states such as **Alzheimer's disease** and **vascular dementia**. These processes are thought to include oxidation of free radicals, calcium homeostasis, and variations in gene expression, mitochondrial dysfunction and alterations in hormone levels (Troller & Valenzuela 2001).

All of these issues have a similar result in that they produce increased levels of cell death as people become older and in some cases this may produce a pathological state. For example hypoestrogenism has been linked to a higher incidence of **Alzheimer's disease** in postmenopausal women (Richards *et al.* 1999). This was given further support by a recent study, which demonstrated that administration of hormone replacement therapy reduced the incidence of alterations in the brain associated with **Alzheimer's disease** and maintained cognitive performance (Maki & Resnick 2000). Levels of homocysteine (a plasma-based amino acid) in the CNS have been demonstrated to increase with age and are indicated as a risk factor for increased incidence of **cardiovascular disease, stroke** and peripheral vascular disease (Perry 1995; Selhub *et al.* 1995).

In terms of brain structure a number of changes have been documented to occur with normal ageing. It has been demonstrated through imaging studies that the lateral ventricles of the brain increase in size, as people get older (Freedman *et al.* 1984; Raz 1996), indicating that atrophy is occurring in the cerebral hemispheres. Magnetic resonance imaging (MRI) studies demonstrate that cerebral volume decreases with age, indicating again that atrophy occurs throughout large regions of the brain and in particular in the cerebral hemispheres (Raz 2000). It has been demonstrated in a number of studies that the front region of the cortex (frontal lobe) shows increased atrophy, as people get older (Cowell *et al.* 1994; Raz *et al.* 1997). In particular it has been identified that while neural cells as a whole are lost, white matter representing the axon (neural) connections between cells are particularly lost. This has again been identified in the frontal and pre-frontal regions of the cortex (Ylikoski *et al.* 1995).

The other area of significant cell loss is the hippocampus in the medial temporal lobe, where like the frontal lobe, cell loss is significant to aspects of cognitive function (Squire 1987).

Changes in myelinated (white matter) areas of the frontal and pre-frontal lobe have been inversely correlated with reduced performance in tasks involving executive function, for example higher planning and organisation of task performance (Valenzuela *et al.* 2000). Speed of information processing seems to be particularly effected in individuals with white matter loss in this area (Ylikoski *et al.* 1993).

The presence of senile plaques in intracellular spaces and neurofibrillary tangles within cells occurs in the ageing brain from the age of 60 onwards; however larger numbers of these are seen in the brains of adults with **Alzheimer's disease** (like Millie in Chapter 5) and also those people with **learning disability** from the age of 50 onwards – like Jean who we met in Chapter 5 (Selkoe 1992; Jones & Ferris 1999).

Neurotransmitters have also been implicated in being involved in the normal ageing process and in some instances linked to pathological states. Neurotransmitters allow the transmission of an action potential across a synapse (from one neurone to the next) and are chemicals released by the terminal part of the neurone. Different neurotransmitters are involved with conduction in different areas of the CNS and PNS.

The neurotransmitter acetylcholine, found in some of the cortical regions is said to impact on learning and memory in people with **Alzheimer's disease** (Op den Velde 1976; Sims *et al.* 1980). It has been suggested that even in normal human ageing, reduction in cholinergic transmission may account for some of the identified decline in learning and memory (Trollor & Valenzuela 2001). Such research has also lead to the use of cholinergic medication to enhance cognitive function in those people with mild **Alzheimer's disease** (Forette & Rockwood 1999).

Dopamine is another neurotransmitter found predominantly in the basal ganglia. Dopamine transmission is required to allow the initiation of movement, which the basal ganglia (lateral to the thalamus) are involved in controlling movement. Reduction in dopamine in the basal ganglia and loss of the striatal cells responsible for its production are associated with **Parkinson's disease**. However studies using positron emission tomography have indicated significant alterations in dopamine neurotransmission with age (Volkow 1996). Further studies have also correlated loss of dopamine producing cells with normal ageing and reduction in ability to perform motor tasks such as finger tapping tests (Volkow *et al.* 1998). Thus significant evidence is provided that reduction in the ability to manufacture dopamine is associated with decreases in motor performance and particularly reaction times. Other neurotransmitters such as serotonin and glutamate also undergo age-related changes and a reduction in the number of receptors available sensitive to them. Changes in the availability of a number of neurotransmitters therefore seem to occur with normal ageing and may be one of the factors producing alterations in brain function, as individuals get older.

The evidence presented suggests that changes in the CNS are a normal product of ageing and are linked to decline in the functional ability of the brain in particular. Gross measures such as reduction in brain volume with age support the hypothesis that normal ageing produces changes in structure, which has implications for reduced CNS function. However it is important to note that recent evidence suggests that the 'normal' ageing brain can show signs of plasticity and recovery (Selkoe 1992; Sofroniew 1997). It is important to consider whether this potential plasticity this can be harnessed in intervention with a client.

Box 6.2 Management of impairment.

Cellular loss seen during normal ageing currently has no specific clinical management and in fact should not significantly affect function unless combined with a pathological state.

Reductions in neurotransmitters such as dopamine can be managed clinically with artificial replacements (L-dopa), but again these are usually only required if a pathological state is reached.

Mr Branch, aged 70, has had **Parkinson's disease** for 15 years, which impairs his concentration and speed of thought processes. Mr Branch will also have the effects for normal ageing as indicated previously, which will affect his CNS function. In most people of Mr Branch's age this would not be significant in their day-to-day activities. However for Mr Branch when this is combined with the effects of his Parkinson's disease this leads to a further limitation in systems function producing the balance problems that Mr Branch suffers with and his increasing tendency to fall.

The peripheral nervous system

The PNS consists of both motor and sensory nerves. The motor nerves synapse with muscles via connections called motor end-plates. Motor nerves are then able to stimulate the muscle to contract. Sensory nerves on the other hand, have more varied connections to different types of sensory receptors. However the principle of these different types of receptors is similar in that they convert mechanical (touch or pressure), thermal (temperature changes), light (as in the eye), chemical (taste or smell) or potentially damaging stimuli (producing pain) into electrical impulses or action potentials for transmission via peripheral sensory nerves to the CNS.

Peripheral nerves are also responsible for connections allowing autonomic responses within the body. Peripheral nerves connect to sweat glands, smooth muscles surrounding veins (allowing venous constriction and dilation) and body hair. This allows these effector organs to be linked to the autonomic nervous system (ANS) and assist in the regulation of body temperature.

An important factor in the function of nerves is the speed at which the nerve can conduct the impulse (or action potential) along its length. A number of body functions depend on this conduction occurring at a fast velocity or speed (see Box 6.3).

A number of electrophysiological studies have demonstrated that the speed at which nerve impulses travel decreases with age, using animal models of human nerve ageing (Dorfman & Bosley 1979; Buchthal et al. 1984). Verdu et al. (2000) also found that the number of myelinated and unmyelinated nerve fibres (in animal models) tend to reduce in the PNS with age, with myelinated nerve fibres being affected more slowly than unmyelinated fibres.

A peripheral nerve injury may cause the loss of motor, sensory and autonomic control of target organs. These deficits may be regained if adequate regrowth of the nerve takes place allowing the nerve to re-connect to the target organ. Parhad et al. (1995) indicate that the ability of peripheral nerves to regenerate following injury is reduced with advancing age. In particular they indicate that the

Box 6.3 Mechanisms to correct balance when tripping over an object.

- In this situation your muscles need to react quickly and in sequence so that you can prevent yourself from falling.
- This requires the CNS to react very quickly to the situation, therefore a number of 'spinal' reflexes are involved and much of the correction may have taken place before the brain is consciously aware of it.
- If this is to take place fast enough, then the speed of conduction in the peripheral nerves must be very fast indeed.
- In Peter's case the speed of nerve conduction would be slightly reduced because of his age. However in the majority of people of this age group this would not be at all significant. But for Peter because this is combined with his Parkinson's disease and it is another factor, which may contribute to his increasing tendency to fall.

production of chemicals which encourage damaged nerves to grow (nerve growth factors) are reduced, as an individual gets older. Again this work is done in animals, but it is thought that a similar mechanism occurs in humans. Therefore, in older people, if injuries occur, then it is likely that the rate and degree of recovery will decrease (Vaughan 1992; Verdu *et al.* 1995).

Voice and speech production

Speech and voice production is a result of the complex co-ordination of sensory and motor processes serving the respiratory, laryngeal, resonatory and articulatory systems. These systems are referred to as the subsystems for speech and provide a framework for describing motor speech production. The subsystems consist of the respiratory, the laryngeal or phonatory, the resonatory and the articulatory systems.

The reader is recommended to refer to anatomy and physiology textbooks to consider the anatomical structures and physiological processes involved in speech production.

Within the larynx, there are a number of tiny, paired cartilages with evidence within the older population of some degree of ossification of the thyroid, cricoid and arytenoid cartilages (Hirano *et al.* 1983). Erosion and calcification of the surfaces of the laryngeal cartilage joints also occurs. This results in less flexibility of movement of the vocal cords, which are responsible for making voice. As a result, this can impact on the perceptual voice quality which can be accentuated in the presence of arthritis (Greene & Mathieson 1989).

Pitch and vocal quality of the produced note (phonation) is also affected by the 'bowing' of shape of the vocal folds. The small intrinsic laryngeal muscles are said to atrophy with the advent of advancing age which affects the strength and resistance of vocal fold movement. This in turn may affect the stability of the note (phonation) (Greene & Mathieson 1989).

- Changes in the structures of the mucosal layer of the vocal folds and changes in the shape of the vocal folds, known as 'Bowing' impacts on the pitch and vocal quality of the note (phonation) (Greene & Mathieson 1989).
- With the advent of advancing age there is evidence of atrophy of the small (intrinsic) muscles of the larynx affecting the strength and resistance of vocal fold movement. This in turn may affect the stability of the vocal note (phonation) (Kahane & Hammons 1991; Greene & Mathieson 1989).

The resonatory system corresponds to the resonance of the voice and speech. In particular it can correspond to the degree of nasal airflow during connected speech (nasality). There can either be too little (hyponasality) which sounds like a blocked nose during a bad cold, or too much nasal airflow (hypernasality) and this is more common in older people. The small structure at the back of the mouth known as the soft palate acts as a shutter system, together with the back wall of the throat (posterior pharyngeal wall), and diverts sound through either the nose or the mouth.

Some sounds require nasal airflow (e.g. 'm') and some sounds requires oral airflow (e.g. 'p'), whilst others require a finely tuned mixture of both (e.g. 'n'). Changes in structures related to ageing, listed below have an effect on this balanced and highly co-ordinated movement:

- Atrophic changes in the oral, pharyngeal and velopharyngeal musculature in addition to the skin and musculature of the face.
- Continued growth of the craniofacial skeleton.
- Descent of the larynx.

(Kahane & Hammons 1991; Benjamin 1988).

Changes within the articulatory system in older people correspond to the movements which are made by the tongue, lips, jaw and palate during speech which are caused by atrophic changes to tongue, jaw, palate and facial muscles (Robertson & Thompson 1987; Murdoch 1998).

The lungs and muscles of respiration (see Chapter 7) have a large part to play in the production of speech and voice. They can be thought of as the power supply to speech. In the young population, speech is produced on expired air. Air is channelled from the lungs to through the trachea and larynx and up through the nasal or oral pharynx, depending on what kind of sound it is. As the air passes through the larynx it sets the vocal cord into motion, which then produces a vibrating column of air, which carries sound. The sound is then shaped by the articulatory system.

Due to the changes in the structures of the respiratory system, which occur with age, there are a number of direct effects, which can be seen on the physiology of speech:

- Reduced expiratory pressure can affect voice quality, making the voice sound breathy, rough and hoarse in quality.
- Increased respiratory effort during speech can have an effect on the rate of speech production and there is a tendency for there to be fewer syllables/words per breath, than in younger counterparts.
- Reduced volume of speech/voice or reduced vocal intensity.
- The reduced respiratory effort can have an impact on the stress and intonation used in conversation.

(Darley *et al.* 1975; Robertson & Thompson 1987).

The vocal cords come together on expiration and vibrate the air coming from the lungs, (like a tuning fork). If they are unable to come together completely, air escape during the production of voice, can have an effect on the quality of the voice. Such changes in voice quality that have been reported in the older population are hoarseness, croak, creak, breathy and rough quality to the voice, increased vocal weakness and fatigue and an altered pitch of the voice, which usually lowers with age. It is important to note however that if there are any changes in the quality of the voice, a referral to a general practitioner is advised especially when there is a history of heavy smoking or drinking. The presence of a carcinoma can have a similar presentation, and therefore every permanent change in the quality of the voice should always be fully investigated.

Finally the tongue has an extremely important role to play in the articulation of sounds. It has a dynamic role in that it has to adapt intricate positions numerous times within a single word. In addition to this it is expected to move at high speeds to keep up with the demands of conversation. Changes in the structures of the articulatory system have an effect on its functioning in older people in the following ways – slower articulation, loss of definition, imprecise articulation and increased number of dysfluencies. It is important to note that alongside the structural and functional impact on motor speech and voice production there are also many **environmental** effects on communication (Robertson & Thompson 1987; Amerman & Parnell 1992).

Mental functions

Deterioration in mental function is seen by many old people as the true marker of the onset of old age and that **dementia** is the only outcome, with the phrase 'you can't teach an old dog new tricks' commonly heard by both young and old alike to describe mental functioning in older age. However a decline in mental functioning into **dementia** is not an inevitable part of old age, but a part of disease processes.

Decline in cognitive function varies, and evidence is sometimes contrary. It must be remembered that older people are a heterogeneous group and therefore evidence has to be considered within this context. Predictors of cognitive change of interest are:

- Lower educational status (associated with faster memory loss and loss of crystallised intelligence).
- Poor midlife lung function (associated with reduction in executive functions).
- Poor general health (including midlife high blood pressure, cholesterol, blood glucose, and body mass) associated with generalised cognitive decline.
- Poor engagement in physical, leisure and mental activities.
                    (Christensen 2001; Gilhooly *et al.* 2003; Verghese *et al.* 2003).

Global mental functions

Consciousness and sleep
Arousal and sleep are seen as opposite ends of a continuum of consciousness, because they have common neurophysiological and neurochemical mechanisms. Therefore these two states will be considered together. Consciousness is not often formally assessed by occupational therapists unless intervening with those with traumatic brain injury (TBI).

Arousal is necessary for most cognitive functions to take place, especially memory, learning and attention. Social and behavioural phenomena also impact on arousal and sleep, with the onset of retirement causing abrupt changes to routine, altered cognitive and physical demands and therefore sleep. However the frontal lobe has an inhibitory role on the ascending reticular arousal system in the brain stem, and therefore any reduction in frontal lobe function with ageing will cause changes in arousal and sleep patterns, as well as a reduction in selective inhibition of information, and therefore reduced function of attention systems (Woodruff-Pak 1997). This under-arousal hypothesis is said to explain a decline in reaction times and psychomotor activity (Birren 1960), but many older people can increase their levels of arousal to those of younger people when required, and can often be over-aroused or anxious as a result (Woodruff-Pak 1997).

Alterations to sleep patterns are well-documented in older people (Kelly 1991; Wolfson & Katzman 1992; Dotinga 2003). The presence of other factors, such as cardiovascular disease, medication or pain also impact on sleep patterns (Dotinga 2003). However it is considered that older people have a more pronounced biphasic circadian rhythm (our internal body clock that determines wakefulness and sleep). This leads them to have a lighter period of sleep during the night from which they are easily aroused, early morning wakening, and afternoon naps. It is thought that the circadian rhythm is controlled by the suprachiasmatic nuclei of the hypothalamus – another area of the brain sensitive to age-related cell death (Hastings 1998). Alterations to sleep are not always inevitable, but sleep disturbances are commonly associated with **depression** (early morning wakening and difficulty falling asleep) and **Alzheimer's disease** (fragmented patterns of sleep, wakefulness at night and sleep during the day). Other sleep problems are sleep apnoea and involuntary leg movements at night experienced by 20–25% of older people which cause frequent arousal (Wolfson & Katzman 1992).

Prescription of hypnotic medication (e.g. benzodiazepines) is problematic in older people. These have only a short-term effect on sleep, but have had a historical tendency to be prescribed repeatedly and long-term, without re-assessment. Because of reduced renal function (see Chapter 7) medication has a longer half-life within the body (see Chapter 8), with an impact on levels of consciousness throughout the day – with the possible impairment of judgement and reaction times. Reduction of benzodiazepines can also induce withdrawal insomnia. Current advice is not to prescribe hypnotics to older people because of their risk of confusion and ataxia (and therefore falls) (British National Formulary 2004). Non-medication techniques should therefore be pursued – including an increase in the daily exposure to daylight, increase in exercise and high carbohydrate meals (Wolfson & Katzman 1992). The opportunity to follow such advice is heavily dependent on individual contextual factors – especially for those older people in long-term residential care.

Levels of consciousness are affected by stimulants such as alcohol and caffeine as well as barbiturates, narcotics and hallucinogens. Whereas the taking of illegal substances may not be a current issue for older people, the increase in alcohol dependency (Alcohol Concern 2002) in older people needs to be considered. Other factors that influence consciousness in older people are:

- Syncope – caused by cardiac disease, hypotension, reflex activity, CNS disease, hypoglycaemia (Lipsitz & Jonsson 1992).

- Epilepsy – where symptoms are commonly mistaken for other diseases in older people (Kilpatrick & Lowe 2002).
- Delirium (acute confusional state) – often undiagnosed, causing impairment in attention, orientation, memory and executive functions (Schuurmans *et al.* 2001).
- General anaesthesia – can cause post-operative cognitive dysfunction and pain (Selwood & Orrell 2004).

Orientation

Orientation to time of day, date and place or season is commonly monitored within cognitive functional assessments of older people. Orientation requires many functions including attention, memory and retention of new information (Zoltan 1996). Disorientation is a symptom of many pathological processes in older people such as **depression, Alzheimer's disease**, and **stroke**. Many of us become disorientated (in its true sense) by getting lost, forgetting today's date; however most people have strategies to resolve this (looking at a watch, a map, diary etc) but this becomes problematic when an individual is consistently disorientated in time, place or person and has an impact on occupational performance, sense of control and self-esteem (Spector *et al.* 2000).

The use of reality orientation programmes has been very popular in the past to orientate clients with **dementia** to time, place or season, but has been criticised more recently (Powell-Proctor & Miller 1982), especially where a mechanised approach has been used. However a recent Cochrane review by Spector *et al.* (2000) has concluded that reality orientation can have beneficial effects on cognition and behaviour in older people with dementia, but the long-term effects are not clear.

Intellect

There is much debate as to whether intellectual ability declines as part of normal ageing or is preserved throughout the lifespan (Goldman & Coté 1991). Definitions of intelligence vary, and an individual's intellectual ability can only be determined by assessment of behaviour. Intellectual functions have been described in terms of crystallised and fluid intelligence, with crystallised intelligence being experience and knowledge of learnt information and facts (numeracy, vocabulary). Fluid intelligence involves the perception of complex relationships, concept formation, abstract thought and reasoning and it is this aspect that is said to decline with age, with crystallised intelligence remaining intact (Christensen 2001). Rabbitt (1997) identified that even though older people may not perform so well on tasks requiring quick problem-solving skills (fluid intelligence) they have the better problem-solving strategies over a longer period of time, because they can utilise past experience and information to help them. In many cultures such ability is seen as wisdom that one aspires to; however in a speed obsessed world wisdom is not deemed as 'better' or worthy of attainment (Rose 2002).

Energy, motivation, personality and temperament

Other global functions that do not seem to dramatically change as part of normal ageing but where changes occur that can be symptoms of pathological processes, are energy and drive (motivation), personality, and temperament. These functions come under frontal lobe control and more specifically the pre-frontal cortex. Damage to this area can range from poor motivation as a key symptom in **depression** and minor impairments such as irritability, reduced motivation and quick loss of temper to a complete change in personality and loss of social inhibition. Such changes are known as 'frontal lobe syndrome' and occur in **stroke**, prolonged **alcoholism**, Korsakoff's syndrome and **Alzheimer's disease** (Woodruff-Pak 1997).

Specific mental functions

Cognitive functions most obviously affected by ageing are the more specific functions of attention and memory. These functions are closely linked and problems in either area prevent effective learning and successful performance of everyday activity.

Attention

The ICF defines attention as 'specific mental functions of focusing on an external stimulus or internal experience for the required period of time' (WHO 2001:53). Attention and memory are inextricably linked, with a dysfunction in either causing problems in **occupational performance**. Attention is not one concept but consists of different types of attention which will be discussed here.

Sustained attention (or vigilance as it is sometimes known) is the maintenance of the ability to focus attention over a period of time (e.g. exams). This tends to be assessed subjectively in the clinical setting, as there are few appropriate tools devised. Perry & Hodges (1999) suggest that the most likely site for this is in the frontoparietal cortex. This requires an adequate level of arousal and sensitivity to different inputs. As older people are said to be in a state of under-arousal (Birren 1960) it is said that sustained attention or vigilance is affected in many tasks, especially as they become more complex (Baddeley *et al.* 1999). This is also said to be problematic in moderate **Alzheimer's disease** and it is contested whether this is affected in earlier stages (Baddeley *et al.* 1999; Perry & Hodges 1999). In **depression** individuals such as Mr Jones have a shorter span of sustained attention, with reduced concentration a common complaint (Butters *et al.* 2000).

Selective attention involves focusing on a single relevant stimulus at one time, ignoring other irrelevant or distracting stimuli. The cortex said to be responsible for selective attention is the posterior parietal cortex and basal ganglia (Perry & Hodges 1999). This requires inhibitory processes to sift out irrelevant stimuli; however cognitive research identifies that cognitive inhibition deteriorates with old age so that older people have more difficulty in suppressing extraneous information (Woodruff-Pak 1997). This is even more noticeable with people with **learning disability** and also in **Alzheimer's disease** and **depression**. Butters *et al.* (2000) suggest that the problem with selective attention with depressed clients is because cognitive resources are taken up by negative thoughts, and that this improves with medication. In **Alzheimer's disease** it is thought that clients have difficulty disengaging and differentiating between stimuli (Perry & Hodges 1999). However an opposite problem is sometimes seen in **Alzheimer's disease** and **stroke** – known as simultanagnosia, where individuals cannot see a picture as a whole, only able to recognise one single object at a time (Zoltan 1996).

Divided attention is the sharing of attention by focusing on more than one relevant stimulus or process at a time. The possible site responsible for this is the pre-frontal cortex and anterior cingulate gyrus (Perry & Hodges 1999). The inability to carry out divided tasks is said to be a problem of the central executive (see following section) and problems with this are well-documented with clients with **Alzheimer's disease** (Baddeley *et al.* 1991; Camicoli *et al.* 1997). Dual tasking is discussed in Chapter 8; it is also considered to be problematic for normal older people, but this may be suggestive of underlying pathology (Rabbitt 1997; Woodruff-Pak 1997).

The concept of a working memory as part of an attentional system was proposed by Baddeley & Hitch in 1974, and has been said to be the 'most significant achievement of human mental evolution' (Goldman-Rakic 1992:73). Working memory consists of a central executive (an attention controlling system) with slave or subsystems for short-term memories known as the visuospatial sketchpad (for visual images) and the phonological loop (for speech-based input). The concept of a working memory replaced the idea of a single short-term memory store. The central executive is said to have access to long-term memory and is said to work as the supervisory attentional system (SAS) as proposed by Norman & Shallice (1980), co-ordinating information from different sources. The SAS is said to be able to override ongoing activities such as in dual tasking (to stop walking while talking, as described in Chapter 8 with Jim) when the SAS is at full capacity. The SAS function is said to be reduced as a result of frontal lobe damage or deterioration (Baddeley *et al.* 1991) and therefore working memory is said to be the most vulnerable cognitive function in normal ageing, especially with the processing of incoming information (Katzman & Terry 1992). Working memory relies on the interaction of the pre-frontal cortex and the hippocampus, with the pre-frontal cortex retrieving facts, events and rules from elsewhere in the brain as well as regulating motor behaviour by initiating, programming, facilitating and cancelling commands to brain structures and the hippocampus to consolidate new associations and learned memory (Goldman-Rakic 1992).

It is therefore important to provide clients with suitable **environments** for learning and performance to take place – ensuring that they are comfortable and not distracted by pain, noise or visual stimuli during assessment and performance especially of new or complex tasks. An awareness of their ability in selective, sustained and divided attention must be taken into account during **occupational performance**.

Memory

A linear decline of memory loss with normal ageing is generally accepted, which accelerates from 70 years onward (Katzman & Terry 1992). Rose (2002) describes memory loss as perhaps the most frightening of impairments, stripping us of our individuality through loss of personal memories, also reducing our ability to perform successfully in a socially interactive and skill-driven world. Memory involves 'the registration, retention and retrieval of information' (Jones & Ferris 1999:212).

Formation of memory traces requires motivation, arousal, perception and attention (Rose 2002) and memory performance and function is believed to be affected by education and occupational class (Marriott *et al.* 2002). Memory and learning are closely linked with the successful storage of learned skills retrieved from memory and tested through observation of behaviour and performance. The mechanisms of memory are not fully understood, but like attention it is considered that there are different types of memory, with different functions. Many older people report memory problems which may not be evident from testing, and memory deficits do not only occur as part of normal ageing (see Table 6.1).

Psychomotor functions and speed of processing

Speed of nerve conduction has been discussed in relation to the PNS; however this is said to impact on slowing of simple motor tasks by a lesser degree than by a reduction in central processing. Performance on timed tasks (reaction time – RT) is said to peak at age 20 and declines thereafter; this decline is more noticeable after age 70 (although some 70-year-olds perform better than 20-year-olds) (Katzman & Terry 1992). Slowing of motor tasks such as writing and sport is relative to previous ability rather than chronological age. Complexity of tasks (discussed in Chapter 8) also impacts on the speed of reaction, with an increase in complexity causing an increase in time in older age groups. However in some instances an increase in time also increases accuracy of performance (Rabbitt 1997). Speed of processing also affects cognitive tasks. It was thought that those individuals with higher intelligence and educational experience performed better than age-equivalents; however Christensen *et al.* (1997) demonstrated that RT tasks were the same for both groups, but the higher intelligence group did better than age-equivalents on verbal tasks of crystallised intelligence. Such a decline in cognitive speed is also associated with white matter changes in the frontal lobe (Christensen 2001).

Increase in reaction time above that expected of a normal older person is seen both in **depression** (Butters *et al.* 2000) and in **Alzheimer's disease** (Perry & Hodges 1999) and seen to be a problem of central processing rather than nerve conduction.

Executive functions

The ICF defines executive functions as higher level cognitive function (WHO 2001:57) and is seen as the most highly developed group of functions in humans – involving planning, abstract thought, decision-making, cognitive flexibility and the use of appropriate behaviours (Woodruff-Pak 1997). These functions are believed to account for most of the cognitive decline in older people (Salthouse *et al.* 2003) and this is most noticeable in clients with **Alzheimer's disease, learning disability, Stroke** and **Parkinson's disease** (Bellelli *et al.* 2002). The function of spontaneous flexibility such as generation of ideas and reactive flexibility to new ideas and situations (known as switching set) are especially impaired in older age (Woodruff-Pak 1997). Such mental inflexibility is said to be due to depletion of dopamine levels in the CNS as part of ageing and particularly **Parkinson's disease**.

Other aspects of executive functions are termed as prospective memory – involving planning, organisation and self-monitoring. Many older adults are said

Table 6.1 Concepts of memory, their function, location and changes with ageing and pathological processes.

Memory type	Function	Area of CNS	Normal ageing	Pathological processes
Short-term memory	Temporary storage of events and information within the past few minutes	Hippocampus, and medial temporal lobe	Some changes with ageing	Noticeable changes in Alzheimer's disease and depression
Long-term memory				
1. Declarative (explicit) memory consisting of:	Directly accessible to conscious recollection			
Episodic memory	Personal experiences, context bound to time and place	Hippocampus of medial temporal lobe, diencephalon	Occurs as part of normal ageing	Korsakoff's syndrome, depression
Semantic memory	Cumulative knowledge of the world, concepts, language	Frontal lobe	More stable and resistant to change	Dementias
2. Procedural (implicit) memory	Learned skills or cognitive operations	Different areas, e.g. motor cortex, cerebellum etc.	More stable and resistant to change	Occurs in TBI, CVA, multi-infarct dementia
Prospective memory	Manipulates and organises memory, rather than acquisition and storage	Medial temporal lobe	Affected in older age	Occurs in depression, dementias
Working memory	A workspace for short-term memories, with a central executive and subsystems	Pre-frontal cortex	Ageing effects occur	Problems in dementias, Parkinson's disease, depression

(Squire 1987; Shimamura 1990; Katzman & Terry 1992; Woodruff-Pak 1997; Stevens & Ripich 1999).

to perform badly on tasks such as remembering future events such as birthdays, appointments or taking medications (Shimamura 1990). The use of external cues such as diaries, calendars and 'post-it' notes are important to compensate for prospective memory loss. Other problems with self-monitoring are socially inappropriate comments, impulsive behaviour and keeping track of conversations – leading to repetition of stories and conversations.

Assessments of executive functions are carried out widely with impairments in this area and are key to a diagnosis of **Alzheimer's disease**, where people complain of problems with everyday tasks such as planning and cooking a meal (like Millie) (Perry & Holmes 1999). However they are criticised for their lack of ecological validity in their relationship to real world tasks (Morris *et al.* 2000) and also for their specificity (Salthouse *et al.* 2003).

Emotion

Whereas positive emotion is more enduring in older people (Carstensen *et al.* 2000), more negative emotions are said to decline with age (Calder *et al.* 2003). However as can be seen in Chapter 5, **depression** is common in older people and is characterised by the negative emotions of sadness, helplessness and loss. A sense of well-being is important in maintaining occupational performances (Borell *et al.* 2001), with the voluntary giving-up of independence (termed 'learned helplessness') being a direct link with poorer cognitive functioning (National Mental Health Association 2003). Other emotional changes seen are those in **Alzheimer's disease** such as inappropriate response and emotional disturbances due to impaired executive functioning.

Perception

Perceptual problems are more commonly associated with older people with **stroke** or TBI. However some changes in perceptual ability do occur with normal ageing. Perception of colour, depth and distance of field all deteriorate with age alongside a reduction in lens accommodation, and retinal illumination (Fozzard *et al.* 1977). Su *et al.* (1995) also identified deterioration in figure ground, visual memory and spatial relationships. A decline in the perception of vertical and horizontal was also noted in older people with **falls** by Tobis *et al.* (1981). All of these will impact on occupational performance in both normal older people and those with **stroke** or TBI.

Like many other aspects of occupational therapy, intervention strategies for adults with perceptual problems do not have a strong evidence base. However, the use of either a remedial approach or the adaptive approach described by Zoltan (1996) will depend heavily on the older person's attentional ability and memory in determining their capacity for learning and retaining new skills.

Language

There are many changes which occur in the structures responsible for processing cognition and language. These changes result in age-related deficits in memory alongside other aspects of cognition, and linguistic skills. Cognition and linguistic skills form the scaffolding upon which language and communication can function. If these are affected there is usually some negative effect on communication experienced. Examples of alterations in neuroanatomical infrastructure associated with ageing include: decreases in brain weight, neuronal cell loss, dendrite atrophy, reduced metabolism and accumulation of neurotransmitter substances (Maxim & Bryan 1994).

The ability to process language in speech, understanding, reading and writing has been investigated a number of times in the ageing population. Older people have been found to have difficulties with naming skills (Bayles & Kaszniak 1987). Cohen (1979) identified that older people have increasing difficulty understanding and producing syntactically complex sentences, but theorised that this was due to the heavy demands placed on working memory. He also concluded that older people have more difficulty drawing inferences from story content and in recalling information from narratives.

Even though the changes in communication skills are relatively small in normal older people, changes in cognition and also hearing acuity will impact on the older person's ability to hold and maintain a conversation. Other neurological diseases such as **stroke, Parkinson's disease** and **dementia** common in older age will cause problems with communication skills (Ryan-Ellen *et al.* 1986).

The sensory systems: structure and function

Sensory modalities change as part of normal ageing, with alterations to smell and taste affecting eating habits and diet in later life (Woodruff-Pak 1997). Quality of life is also affected by alterations to touch, vibration, sight, hearing and balance as part of normal ageing (Woodruff-Pak 1997).

Touch

Touch is not only affected by poor circulation causing occlusion of the small capillaries under the surface of the skin, but also by the reduction of touch receptors (Meissner's corpuscles) form the age of 50 onwards (Woodruff-Pak 1997). This impacts on hand function and grip strength in older age (Shumway-Cook & Woollacott 2001).

Pain

The CNS in relation to ageing has been discussed and the peripheral (PNS) sensory receptors detecting mechanical (touch or pressure), thermal (temperature changes) and damage stimuli (producing pain) have also been mentioned. However one issue that involves both central systems and peripheral systems is that of pain. Pain is an important sensory function, which protects the body from possible injury. However in many cases it can be very distressing to the individual, which may in itself cause significant activity limitation. In some cases pain responses may be out of proportion to the nature of the stimulus presented to the body and again cause activity limitation.

Pain sensation is transmitted to the CNS via peripheral nerves, which undergo some changes with age. This can lead to a reduction in the transmission frequency and rate of pain-related sensation in older people. However a study by Harkins (1996) found no age-related alterations in pain perception. Moreover pain is often under-reported in older people, not because they feel less pain, but because they fear that more pain may indicate progression of disease (Nishikawa & Ferrell 1993; Ferrell 1996). Because of the diseases that are more common in older age, persistent pain is more prevalent. It is often accepted as part of the ageing process by both older people and medical professionals working with them, and as a consequence of this is often left unmanaged. Therefore because older people may be less likely to voluntarily report pain, professionals working in this area need to be aware of this issue and be proactive in pain management.

The eye

The eye as a sensory organ is another receptor allowing perception of our **environment**. However the visualisation of the environment requires many processes to be meaningful and useful. The eye is anatomically and developmentally closely related to the brain. Information from the eye is transmitted to the brain via the optic nerve. Visual information is then interpreted by the occipital lobe allowing the brain to form a perception of the visual environment.

Before reading further it would be useful to review the general structure and function of the eye, in particular the anatomy and principal functions.

Deterioration in visual acuity is one of the most common sensory changes occurring with advancing age, with one in five over 75-year-olds having a visual impairment (Philp 2003). This is often seen when individuals are looking at objects in their immediate 'close' environment. It is also common, as individuals get older, for some deterioration to occur to the corneal layer of the eye. Cell death in this area can cause a decrease in the ability of the cornea to allow light into the eye and cataract is not uncommon. Other impairments have also been identified such as spatial discrimination, restriction in upward gaze and the reduction in ability to 'track' (follow) moving object.

The ear

The ear provides recognition of auditory stimuli and also forms one of the key organs for orientating the body in space thus contributing to balance. When discussing the anatomy of the ear we usually refer to three regions: the outer (external) ear; the middle ear; and inner (internal) ear or labyrinth.

Before reading further it would be useful to review the general structure and function of the ear, in particular the anatomy and principal functions of external, middle and inner ear.

The inner ear provides two main functions, hearing and balance information. The ageing process can affect both of these functions. Difficulties in hearing in older people are well-documented in the literature and are also a well-known factor to the general public. Hearing loss related to ageing is known as presbycusis and is the most common hearing disorder (National Institute of Ageing 2002). Presbycusis is caused by a combination of intrinsic and extrinsic factors. Intrinsic factors affecting hearing may be related to apoptosis in some of the cells related to the nerve conduction to the brain. They may also relate to cell loss and death in the specialist hair cells (stereocilia) producing an inability of the system to detect sounds at certain frequencies. The blood (vascular) supply to the inner ear may deteriorate with age, which may contribute to loss of neural cells or stereocilia. Thickening of the tympanic membrane, loss of elasticity in the ossicular chains and atrophy of the cochlea all impair hearing (Zoltan 1996). Extrinsic factors, which may contribute to this process, include issues such as exposure to chronic noise (accounting for the largest single reason for hearing impairment in older people). Functionally this can result in deterioration in hearing at certain frequencies and difficulty in following conversation and speech in unfavourable listening conditions.

Balance

In a similar way to the cellular deterioration of auditory structures, vestibular structures of the inner ear are also susceptible to cellular deterioration. The saccule, utricle and semicircular canals rely on specialist sensory cells, which are similar to stereocilia and indicate the movement of fluid in these structures, providing information regarding the body's position in space. Cell loss is seen with increasing age in these structures and leads to a decrease in the response time to balance perturbations registered by structures of the inner ear. This is also linked to cellular loss in the cerebellum and higher brain centres involved with balance.

Deterioration in the inner ear structures involved with balance should be considered alongside reduced conduction velocities in the PNS and the reduction in sensitivity of sensory receptors. Joint position receptors (proprioceptors), muscle spindles and skin pressure receptors all need increased stimulus before firing, as individuals get older. This means that body position information from joint positions, muscle length and skin pressure are all slightly reduced. The CNS correlates this information with body position information from the structures of the inner ear and with information from the visual system. These three systems then work together to produce functional balance and correction of balance when perturbations (loss of balance) occur.

The deficits in balance information from the inner ear and the structures of the peripheral sensory systems are actually quite small according to most studies (Gaeta *et al.* 2003; Gates *et al.* 2002). However the combined effect of these slight

Box 6.4

> - With a partner, take it in turns to observe each other for approximately 30 seconds in quiet standing, firstly with the eyes open and then with the eyes shut.
> - What do you observe?

deteriorations in structure leads to a cumulative effect in terms of reduced systems function. At most activity levels these minor alterations in function will not be significant; however when the system is challenged, this can lead to decreased ability to deal with situations which require balance correction. When this is then linked to deterioration in vision more significant problems may be evident.

The visual system is said to dominate over the proprioceptive and vestibular systems in quiet standing, when normal subjects are observed to increase their anteroposterior sway (known as postural sway) with the eyes shut. An increase in postural sway is also observed in quiet standing with the eyes open by those people with poor visual acuity, young children and also older people. Balance correction is required in a number of different circumstances in everyday activity. Shumway-Cook & Woollacott (2001) describe two different types of balance control – reactive and proactive which are dependent upon constant postural adjustments and adaptation, equilibrium, righting and protective reactions. Reactive control of balance is required in both quiet standing and sitting or when standing still on a moving platform such as a bus and reacting to a sudden jolt or perturbation. Proactive control of balance is required where postural adjustments are made in advance of a potentially destabilising situation, such as hanging clothes on a washing line, or picking up a heavy shopping basket. In walking, both types of balance control are required – to avoid tripping over an obstacle on the floor or regaining one's balance as a result of a trip. These situations place increased pressure on the balance control systems. Reduction in postural balance occurs gradually with ageing, but a decline is most noticeable during the sixth decade of life (Shepard 1978). Deterioration in the combined factors producing a reduction in postural balance, lead to an increased risk of falls as already described in Chapter 5.

Summary

This chapter has considered those body functions and structures primarily related to the central and peripheral nervous systems. Impairments of these systems both in normal ageing and also in pathological states such as stroke, Parkinson's disease and dementia impact not only on motor skills but the more complex and higher cognitive and language functions. Many of these are still not fully understood and it is only more recently since the more common usage of PET and MRI scanning those theoretical concepts about human functioning and the ageing process can be scrutinised.

References

Alcohol Concern (2002) Alcohol misuse among older people. *Acquire* Autumn.

American Occupational Therapy Association (2002) Occupational therapy practice framework: domain and process. *American Journal of Occupational Therapy* 56(6), 609–639.

Amerman J & Parnell M (1992) Speech timing strategies in elderly adults. *Journal of Phonetics* 20(1), 65–76.

Baddeley AD, Bressi S, Della Salla S, Logie R, Soinnler H (1991) The decline of working memory in Alzheimer's disease. *Brain* 114(6), 2521–2542.

Baddeley AD, Cocchini G, Della Sala S, Logie RH, Spinnler H (1999) Working memory and vigilance: evidence form normal ageing and Alzheimer's disease. *Brain and Cognition* 41(1), 87–108.

Bayles K & Kaszniak A (1987) *Communication and Cognition in Normal Ageing and Dementia*. Boston: Little, Brown and Co.

Bellelli G, Lucchi E, Cipriani G (2002) Executive dysfunction and depressive symptoms in cerebrovascular disease (Letter). *Journal of Neurology, Neurosurgery and Psychiatry* 73(4), 460–464.

Benjamin B (1988) Changes in speech production and linguistic behaviours with ageing. In: Shadden B (ed.) *Communication Behaviour and Ageing: A Sourcebook for Clinicians*. Baltimore: Williams & Wilkins, pp. 163–181.

Birren JE (1960) Behavioural theories of ageing. In: Shock NW (ed.) *Ageing – Some Social and Biological Aspects*. Washington DC: American Association for the Advancement for Science.

Borell L, Lilja M, Sviden GA, Sadlo G (2001) Occupations and signs of reduced hope: an explorative study of older adults with functional impairments. *American Journal of Occupational Therapy* 55(3), 311–316.

British National Formulary (2004) *BNF No. 47* (March 2004). London: British Medical Association and Royal Pharmaceutical Society of Great Britain.

Buchthal F, Rosenfalck A, Behse F (1984) Sensory potentials of normal and diseased nerves. In: Dyck PJ, Thomas PK, Lambert EH, Burge R (eds). *Peripheral Neuropathy*. Philadelphia: WB Saunders, pp. 981–1105.

Butters MA, Mulsant BH, Hagerty BM, Therrien B, Wiliams RA (2000) Changes in attention and short processing speed mediate cognitive impairments in geriatric depression. *Psychological Medicine* 30(3), 679–691.

Calder AJ, Keane J, Manly T *et al.* (2003) Facial expression recognition across the adult lifespan. *Neuropsychologica* 41(2), 195–202.

Camicoli R, Howieson D, Lehman S, Kaye J (1997) Talking while walking: the effect of a dual task in ageing and Alzheimer's disease. *Neurology* 48(4), 955–958.

Carstensen LL, Pasupathi M, Mayr U, Nesselroade J (2000) Emotional experience in everyday life across the adult lifespan. *Journal of Personality and Social Psychology* 79(4), 644–655.

Christensen H, Henderson AS, Griffiths K, Levings C (1997) Does ageing inevitably lead to declines in cognitive performance? A longitudinal study of elite academics. *Personality and Individual Differences* 23(1), 67–78.

Christensen H (2001) What cognitive changes can be expected with normal ageing? *Australian and New Zealand Journal of Psychiatry* 35(6), 768–775.

Cohen G (1979) Language comprehension in old age. *Cognitive Psychology* 11(4), 412–429.

Cowell PE, Tuetsky BI, Gur RC, Grossman RI, Shtasel DR, Gur RE (1994) Sex differences in ageing of the human frontal and temporal lobes. *Journal of Neuroscience* 14(8), 4748–4755.

Darley FL, Aronson AE, Brown JR (1975) *Motor Speech Disorders*. Philadelphia: WB Saunders.

Dorfman LJ & Bosley TM (1979) Age related changes in peripheral and central nerve conduction in man. *Neurology* 29(1), 38–44.

Dotinga R (2003) *For Many Seniors, Sleep is an Elusive Dream*. Health on the Net Foundation. Accessed 09.03.2004. http://www.hon.ch/News?HSN/512493.htm

Ferrell BA (1996) Overview of ageing and pain. In: Ferrell BR & Ferrell BA (eds). *Pain in the Elderly*. Seattle: IASP, pp. 1–10.

Fillenbaum GG, Landerman LR, Blazer DG, Saunders AM, Harris TB, Launer LJ (2001) The relationship of APOE genotype to cognitive functioning in older African–American and Caucasian community residents. *Journal of the American Geriatrics Society* 49(9): 1148–1155.

Forette F & Rockwood K (1999) Therapeutic intervention in dementia. In: Wilcock GK, Bucks RS, Rockwood K (eds). *Diagnosis and Management of Dementia: A Manual for Memory Disorders Teams*. Oxford: Oxford University Press, pp. 294–310.

Fozzard J, Wolf E, Bell B, McFarland R, Podolsky S (1977) Visual perception and communication. In: Birren J & Schaie K (eds). *Handbook of Psychology of Ageing*. New York: Van Nostrand Reihold.

Freedman M, Knoefel J, Naeser M (1984) Computerized axial tomography in ageing. In: Albert M (ed.) *Clinical Neurology of Ageing*. Oxford: University Press.

Gaeta H, Friedman D, Ritter W (2003) Auditory selective attention in young and elderly adults: the selection of single versus conjoint features. *Psychophysiology* 40(3), 389–406.

Gates GA, Beiser A, Rees TS, D'Agostino RB, Wolf PA (2002) Central auditory dysfunction may precede the onset of clinical dementia in people with probable Alzheimer's disease. *Journal of the American Geriatrics Society* 50(3), 482–488.

Gilhooly M, Phillips L, Gilhooly K, Hanlon P (2003) *Quality of Life and Real Life Cognitive Functioning*. Economic Social Research Council Growing Older Programme. Accessed 06.03.2004. http://www.shef.ac.uk/uni/projects/gop/MaryGilQOL_F15.pdf

Goldman J & Coté L (1991) Ageing of the brain: dementia of the Alzheimer's type. In: Kandel ER, Schwartz JH, Jessell TM (eds). *Principles of Neural Science*, 3rd edn. Connecticut, Prentice-Hall International, pp. 974–982.

Goldman-Rakic PS (1992) Working memory and the mind. *Scientific American* 9, 73–79.

Greene L & Mathieson ML (1989) *The Voice and its Disorders*, 5th edn. San Diego, CA: Singular Publishing Group.

Harkins SW (1996) Geriatric pain. Pain perceptions in the old. *Clinical Geriatric Medicine* 12(3), 435–459.

Hastings M (1998) The brain, circadian rhythms, and clock genes. *British Medical Journal* 317, 1704–1707.

Hirano M, Kurita S, Nakashima T (1983) Growth development and ageing of the human vocal folds. In: Bless DM & Abbs JH (eds). *Vocal Fold Physiology*. San Diego: College Hill Press.

Joaquin AM & Gollapudi S (2001) Functional decline in ageing and disease: a role for apoptosis. *Journal of the American Geriatrics Society* 49(9), 1234–1240.

Jones RW & Ferris SH (1999) Age-related memory and cognitive decline. In: Wilcock GK, Bucks RS, Rockwood K (eds). *Diagnosis and Management of Dementia: A Manual for Memory Disorders Teams*. Oxford: Oxford University Press, pp. 211–230.

Kahane J & Hammons J (1991) Developmental changes in the particular cartilage of the cricoarytenoid joint. In: Baer T, Sasaki C, Harris J (eds). *Laryngeal Function in Phonation and Respiration*. San Diego: Singular Publishing Group, pp. 14–24.

Katzman R & Terry R (1992) Normal ageing of the nervous system. In: Katzman R & Rowe JW (eds). *Principles of Geriatric Neurology*. Philadelphia: FA Davis, pp. 18–58.

Kelly DD (1991) Disorders of sleep and consciousness. In: Kandel ER, Schwartz JH, Jessell TM (eds). *Principles of Neural Science*, 3rd edn. Connecticut: Prentice-Hall International, pp. 808–819.

Kilpatrick CJ & Lowe AJ (2002) Management of epilepsy in older people. *Journal of Pharmacy Practice and Research* 32(2), 110–114.

Law M & Baum C (2001) Measurement in occupational therapy. In: Law M, Baum C & Dunn W (eds). *Measuring Occupational Performance: Supporting Best Practice in Occupational Therapy*. Thorofare: Slack, pp. 3–19.

Lipsitz LA & Jonsson PV (1992) *Transient Loss of Consciousness*. In: Katzman R & Rowe JW (eds). *Principles of Geriatric Neurology*. Philadelphia: FA Davis, pp. 300–313.

Maki P & Resnick S (2000) Longitudinal effects of oestrogen replacement therapy on PET cerebral blood flow and cognition. *Neurobiology and Ageing* 21(2), 373–383.

Marriot M, Banks J, Blundell R, Lessof C, Nazroo J (2002) *English Longitudinal Study of Ageing – Health, Wealth and Lifestyles of the Older Population in England*. London: Institute for Fiscal Studies.

Maxim J & Bryan K (1994) *Language in the Elderly, A Clinical Perspective*. London: Singular Publishing.

Morris RG, Worsley C, Matthews D (2000) Neuropsychological assessment in older people: old principles and new directions. *Advances of Psychiatric Treatment* 6(5), 362–372.

Murdoch E (1998) *Dysarthria: A Physiological Approach to Assessment and Treatment*. Cheltenham: Stanley Thornes.

National Institute of Ageing (2002) *Hearing Loss*. Accessed 25.05.2005. http://www.niapublications.org/engagepage p

National Mental Health Association (2003) *Well into your Future: Maintaining Mental Health*. Accessed 26.04.2004 http://www.nmha.org/infoctr/factsheets/index.cfm#elderly

Nishikawa ST & Ferrell BA (1993) Pain assessment in the elderly. *Clinical Geriatric Issues in Long Term Care* 1, 15–28.

Norman DA & Shallice T (1980) *Attention and Action: Willed and Automatic Control of Behaviour*. GHIP Report 99. San Diego: University of California.

Op den Velde W (1976) Some cerebral proteins and enzyme systems in Alzheimer's presenile and senile dementia. *Journal of the American Geriatrics Society* 24(1), 12–16.

Parhad IM, Scott JN, Cellars LA, Bains JS, Kerkoski CA, Clark AW (1995) Axonal atrophy in ageing is associated with a decline in neurofilament gene expression. *Journal of Neuroscience Research* 41(3), 355–366.

Perry I (1995) Prospective study of serum total homocysteine concentration and risk of stoke in middle-aged British men. *Lancet* 346, 1395–1398.

Perry RJ & Hodges JR (1999) Attention and executive deficits in Alzheimer's disease: a critical review. *Brain* 122(3), 383–404.

Philp I (2003) Improving the way health and social care organisations provide services for older people with sight problems. London: RNIB.

Powell-Proctor L, Miller E (1982) Reality orientation: a critical appraisal. *British Journal of Psychiatry* 140, 457–463.

Rabbitt P (1997) Ageing and human skill: a 40th anniversary. *Ergonomics* 40(10), 962–981.

Raz N (1996) *Neuroanatomy of the Ageing Brain: Evidence from Structural MRI.* In: Bigler E (ed.) *Neuroimaging II: Clinical Applications.* New York: Academic Press, pp. 153–182.

Raz N (2000) Ageing of the brain and its influence on cognitive performance: integration of structural and functional findings. In: Craik F, Salthouse T (eds). *The Handbook of Ageing and Cognition.* New Jersey: Lawrence Erlbaum, pp. 1–90.

Raz N, Gunning FM, Head D *et al.* (1997) Selective ageing of human cerebral cortex observation in vivo: differential vulnerability of the pre-frontal grey matter. *Cerebral Cortex* 7(3), 268–282.

Richards M, Kuh D, Hardy R (1999) Lifetime cognitive function and timing of the natural menopause. *Neurology* 53(2), 308–314.

Robertson J & Thompson S (1987) *Working with Dysarthric Clients: A Practical Guide to Therapy for Dysarthria.* Austin, TX: Pro Ed.

Rose SP (2002) Smart drugs: do they work? Are they ethical? Will they be legal? *Nature Reviews/Neuroscience* 3(12), 975–979.

Ryan-Ellen B, Giles H, Bartolucci G, Henwood K (1986) Psycholinguistic and social psychological components of communication by and with the elderly. *Language and Communication* 6(1–2), 1–24.

Salthouse TA, Atkinson TM, Berish DE (2003) Executive functioning as a potential mediator of age-related cognitive decline in normal adults. *Journal of Experimental Psychology* 132(4), 566–594.

Savory J, Rao JK, Huang Y, Letada PR, Herman MM (1999) Age-related hippocampal changes in Bcl-2 Bax ratio, oxidative stress, redox-active and apoptosis associated with aluminium-induced neurodegeneration: increased susceptibility with ageing. *Neurotoxicology* 20(5), 805–817.

Schuurmans MJ, Duursma SA, Shortridge-Baggett LM (2001) Early recognition of delirium: a review of the literature. *Journal of Clinical Nursing* 10(6), 721–729.

Selkoe DJ (1992) Ageing brain, ageing mind. *Scientific American* 267(3), 134–142.

Selhub J, Jacques PF, Bostom AG (1995) Association between plasma homocysteine concentrations and extra cranial carotid-artery stenosis. *New England Journal of Medicine* 332(5), 286–291.

Selwood A & Orrell M (2004) Long term cognitive dysfunction in older people after non-cardiac surgery. *British Medical Journal* 328, 120–121.

Shepard RJ (1978) *Physical Activity and Ageing.* Chicago, IL: Yearbook Medical Publishers.

Shimamura AP (1990) Ageing and memory disorders: a neuropsychological analysis. In: Howe ML, Stones MJ, Brainerd CJ (eds). *Cognitive and Behavioural Performance Factors in Atypical Ageing.* New York: Springer, pp. 37–65.

Shumway-Cook A & Woollacott MH (2001) *Motor Control: Theory and Applications,* 2nd edn. Baltimore: Lippincott, Williams & Wilkins.

Sims N, Bowen D, Smith C (1980) Glucose metabolism and acetylcholine synthesis in relation to neuronal activity in Alzheimer's disease. *Lancet* 1, 333–336.

Sofroniew MV (1997) Cellular recovery. In: Greenwood R, Barnes MP, McMillan TM, Ward CD (1997) *Neurological Rehabilitation.* Hove: Psychology Press, pp. 67–84.

Spector A, Orrell M, Davies S, Woods B (2000) *Reality Orientation for Dementia* (Cochrane Review). The Cochrane Library, Issue 2, 2004. Chichester, UK: John Wiley.

Squire A (1987) *Memory and Brain.* New York: Oxford University Press.

Stevens S & Ripich D (1999) The role of the speech and language therapist. In: Wilcock GK, Bucks RS & Rockwood K (eds). *Diagnosis and Management of Dementia: A Manual for Memory Disorders Teams*. Oxford: Oxford University Press, pp. 137–157.

Su CY, Chien TH, Cheng KF, Lin TY (1995) Performance of older adults with and without cerebrovascular accident on the test of visual perceptual skills. *American Journal of Occupational Therapy* 49(6), 491–499.

Tobis JS, Nayak L, Hoehler F (1981) Visual perception of verticality and horizontality among elderly fallers. *Archives of Physical Medicine and Rehabilitation* 62(12), 619–622.

Troller JN & Valenzuela MJ (2001) Brain Ageing on the new millennium. *Australian and New Zealand Journal of Psychiatry* 35(6), 788–805.

Valenzuela MJ, Sachdev PS, Wen W, Shnier R, Brodaty H, Gillies D (2000) Dual voxel proton magnetic resonance spectroscopy in the healthy elderly: subcortico-frontal axonal N-acetylaspartate levels are correlated with fluid cognitive abilities independent of structural brain changes. *Neuroimage* 12(6), 747–756.

Vaughan DW (1992) Effects of advancing age on peripheral nerve regeneration. *Journal of Comparative Neurology* 323(2), 219–237.

Verdu E, Buti M, Navarro X (1995) The effect of ageing on efferent nerve fibre regeneration in mice. *Brain Research* 696(1–2), 76–82.

Verdu E, Celballos D, Vilches JJ, Xavier N (2000) Influence of ageing on peripheral nerve function and regeneration. *Journal of the Peripheral Nervous System* 5(4), 191–208.

Verghese J, Lipton RB, Katz MJ *et al.* (2003) Leisure activities and the risk of dementia in the elderly. *New England Journal of Medicine* 348(25), 2508–2516.

Volkow N (1996) Measuring age-related changes in DA D2 receptors with [11C] raclopride and with [18F] N-methylspiroperidol. *Psychiatry Research* 67(1), 11–16.

Volkow N, Gur R, Wang GJ (1998) Association between decline in brain dopamine activity with age and cognitive and motor impairment in healthy individuals. *American Journal of Psychiatry* 155(3), 344–349.

Volloch V, Mosser DD, Massie B, Sherman MY (1998) Reduced thermotolerance in aged cells results from a loss of an hsp72-mediated control of JNK signalling pathway. *Cell Stress Chaperones* 3(4), 265–271.

World Health Organisation (2001) *The International Classification of Functioning Disability and Health*. Geneva: WHO.

Wolfson L & Katzman R (1992) The neurologic consultation at 80 II: some specific disorders observed in the elderly. In: Katzman R & Rowe JW (eds). *Principles of Geriatric Neurology*. Philadelphia: FA Davis, pp. 339–355.

Woodruff-Pak DS (1997) *The Neuropsychology of Ageing*. Malden, USA: Blackwell Publishing.

Ylikoski R, Ylikoski A, Erkinjuntti T, Sulkava R, Raininko R, Tilvis R (1993) White matter changes in healthy elderly persons correlate with attention and speed of mental processing. *Archives of Neurology* 50(8), 818–824.

Ylikoski A, Erkinjuntti T, Raininko R, Sarna S, Sulkava R, Tilvis R (1995) White matter hyperintensities on MRI in the neurologically non-diseased elderly: analysis of cohorts of consecutive subjects aged 55–85 years living at home. *Stroke* 26(7), 1171–1177.

Zoltan B (1996) *Vision, Perception and Cognition: A Manual for the Evaluation and Treatment of the Neurologically Impaired Adult*, 3rd edn. New Jersey: Slack.

Chapter 7

BODY STRUCTURES AND BODY FUNCTIONS: PART 2

Linda Gnanasekaran and Anne McIntyre

Introduction

Ageing is an inevitable consequence of the passage of time interacting with biology. The ageing process is characterised by change, largely decremental, in the anatomical structures and physiological functions of the body. These changes are most frequently viewed as negative, seeming to manifest as loss – of capacity or potential for extremes of human endeavour, of physical attractiveness, and of health. A young person may perceive the behaviours and lifestyle of an older person to result from impairments of function, giving rise to **activity limitations** and **participation restrictions**. For older people, however, behaviour and lifestyle differences may represent adaptive changes, forming part of a process of accommodation of habits, activities and roles to the gradually changing capacities and functions of the body. Change is not entirely decremental, and in some instances, as will be seen in this chapter, ageing within a body system sees a trade-off between component structures or functions with little net change to overall effectiveness.

For this chapter, a basic knowledge of anatomy and physiology of the body systems is assumed. The reader is therefore recommended to consult one of the many anatomy and physiology texts available for students of the health professions.

All body systems are essential for homeostasis. Those which impact primarily upon occupational performance are those systems which directly affect the interaction of the person with his/her physical and social environments, i.e. the cardiovascular, respiratory, neuromuscular and musculoskeletal. Less direct in their role and impact are those systems which support homeostasis, maintain biological integrity and mediate autonomic processes i.e. the endocrine, immune, digestive, reproductive, excretory and integumentary systems.

As in Chapter 6, the sections of this chapter follow the framework of the ICF (WHO 2001) and those considered are listed in Box 7.1.

Age-related changes in any one system have the potential to influence functioning in other systems, and alter the body's response to illness or injury. Hence trauma or an illness event happening to an older person may give rise to further impairment and deterioration in health, whereas a younger person may recover quickly and fully. This increased vulnerability to complications and reduced recovery

Box 7.1

- Structures and functions of the integumentary system.
- Structures and functions of the cardiovascular, respiratory and immune system.
- Structures and functions of the neuromusculoskeletal system.
- Structures and functions of the digestive, metabolic and endocrine system.
- Structures and functions of the genito-urinary and reproductive systems.

reinforces the need for therapists to understand the interrelatedness of systems and the influence of age-related change. Table 7.1 illustrates this, using an example of an elderly person suffering a fractured tibia and fibula with subsequent immobilisation of the limb.

Table 7.1 Example of the impact of age-related changes upon body systems following trauma.

Normal age-related changes to body structures/ functions	Traumatic event	Changes to body structures/ functions arising from traumatic event	Interaction of normal age-related changes with post-traumatic changes
1. Progressive loss of fast-twitch anaerobic muscle fibres.	A fall from a bicycle, resulting in fractured tibia and fibula. Immobilised from above knee to ankle, non-weight bearing.	1. Muscle atrophy, particularly slow-twitch aerobic fibres in affected limb.	1. More pronounced loss of muscle bulk, strength and endurance. Easily fatigued. Wastage and weakness contribute to joint instability and slower (or failure to) return to pre-fracture strength.
2. Reduced thyroid hormone production (lower metabolic rate).		2. Increased local metabolic activity needed for tissue repair.	2. Slower tissue repair.
3. Resorption of calcium from bone (reduced calcitonin, increased parathyroid production).		3. Decreased physical activity leading to reduced calcitonin and increased parathyroid production.	3. Accelerated general loss of bone mass and density, slower bone repair. Increased risk of osteoporosis.
4. Reduced absorption of calcium from gut.		4. Increased local demand for calcium for osteoblast activity.	4. Slower bone repair.
5. Thickening and stiffening of synovial joint capsules.		5. Immobility of lower limb joint leading to stiffness and capsule changes.	5. More pronounced joint stiffness, higher possibility of permanent reduction in joint range of movement.

The integumentary system

Arguably the most visible signs of ageing are manifest in changes to the skin and one of its accessory structures, hair. The skin is the largest organ of the body, its principle functions being as a physical barrier against the external environment, and an essential medium for sensory information about the effects of the external **physical environment** upon the body. It protects underlying structures, regulates temperature, provides insulation and shock absorption, water proofing, secretion of waste, synthesis of vitamin D, production of chemicals to prevent infection, and protection against harmful light waves.

Age-related changes to the skin:

- Collagen fibres in the dermis progressively stiffen and break apart. They reduce in number, becoming tangled and disorganised.
- Elastic fibres lose elasticity and clump together.
- Fewer of both types of fibre are produced, so that degeneration exceeds new production.
- Langerhans cells decrease in number and immune responsiveness decreases (see the Immune system, p. 139).
- Sebaceous and sweat glands reduce in number and productiveness. Skin therefore becomes drier, more liable to break, and less able to perform its cooling function.
- Keratinocyte production slows, skin becomes thinner.
- Melanocytes reduce; hair loses pigmentation and skin develops uneven pigmentation.
- The adipose layer becomes thinner.
- Walls of blood vessels stiffen and become less permeable.
- Growth of hair and nails slows.

The skin generally becomes thinner, drier and less elastic; therefore it is more easily damaged. Shock absorbing and cushioning properties are reduced. Temperature regulating (insulating and cooling) properties are reduced. Reduced secretions mean that the skin is less hostile to microbes, and bacteria might more easily enter the skin and hence the bloodstream. Healing is slower and there is a greater susceptibility to sun damage and to neoplasms.

The appearance and texture of integumentary tissues provides a visible signal to the self and others, not only of the health status of the tissue, but often of the physical health and psychological state of the individual as a whole. The rich supply of blood vessels to the skin means that states of emotional arousal, triggering autonomic nervous system activity, rapidly produce significant circulatory change with consequent change to skin colouration. States of ill health (e.g. hypothermia, anaemia, or hypotension), result in reduced blood flow to the skin, to preserve core body temperature or maintain adequate circulatory supply to essential organs such as the heart and brain. Hence the skin can suffer as a secondary consequence of diseases of other organs/systems, and can convey signs of health status to the careful observer. Indeed the skin may betray the presence of health problems that would otherwise be asymptomatic, or easily hidden from view, such as hypertension or anorexia nervosa (by the presence of lanugo, a soft downy hair growing on the body).

Primary disorders and diseases of the skin include infections (e.g. impetigo), allergies (e.g. hives), neoplasms (e.g. warts, cancers), and traumatic damage such as cuts and burns. The older adult is as much at risk of these disorders as at any other age, but susceptibility to some may increase as a direct result of longevity (cumulative total exposure to sunlight increases the risk of malignant melanoma), and of the declining strength and resilience of the skin (increasing age is again positively correlated with risk of developing decubitus ulcers if subjected to prolonged pressure). Skin breakdown may also occur as a result of diseases of other systems (infectious organisms may take hold and result in serious damage or even death if the circulatory or immune systems are compromised, and cannot effectively combat the invasion, as in **diabetes** or AIDS, and the infection becomes systemic). Finally, side effects of medication may have long-term and permanent effects upon the skin, such as corticosteroids (collagen breakdown and thinning of the skin), or photosensitivity reactions.

Therefore the skin can be a useful indicator of health status, a primary target of disease or damage, or may suffer significant secondary effects of disease elsewhere in the body. Age-related changes have the overall effect of reducing the effectiveness of the skin across all of its functions, and therefore throughout the occupational therapy process the structural and functional integrity of this organ/system may be both a target of intervention and an important secondary consideration.

Examination of the skin should form a routine part of any physical assessment – its colour, texture, moistness, temperature and blood supply, any signs of damage or infection, known sensitivities (e.g. to plasters) or allergens. Attention to medication is also important to be aware of signs of possible adverse reactions, or to know to take precautions against interactions of drugs with for example, exposure to sunlight.

Pressure risk assessment, together with a visual assessment of known pressure risk areas of the body, may do much to prevent unnecessary and avoidable decubitus ulcer formation. Once such an ulcer develops, it renders an individual vulnerable to infection, as well as being a source of pain and taking weeks or months to heal.

In some cases the skin is a primary focus of intervention such as in the treatment of burns. In others, knowledge of its structure, functions, and the changes that occur with advancing age, will lead to modifications of planned treatment, or adjustment of certain parameters of intervention. The poorer thermal regulating properties of older skin could mean increasing the room temperature during treatment sessions to minimise heat loss, or taking care to reduce sun exposure during outdoor activities.

Trauma to the skin is more likely to lead to bruising, and will be more painful if the adipose layer is minimal. Reduced or delayed sensory processing from cutaneous receptors, and/or slowed motor response times further add to the risks of sustaining damage to the skin from activities such as cooking, gardening or sewing.

Similarly, the wearing of a prosthesis or orthosis might result in skin breakdown more easily in an older person whose skin is less elastic, less resilient and less padded.

Pre-existing conditions such as **heart failure** or **respiratory disease** will seriously compromise the blood supply to, and healing capabilities of skin, over and above age-related changes. The lower limbs will be particularly prone to skin breakdown in the presence of oedema or impaired arterial supply, and so the affected individual must learn and incorporate skin care into daily life and routines. Visual checking, good skin hygiene, avoidance of extremes of temperature, protecting the limbs from knocks and cuts, and aiding fluid circulation through exercise and limb elevation, will all aid good integumentary health in such cases.

Finally it is important to bear in mind that skin also has a communication function. Most obviously it can indicate emotional state (blushing, or pallor) but the appearance of unexplained tissue trauma or bruising might indicate that an older person is, for example, experiencing falls but not wanting to admit to it, may be subject to physical abuse, or may be self-harming. Any skin damage for which a cause has not been identified must be investigated carefully and sensitively.

The cardiovascular system

The cardiovascular system – heart, blood vessels and blood – is the transport system through which all cells, tissues and organs and systems of the body receive the substances essential to their survival, growth and function, and which ensures the maintenance of an optimal fluid environment within the body for all metabolic processes. It is also a communication system by which chemical messengers travel from their point of production to their target tissues, to alter activity within those tissues. The behaviour of the cardiovascular system therefore impacts upon and can modify the activity of every other tissue/organ/system within the body, and any change within it will have consequences for the health and functioning of the organism as a whole.

Ageing affects all components of the system, but as with many body structures and functions, the cardiovascular system has considerable reserve capacity, which in normal health will mean that ageing per se has negligible impact upon its efficiency and effectiveness. Of more significance, is the incidence and prevalence of pathological change, which is highly correlated with increasing age and certain lifestyle factors. It is the interrelationship of age-related change and pathology which raises significant concerns for functioning and cardiovascular health. Principle (normal) age-related changes within the system are identified in Box 7.2.

Changes in other systems can also have a compounding or cumulative effect. As discussed below, chronic respiratory disease with extensive damage to lung tissue will impair pulmonary blood flow, and could cause a backlog of blood in the right heart, leading to right heart failure.

Reduction in cardiovascular efficiency may have consequences for all body systems, in that there will be a reduction in oxygen and nutrient supply, in waste clearance, and lessened ability to respond to sudden changes in demand from

Box 7.2 Age-related changes in the cardiovascular system.

Heart
Conduction system: Fibrotic change in the fibres slows the rate of cardiac impulses and can give rise to irregularities.
The myocardium: Becomes less elastic and more fibrous. Contraction is less efficient with less response variability. The mass and volume of fibres decreases.
Valves: Become stiffer and less pliable.

Blood vessels
Decrease in elasticity, increased stiffness and rigidity, loss of distensibility.
The reservoir capacity of the venous system decreases.
Arterial BP increases.
Lowered responsiveness of smooth muscle to neural and hormonal influences.

Blood
Decreased production of erythrocytes; reduced oxygen carrying capacity.
Lowered white cell count; reduced production of T and B-lymphocytes – poorer immune response.
Increased systemic BP impacts upon diffusion and bulk flow into and out of tissues.

tissues. Thermostatic regulation may be less effective. Wound healing and tissue repair may be slowed, with poorer immune responses to infections. Fluid volume adjustments in response to position change relative to gravity (orthostatic adjustment) may be slower.

Cardiovascular pathologies are amongst the most prevalent disorders affecting the older age group in western societies. Table 7.2 illustrates the rise across a range of such conditions with age.

The risk of much cardiovascular disease can be reduced with attention to known modifiable factors, and those with diagnosed and established pathology are invariably advised to make important lifestyle adjustments, which will help to slow or halt progression of a disease (e.g. lose weight, stop smoking, increase exercise, make dietary changes). This is not always easily done, if one considers that older

Table 7.2 Prevalence rates per 10 000 population for diseases of the circulatory system by age 1991–92. England and Wales (male and female figures combined).

Age	15–24	25–44	45–64	65–74	75+
Uncomplicated hypertension	10	98	812	1637	981
Acute myocardial infarction	0	4	47	115	152
Angina pectoris	0	11	195	472	507
Stroke	2	4	59	225	537

(British Heart Foundation Statistics 2004).

people frequently have other conditions (e.g. **osteoarthritis**) or limitations (e.g. financial) which prevent them from taking action, or are being asked to change habits that have been with them throughout adult life, or are a source of pleasure, and are very difficult to forgo or change.

The interrelationship of different body systems, and of pathology with ageing, is particularly pertinent when considering the cardiovascular system and the effect of immobility. Absence of, or greatly reduced, physical activity leads to atrophy of muscle fibres, reduced muscle metabolism, reduced joint movements, stability and strength. Cardiac output decreases in the absence of demand from the muscles. Venous return is less efficient as the skeletal muscle pump is not active, with the risk of venous thrombosis. Peripheral tissues may become oedematous. As muscles atrophy, so their capillary beds shrink, reducing their blood supply. Even a short period of immobility (a week in bed due to illness, a period of hospitalisation) will quickly lead to changes occurring, which combine with age-related changes, and any will present pathology, to compromise the circulatory system and its ability to respond to increased activity demands. Cardiac deconditioning may occur, and with the identified musculoskeletal changes, the person's ability to resume normal levels of activity may be seriously impaired.

Immobility therefore represents a challenge to the cardiovascular system. Pathology within the system compounds any stresses and makes further deterioration more likely. A failing heart may not be able to respond adequately to increased activity demands following a period of immobilisation. Atherosclerotic vessels tend to be stiff and unable to alter diameter and so blood pressure homeostasis will be more difficult to achieve, carrying increased risks of stroke, organ failure, or postural hypotension. Increased blood viscosity makes it more likely to clot in conditions of sluggish circulation or in diseased vessels.

The prevalence of cardiovascular disorders in the older population means that all therapists will work with older people with some cardiovascular pathology, whether or not that is the reason for their presenting difficulties. Even if working with individuals who have no apparent or clinically diagnosed pathology, initial assessment should include measures of levels of physical activity, diet, and lifestyle factors that may have a bearing on cardiovascular health. Tolerance for exercise and exertion, and the person's capacity to meet and recover from physically demanding tasks, should be ascertained. Many people will be functioning within narrowed margins of cardiovascular responsiveness and capacity. Periods of ill health, or hospitalisation for surgery or treatment of other conditions will impact upon a system that may not have been challenged for some time. It is therefore important for that degree of impact to be identified and taken into account when planning rehabilitation or other interventions. A combination of interview, screening for symptoms and signs of cardiovascular limitation or distress, and observation of ADLs, will provide early indications if function is compromised. Activity–rest balance, diet, sleep quality and quantity, and habits such as smoking or drinking should be explored. Episodes of breathlessness, excessive fatigue, dizziness or fainting, complaints of feeling unwell or weak, of chest or arm pain, skin colour changes, or any other indications of cardiovascular dysfunction should be investigated.

In addition to assessment, the therapist must incorporate risk management and precautionary measures into therapeutic interventions. Some activities and tasks may be contraindicated. The reader is referred to Chapter 5 and other therapy texts, for information about cardiac rehabilitation (Trombly & Radomski 2002; Crepeau *et al.* 2003) but the following are some considerations in relation to age-related aspects of cardiovascular function, and occupational interventions:

- **Awareness of delayed or impaired orthostatic adjustment:** careful preparation for transfers or other major positional changes need to be made, with education of client and carer of prevention and management of postural hypotension.
- **Knowledge of psychological and physical stress responses including:**
  - Knowledge of the impact of sympathetic arousal on the cardiovascular system (increased cardiac output, vasoconstriction, increased BP and increased venous return).
  - Avoidance of anxiety and distress.
  - Provision of timely and appropriate information, and reassurance.
  - Techniques to aid relaxation and restful sleep may be beneficial.
- **Attention to environmental stressors** – extremes of temperature, or sudden changes, triggering peripheral circulatory adjustments (vasoconstriction or dilation) impacting upon blood pressure and blood supply to peripheral tissues. The heart will be less efficient in its response to altered demand.
- **Compounding factors:**
  - Pathology and/or impairment of other body systems.
  - Emotional distress can trigger cardiac arrhythmias.
  - Lung diseases.
  - Musculoskeletal problems adversely affect the circulation.
  - Medications carry the risk of cardiovascular side effects, including iatrogenic cardiovascular problems.
- **Occupational deprivation and inactivity:** inability, unwillingness, or lack of opportunity to engage in activities, roles, and community life will impact upon cardiovascular functioning.
  - Reduced mobility and physical inactivity.
  - Affective states also impact, mediated by hypothalamic function and the balance between sympathetic and parasympathetic activity.
- **The development or continuation of habits** (e.g. tobacco smoking, excessive drinking, poor diet).

The respiratory system

The respiratory system provides the structures and mechanisms by which gaseous exchange occurs between the atmosphere and the blood: oxygen is obtained, carbon dioxide is removed, and an appropriate balance is maintained between the two. Blood gas homeostasis is essential to the functioning of all body structures and systems, and so the functioning of the respiratory system is closely bound up with that of the cardiovascular system, which must deliver blood to the lungs, and then transport it around the body.

The respiratory system is conventionally described as having two components – the upper respiratory tract (URT), consisting of nose, pharynx, and associated structures (as discussed in Chapter 6) and the lower respiratory tract (LRT), comprising the larynx, trachea, bronchi and lungs (Tortora & Grabowski 2003). This description however, belies the reliance of these structures upon other body systems for their functioning. The ICF (WHO 2001) more accurately includes the thoracic cage, intercostal muscles, diaphragm, and accessory muscles, which cause lung expansion (inspiration) and assist their deflation (expiration).

Ageing affects the respiratory system through changes in the tissues of the airways, lung parenchyma, musculoskeletal components (rib cage, thoracic muscles, abdominal muscles) and nervous system components. Cardiovascular decline or pathology also impacts upon efficiency of gaseous exchange, and may accelerate lung deterioration, as discussed below (pathology and ageing).

The trachea and bronchii undergo little change, but the smaller airways become less elastic. The alveoli become more fibrous and less elastic, so degree of recoil on expiration reduces, and residual air volume (the air left in the lungs at the end of expiration) increases. Both the alveolar surface areas, and the pulmonary capillary bed, are thought to decline (Bonder & Wagner 2001). Changes to the musculoskeletal system (joint stiffness, muscle fibre atrophy, calcification of costal cartilages) reduce the amount of movement of the chest wall during breathing. Loss of abdominal muscle strength makes coughing less effective. Reduction of sensorineural effectiveness may reduce strength of protective reflex responses, and lead to less efficient adjustment of breathing patterns in response to blood–gas changes. Cardiovascular disease – atherosclerosis of the aorta and carotid vessels, or impaired brainstem blood supply may contribute to this.

The net consequence of ageing is a decline in efficiency. The lungs deflate less well and the chest wall and diaphragm move less and so overall airflow decreases. With a greater residual volume of air in the lungs, coupled with decreased alveolar surface and capillary density, gaseous exchange is less efficient.

For a person in good health, the impact of these changes may be minimal. Respiration can vary by rate as well as volume, and so slightly increased breathing rate may compensate for reduced volume. Inactivity or restricted mobility will compound ageing, and so maintenance of **activity** and exercise becomes important for maintaining muscle strength and joint range of movement, hence countering the decreased elasticity of the lungs. Physical activity is also important for cardiovascular fitness, which in turn will help maintain pulmonary efficiency.

There will be an increased vulnerability to pathogens; the ciliary action of the epithelium decreases with age, and the alveolar macrophages become less active, therefore non-specific resistance to disease decreases. Ageing of the immune system means less effective specific immune responses, and so infections are more likely to occur, and with greater severity. Again lack of physical activity may compound this situation. Stagnant air and moisture remain in the alveoli, because of greater residual volume, creating ideal conditions for bacterial growth. Heart failure, causing pulmonary congestion, has a similar effect. Hence, an important precaution for older people and those with respiratory or cardiac disease is to receive influenza vaccinations each winter to protect against possible complications.

The greatest threat to respiratory health continues to be **environmental**; from the contents of the air we inhale. Active (i.e. deliberate) and passive inhalation of tobacco smoke, exposure to irritant particles and substances in the work place (e.g. cotton mills, sawmills, bakeries, coalmines), exposure to noxious gases (e.g. from mistakes made in chlorine treatment of swimming pools) and general atmospheric pollutants have a cumulatively damaging effect upon the protective mechanisms of the airways, and the delicate lung parenchyma (see Chapter 10).

The healthy and active older adult should demonstrate little observable difference in pulmonary function from a younger adult. Persistent cough, excessive production of mucus or bloodstained sputum, wheezing, breathlessness at rest or with mild exertion, or pain, will be as abnormal in healthy old age as at younger ages, and should be investigated. Where pulmonary or cardiovascular disease is present, respiratory function will be impaired, and this must be taken into account.

The symptoms (e.g. coughing, dyspnoea) of respiratory disease are distressing and physically exhausting in themselves. The extra mechanical work to effectively inflate and deflate diseased lungs demanded of musculoskeletal structures that are stiffer and less effective themselves, increases the energy demand of breathing. Expiration tends to be prolonged with rapid shallow breaths to minimise the metabolic costs to the muscles. Hypoxia and hypercarbia alter the chemical balance of the blood, affecting metabolism in all cells. Individuals will have limited capacity and tolerance for activity, experience fatigue, and possibly mild cognitive deficits. Depression will be common. Excess load on the heart, coupled with myocardial hypoxia may precipitate heart failure. Even eating a meal may be difficult, as it will interfere with breathing rhythm, and the metabolic requirements of digestion will increase oxygen demand.

The immune system

The immune system is concerned with protecting the body against foreign substances (pathogens), through the action of non-specific and specific immune mechanisms. This involves cell and antibody-mediated responses, the functions of lymph, lymphatic vessels and lymph nodes.

Other, innate and non-specific defenses operate to protect the body and/or remove pathogens as a first line of defence, for example the nasal mucosa and cilia, and the skin. These are not components of the immune system and are identified in this chapter as parts of the systems to which they belong (e.g. respiratory system, integumentary system).

Non-specific immune mechanisms include anti-microbial proteins, natural killer cells and phagocytes. These are carried in the blood, and are capable of diffusing into tissues.

Inflammation is a general response to tissue damage, and fever (pyrexia) is a response to the presence of certain toxins in the body, which can have the effect of inhibiting viral or bacterial activity. Specific resistance involves the production of cells and antibodies able to recognise and destroy specific antigens, and so requires mechanisms to monitor and detect their presence and respond rapidly to them.

Age-related changes to the immune system (immunosenescence) structure and function can be considered as primary, affecting the immune tissues and organs directly, or secondary, occurring in other systems but impacting upon immune functioning.

Secondary changes affect systems involved in first-line defence, and systems which support immune function. Ageing of the skin (thinner, drier, fewer secretions) and other barriers allows pathogens to breach these defences more easily, so increasing the number of challenges to both the non-specific and specific immune mechanisms, at a time when these mechanisms are themselves becoming less efficient. Changes to haemodynamics (blood pressure, flow, resistance etc) because of ageing of the cardiovascular system will affect the circulation of lymphocytes and platelets, and the movement of fluid, cells and particles between capillaries, interstitial spaces, and lymphatic vessels.

Primary changes within the immune system include:

- Atrophy of the thymus gland (commences at puberty and continues into old age).
- Falling concentrations of T-cells and reduced responsiveness to antigens.
- Reduced responsiveness of B-cells and impaired antibody production.
- Increased risk of autoimmune responses (B-cell response to self-antigen not so effectively eliminated).
- Altered inflammatory response, and longer wound healing time.

                    (Kirkwood & Ritter 1997, Horan & Ashcroft 1997).

As with other body systems, there are wide individual variations in immune system effectiveness and rate of decline. Nutrition, cardiovascular and musculoskeletal health, heredity and environment will impact upon immune function. In general, ageing will not necessarily compromise the homeostatic function and general competence of the immune system, but older individuals may be less able to withstand pathogenic stresses imposed upon it.

As a consequence of age-related changes, immunisation becomes less effective. However, vaccination against influenza for example, is advised for older people in order to boost their protection against such viruses which carry a much higher risk of complications such as chest infections and increased cardiac workload.

With age there is undoubtedly an increase in the incidence of infections, autoimmune disorders and neoplasms. Adaptive responses to physical stressors such as temperature extremes, exercise and fluid balance disturbance take longer, and recovery to a homeostatic baseline also takes longer to achieve (Herbert 1991).

Crucially, stressful events are commonplace in old age, whether it be illness events and hospitalisation, bereavement or isolation, financial or housing worries, or caring for a disabled relative. Suppressed immune function is associated with sustained stress levels of cortisol circulating in the bloodstream, and also with exposure to negative emotional experiences (distress) and chronic or recurrent stressful events. It also results in lowered resistance to new infections and likely reactivation of latent viruses such as varicella zoster, causing shingles (Lovallo 1997).

A study of older people caring for spouses with **Alzheimer's disease** found a correlation between degree of distress, low social support, and levels of cellular immunity. The same group experienced more respiratory tract infections and slower wound healing, than older non-carers (Kiecolt-Glaser *et al.* 1995). *(For a fuller discussion of the relationship between immune function and stress, see Lovallo 1997.)*

There are three basic types of pathological dysfunction which affect the immune system: allergic reactions, autoimmune responses (loss of self-tolerance) and failure or reduced ability to mount effective responses to pathogens and antigens.

However, the immune system presents one example where ageing can confer benefit to the individual. Reduced levels of T and B-lymphocytes can weaken allergic responses (to harmless substances) and also reduces the likelihood of organ or tissue rejection following transplantation. Nevertheless, with a reduced ability to fight off infections, and decreased immune surveillance, the older person is more vulnerable to development and growth of tumourous tissue, and is more severely affected by viruses and bacteria, with longer recovery periods and increased susceptibility to secondary complications.

With age, the efficiency with which self-reactive T and B-cells are inactivated becomes less, with a greater risk of autoimmune responses developing. However, T and B-cells become less responsive with ageing and so there is some mutual cancelling out. Autoimmune diseases most commonly arise in earlier life, and in some autoimmune diseases there is a reduction in disease activity in later life (**rheumatoid arthritis** for example) and inflammatory activity may subside.

Immune suppression may be a deliberate aim of drug treatment (for organ/tissue grafting for example) or the result of disease, most typically the human immunodeficiency virus (HIV). With the basic mechanisms of immune surveillance and responsiveness suppressed, the organism becomes vulnerable to a wide range of opportunistic infections and neoplastic growth (for example, as in AIDS). The improvement in medical treatments, particularly for HIV and AIDS, means that more people will survive into older age and experience then, the problems of opportunistic infections and their secondary complications.

Pathology in other systems can impact upon immune function, perhaps most significantly the cardiovascular system. Right heart failure, for example, will cause congestion of the venous system, forcing excess fluid to leak from capillaries into tissues (most notably in the legs and feet due to gravity), causing oedema. This impairment of circulation and excess interstitial fluid makes normal diffusion of substances in and out of cells difficult, and slows immune reactions in areas of damage or infection. Pathogens that may enter through damaged skin cannot be contained or destroyed effectively, and ulcers may develop on the legs. Lymphatic vessels cannot drain fluid away efficiently because they too ultimately drain back in to the great veins, which are congested.

Immune status and immune function are not primary targets of occupational assessment or interventions, but are factors that require consideration with any older person, and particularly where immunity is known to be compromised, or abnormal in some way. Therefore the occupational therapy process should be dictated by good professional standards of care and practice, and knowledge of and adherence to health and safety guidelines and requirements.

Where a person has an identified pathology such as HIV/AIDS, is a known carrier of a virus harmful to others (e.g. hepatitis) or is on immuno-suppressing medication, the risks to the individual, the therapist, or others, must be assessed and appropriate protocols and precautions followed. All hospitals and services dealing with such people should have appropriate procedures in place, and therapists must be cognisant with them (see Chapter 4).

Screening and assessment procedures should incorporate information gathering that will identify particular immune considerations, including allergies, cardiac disease and predispositions to particular conditions such as bronchitis.

As identified and discussed above, there are many factors which have a bearing upon immune functioning. So whilst it can be argued that immune function is not a prime consideration for occupational therapy, it must equally be recognised that occupational therapists can do much to help to support or strengthen immune functioning because of the general health effects of occupational therapy interventions. Table 7.3 below identifies some common occupational interventions and identifies their benefits to immune system functioning.

Table 7.3 Benefits to immune system functioning of occupational interventions.

Occupational intervention	Immune system benefit
Relaxation training/stress management	Reduction in blood cortisol levels; immune responsiveness improved.
Self-care: washing/bathing	Improved hygiene, skin defences supported, reduced pathogenic threat.
Self-care: feeding	Improved nutrition and hydration, improved immune function.
Domestic ADL: cooking skills	Improved nutritional intake, improved immune function.
Environmental adaptation for access	Easier mobility, increased physical activity: improved blood circulation and muscle action (lymphatic drainage and wound healing).
Wheelchair provision, seating and support systems	Prevention of pressure sores, maintaining circulation. Reduces risk of infection and oedema.

The neuromusculoskeletal system

The production of purposeful movement requires neural processing and motor output, a responsive muscle system, and an articulated bony framework for muscle forces to act upon. Hence the central and peripheral nervous systems (CNS and

PNS), skeletal muscles, and the skeletal system form the essential component structures for this function.

Movement is immensely variable, from the delicate and subtle movements of facial expressions, to the massive force generated by a weight lifter. Muscle action is the medium through which we express ourselves and communicate (speech, expression, gesture), interact with the **environment** and meet our needs. All individuals have characteristic movement patterns and habits, and movement and postures also alter with age.

Bone and muscle tissue have important metabolic and homeostatic functions as well as their roles in movement and stability of the body. For example, bone is an important mineral store and acts as a buffer against fluctuating blood levels of calcium. Muscle is an important generator of heat, assists blood circulation and lymph drainage, and in circumstances of nutritional deficit provides a protein source to the body. The forces generated by muscles acting on bone stimulate bone growth and so movement is important for bone density and strength.

In Chapter 6 many aspects of nervous system functioning were discussed, and the reader should bear in mind the content of that chapter while considering ageing and the motor system. Large areas of the brain are involved directly or indirectly in movement production. Therefore general changes in brain structure or function will impact upon motor processes and movement. Deterioration of sensory, integrative, cognitive and perceptual functions will affect reflex responses and quality and effectiveness of voluntary movements. Deterioration of subcortical and brainstem structures will affect reflexes, tone and postural mechanisms.

It can be very difficult to separate out the neural contribution to decline in movement functions from the muscular contribution. Movement results from CNS output to lower motor neurones (LMNs), their communication with muscle fibres at the neuromuscular junction, and the consequent contractile behaviour of the muscle fibres. Movement quality and quantity derives from the integrity and health of all these structures and processes.

There is evidence that the number of LMNs declines with age. As a result there are fewer functional motor units, and these tend to increase in size, i.e. collateral branches of surviving axons innervate nearby muscle fibres that have lost their original innervation and so individual LMNs control more muscle fibres each (Harridge & Young 1998).

At the same time, the overall number of skeletal muscle fibres reduces, (known as sarcopaenia) and it is suggested that older muscle fibres exhibit poorer quality; e.g. may be weaker for their given size. The relative proportions of muscle fibre types within any given muscle may also alter with advancing years, with a decline in the proportion of Type II fibres (slow twitch, aerobic, fatigue resistant). This changes the contraction characteristics and lowers the fatigue resistance of the muscle (Harridge & Young 1998).

It is important to remember that cardiovascular and respiratory function will affect muscle performance through the efficiency and quality of blood supply and waste removal. In turn, decline in skeletal muscle function will impact upon respiratory efficiency through reduction in inhalatory and exhalatory movements of the thorax.

Bone tissue is affected both in the mineral component (hardness), and the collagen matrix (tensile strength). Through childhood and youth, mineral deposition exceeds resorption (though influenced by diet and exercise), and so bone increases in density and strength. With advancing years, resorption exceeds deposition, and so bone density decreases by approximately 1% each year. Protein synthesis also decreases, hence the collagen matrix deteriorates and bones become more brittle. In women, the menopause, with its associated decrease in oestrogen levels, accelerates the process with increased risk of **osteoporosis** (see Chapter 5). Bone mineral density (BMD) is increased by regular progressive exercise and the skeleton can respond and increase BMD up until the eighth decade, therefore exercise to counteract the 1% loss is worthwhile (Bassey 2001).

Joint structures and tissues include the articulating surfaces of the bones, cartilages, synovial membranes and synovial fluid, joint capsules, ligaments and other connective tissues. Age-related changes arise from connective tissue changes whereby the joint capsule and ligaments stiffen and lose elasticity and some shortening of fibres occurs. Synovial fluid production decreases and cartilage thins. **Osteoarthritis**, although a recognised joint pathology, may be at least partially attributable to the ageing process. The combination of wear and tear with age-related tissue changes means that virtually all people over the age of 70 have some degree of **osteoarthritic** change (Tortora & Grabowski 2003).

The organisation, flexibility and capacity of the neuromusculoskeletal system means that throughout life and into old age, new motor skills and movement abilities can be developed and learned. However, the general impact of ageing on all the component structures tends towards decline in function, but once again this is immensely variable between individuals and highly dependent upon past and present health status, and (as will be seen later) activity levels. As with our earlier consideration of the immune system, it is perhaps more salient to consider normal age-related changes in relation to risk, vulnerability, and the capacity to withstand stresses – physiological and mechanical in this case.

Functionally, the ageing adult will experience:

- A decline in muscle strength and mass (sarcopaenia).
- A decline in endurance (reduced fatigue resistance).
- Reduced joint flexibility.
- Changes in postural alignment (increased spinal flexion).
- Concomitant changes to gait, posture and equilibrium demands.
- Slowed reaction times to sensory stimuli including balance disturbance.
- Reduced bone density and tensile strength (prone to fracture).
- Slower tissue healing.
- Impaired heat generation and retention due to decreased muscle mass and metabolic activity.
- Poorer venous return due to decreased muscle tissue.

The loss of soft tissues (muscle and fat) reduces cushioning, and this coupled with bone changes increases the risk of more severe damage from falls and other impact events. The reduced flexibility of joints renders the soft tissues more prone to strains and sprains, and the avascular nature of ligaments and tendons make them more prone to rupture under sudden or excessive force, and very slow to heal.

There are numerous pathological changes that can affect one or all of the component subsystems (neural, muscular and skeletal) and impact upon movement related and homeostatic functions. Many, if not all, such pathologies, though frequently associated or more common with ageing, are not unique to later life, such as **stroke, osteoarthritis,** or **Parkinson's disease.** Our consideration here then, must be about the interrelationship of these pathologies with ageing and the consequent impact upon the person affected.

A further, and very important consideration in all situations where mobility is compromised, is the interplay between the consequences of reduced mobility, the ageing process, and functional ability in general (see Chapter 8). Such interplay often leads to the establishment of a cycle of decreased activity and increasing impairment, arising from some original pathology, but not dependent upon it. This has the effect of intensifying or accelerating deterioration of structure and function. To illustrate this process, the case of Mrs Robinson in Box 7.3 (p. 146) identifies how ageing, pathology and functional limitation create a cycle of deterioration.

By considering Mrs Robinson's story it becomes apparent that occupational assessment must be comprehensive whenever mobility and movement functions are compromised. It could be argued that every body structure and body function affects, and is affected by, movement. It is even known and accepted that physical exercise beneficially affects mood due to the stimulatory effect upon endorphin release in the brain. Hence assessment of functions at impairment level, such as mood, cognition, sensory function, motor function, joint range of movement, muscle function, is relevant. **Activity** and occupational assessment are also vital to determine habits, patterns, routines, task demands and the individual's capacity and performance abilities.

In terms of interventions, while one could argue that any movement is beneficial to the individual, movement that occurs within occupational contexts is particularly so because it has value, meaning and is goal related. Therefore occupations and activities provide both motivations and rewards for movement, while serving as means to movement itself.

One occupational goal should always be automatically included in any intervention with any person who has restricted mobility and movement difficulties, that is, to seek ways to maintain, if not improve upon, levels of physical activity within daily routines. This should incorporate attention to joint range of movement, quality and quantity of muscle work, application of forces through the skeleton, and variations in posture and positioning throughout the day. Not to do so, as has been illustrated in Box 7.3, leaves the way open to further, possibly avoidable, deterioration.

The digestive system

The ICF considers the structure and functions of the digestive system to involve ingestion and digestion of food and elimination of waste (WHO 2001). Ageing itself

Box 7.3 Mrs Robinson with osteoarthritis of the knees.

Mrs Robinson, aged 77 has **osteoarthritis** of both knees. She has the following impairments:

Reduced movement of knee joints, especially into flexion, due to joint surface damage, osteophyte formation, thickening and stiffening of joint capsule, and pain on movement.

Acitivity limitations:

Limited amount of walking, and frequency of standing up and sitting down, during a day because of pain.

Sits in an armchair with legs raised on a stool to limit flexion.

When climbing steps and stairs she leads with the less affected leg to avoid flexing the other knee.

She experiences difficulty with getting in and out of the bath, car, and with sitting and standing when using the toilet.

When walking Mrs Robinson does not adequately flex her knees and so brushes the floor with her feet and is at risk of catching her toe and stumbling.

Functional and systemic consequences:

Habitual avoidance of fullest possible range of movement at the knees encourages joint capsule stiffening and shortening of the fibres on the extensor aspect of the knee.

Limited joint movement reduces the circulation of synovial fluid which reduces nourishment of the cartilages.

Both flexor and extensor muscles of the knee are used less, leading to muscle atrophy and loss of sarcomeres (fibre shortening).

Blood supply to the muscles is reduced due to the reduced contraction activity. General reduction in activity (mobility) and exercise contributes to reduced respiratory capacity, and cardiac deconditioning.

Venous return will be less efficient.

Lack of mechanical stress upon bones will increase calcium resorbtion and the risk of osteoporotic change.

Reduced muscle activity will impair heat production.

A decline in cardiorespiratory fitness makes her more vulnerable to chest infections.

is said not to cause problems of the digestive system as it has a large functional reserve capacity. Nutrition and diet are important throughout the lifespan to maintain health and this is especially true in older age (see Chapter 8). However many older people are often at nutritional risk because of impaired ingestion, digestion, absorption and utilisation of nutrients because of chronic disease and drug–nutrient interactions.

As discussed in Chapter 6, sensation of smell and taste are reduced not only as part of the normal ageing process (Woodruff-Pak 1997) but also by medication and some diseases. The importance of tasting food to avoid food poisoning is of great importance for health but also to control sugar and salt intake (Ministry of Health 1996). The ability to chew food is important as many older people with poor dentition avoid eating fresh fruit and vegetables to maintain a balanced and varied diet. For many older people with few of their own teeth well-fitting dentures are crucial to chew and masticate food sufficiently and to maintain an appropriate calorie intake. Those older people with stroke or bulbar palsy may find it difficult to have well-fitting dentures. For many older people loss of teeth is caused by periodontal disease because of poor oral hygiene and therefore regular, efficient cleaning and brushing of teeth and gums is important to optimise nutritional intake. A reduced production of saliva and a dry mouth is often associated with ageing which also affects chewing and consequent swallowing of food; however these symptoms are often induced by medication or as a result of interventions such as radiotherapy (Phillips 2003).

There is conflicting evidence for swallowing difficulties in normal ageing (known as presbyphagia) (Leslie *et al.* 2003; Beers & Berkow [no date]); however this is often compromised by central nervous system disturbances following a stroke, **Parkinson's disease**, or bulbar palsy (known as dysphagia), because of impairment to the swallowing reflex. Such swallowing difficulties are identified in 60% of clients with **stroke** and are consequently linked to the incidence of chest infection in this client group. Swallowing is a complex action involving the appropriate cessation of respiration and closure of the airways. Any problems therefore need thorough and rapid investigation to ensure appropriate nutritional intake, homeostasis and prevention of aspiration of food into the lungs.

Atrophy of the stomach mucosa occurs in a third of older people over 60 (Horwarth 2002) causing a reduction in the secretion of gastric acid, pepsin and intrinsic factor. These cause a reduction in the absorption of vitamin B_{12}, folate, calcium and iron – with deficiencies in vitamin B_{12} and folate being associated with reduced cognitive function and immunity, calcium with bone density and iron with iron deficiency anaemia (Phillips 2003). Malabsorption of calcium is also associated with a deficiency of vitamin D. Ageing is also associated with a slowing of gastric emptying which prolongs the sensation of meal-induced fullness, and may lead to anorexia and weight loss. Alterations to levels of leptin and cholecystokinin which are gastrointestinal hormones also cause the sensation of satiety in response to fat in older people, causing the 'anorexia of ageing' (Morley 2003).

The pancreas is affected by ageing with a reduction in the pancreatic enzyme impairing the digestion of fats. However more common changes in the pancreas are noted such as a reduction in overall weight, and fibrosis of the pancreatic lobes. Ageing is commonly associated with reduced insulin efficiency and therefore with glucose intolerance and non-insulin dependant **diabetes** mellitus (NIDDM).

The liver is said to have a progressive decline of volume and blood flow with increasing age. Whereas these may not have much impact on normal liver function it may cause slower elimination of some medications from the body. However more age-related changes occur in the gall bladder, which concentrates and secretes bile acids; these make fats present in the intestine soluble and more easily digested. A reduction in the secretion of these acids probably leads to the higher incidence of gall stones in older people which may lead to the need for surgical removal in cases of severe upper abdominal pain, pancreatitis and jaundice (Bateson 1999).

Changes in the small and large intestine do not seem to occur with ageing, so that the motility of food and waste through these organs is not affected. However many older people do complain of changes to bowel habits with increasing age, such as constipation or more distressingly faecal incontinence. Constipation can be difficult to determine as this has different connotations for different people. Whereas current older people were given laxatives as children to 'keep them regular' the emphasis of daily defaecation is no longer in vogue. Faecal incontinence is more distressing and occurs in 7% of over 65-year-olds. It is the second most common reason for admission to residential care, with a third of older residents in care homes faecally incontinent (Kamm 1998).

Faecal incontinence can either be seen as 'an inevitable consequence of old age or as a failure of medical and nursing management' (Allen 1998:62). It causes embarrassment, humiliation and fear in an older person – proof of regression into a second childhood and many who suffer from it curtail both physical and social activity. For many carers it is the 'last straw' in their ability to cope with an older relative. Causes of faecal incontinence are:

- Constipation with overflow.
- Faecal impaction.
- Colo-rectal disease (irritable bowel syndrome).
- Diarrhoea.
- Drug-induced.
- Impaired absorption of food and constituents by stomach, small or large intestine.
- Gastrointestinal infection.
- Neurogenic incontinence (reduced cortical inhibition – common in dementia).
- Environmental (poor mobility, inability to get to toilet, cope with clothing etc).

As occupational therapists, an awareness of impairment of digestive function in older age is important. Advice may be given to older people about nutritional intake and supplementation, as well as ensuring that they can eat adequately and safely. This may be done either through the simple provision of modified cutlery or a non-slip mat, as well as improving positioning, and co-working with a speech and language therapist with a client with swallowing difficulties. The reinforcement and facilitation through the use of assistive products of good oral hygiene is also important. An awareness of the interaction of medications with the digestive system and possible causes of constipation and faecal incontinence are crucial, especially where **environmental factors** may be a barrier.

Weight maintenance

Whilst obesity remains to be a debated health-care issue, under-nourishment in older people is not given high media priority. An alarming 40% of the patients admitted to hospital and 10% of patients in the community are under-nourished (Royal College of Physicians 2002). Groups of older people that appear to be most at risk are older people in care homes (DH 1998) and those with long-standing illness (Margetts *et al.* 2003). Other risk factors include dysphagia, slow eating, low protein intake, poor appetite, presence of a feeding tube and age (Keller 1993). Poor nutritional intake can hinder recovery from illness and is an associated risk factor for skin ulceration and also thermoregulation. Reduced calorie intake as part of a reduction of energy needs also means that older people need to eat foods with high nutritional value to compensate for this lower intake (Phillips 2003). For many older people eating well and poor nutritional status may also be affected by:

- Early satiety due to slow movement of food through the stomach.
- Reduction in vitamin D because of poor exposure to sunlight (Reid *et al.* 1986).
- Low social status and monetary income.
- Living alone leading to greater preference for easy-to-prepare foods and less fresh fruit and vegetables (Horwath 1989a).
- Lack of social contact, recent bereavement, being less socially and physically active.
                    (Krondl *et al.* 1982; Walker & Beauchene 1991).

Other factors having an impact are:

- Disability.
- Lack of transport.
- Shopping difficulties.
- Depression.
- Poor life satisfaction.
- Specific stressful life events.
- Negative attitudes towards eating or nutrition.
- External locus of control.
                                        (Horwath 1989b).

Occupational therapists have an important role collaborating with dieticians and **health promotion** experts to advise on food budgeting and planning low-cost nutritious meals, including enjoyable food preparation 'for one'. Provision of opportunity to eat with and to cook for others e.g. at luncheon clubs, restaurants, 'pop-in' cafes and encouragement of older people to use the Internet for food shopping and recipe selection can also be part of the occupational therapist's role.

Metabolism

Metabolism is defined as 'the regulation of essential components of the body such as carbohydrates, proteins and fats, the conversion of one to another and their breakdown into energy' (WHO 2001:85). Basal (or resting) metabolic rate (BMR) is the rate of energy expenditure required to keep the body functioning at rest. This is said to decline with ageing with the BMR of a 70-year-old being 9–12% lower than of a 30-year-old. The reduction in BMR is mainly caused by reduction in lean body mass due to muscle loss (Phillips 2003). Such a decline in BMR impacts on calorie intake and weight regulation. Metabolism of minerals is also affected in ageing, with some loss of bone density due to removal of minerals and collagen matrix, as part of normal ageing; however, more accelerated loss is associated with **osteoporosis**, as already discussed.

Water and electrolyte balance are controlled by thirst, hunger and renal functions, which all change with normal ageing. These changes do not impact upon the body's homeostasis in normal events, but puts an older person on a 'knife-edge' of control so that an infection, changes in weather, or use of medications can cause an imbalance of water and electrolytes within the body (Allen 1998). Older people have a delayed and less intense response to thirst, which inhibits water intake. Dehydration is the most common cause of water and electrolyte imbalance in older people and in mild cases can cause dry skin, cognitive changes, lethargy or syncope, but can in extreme situations lead to **stroke, heart attack** or renal failure. It is therefore necessary for older people to be encouraged to drink not only plenty of water but also to replenish sodium levels at times of illness or hot weather to prevent serious consequences of dehydration.

Thermoregulation

Regulation of body heat to prevent either hypothermia or hyperthermia in older people is crucial to prevent pathological events within body functions or structures, including exacerbation of existing conditions or even death. Thermoregulation is a finely tuned process maintaining the core temperature at the optimal level for the body's biochemical processes to take place (Worfolk 1997). Regulation of body heat is carried by both intrinsic and extrinsic means, with intrinsic regulation through functioning of the cardiovascular, respiratory, neuromuscular, digestive and endocrine systems and extrinsically with nutrition and medication (Knies 1996).

As discussed in previous sections, much of the body's heat is generated as a by-product of metabolism in the organs and muscles and regulated by the hypothalamus through neuroendocrine and autonomic nervous system mechanisms. Most of these organs and systems have declining activity from the age of 70 onwards. Loss of subcutaneous fat, reduced vasoconstriction and ability to shiver (due to loss of muscle mass) all impact on maintenance and response to heat changes. Response to body temperature changes is also impaired with the ageing process (more so in 80+ year-olds and the very frail) with reduction in the number of thermal, chemical and mechanical receptors, and also a reduced sensitivity, perception and processing of changes in both body and **environmental** temperatures (see Chapter 10).

A reduced ability to sweat in high ambient temperatures and a reduced thirst sensation can lead to heat stroke if poorly monitored. An increased cardiovascular activity to release heat through radiation from vasodilatation of skin capillaries (which may be less in number or atherosclerotic) results in increased cardiac output and is often the cause of death rather than the exposure to higher ambient temperatures (Wilmshurst 1994). Attention should be paid to the types of clothing worn (light and loose fitting) and avoidance of unnecessary exertion (Keatinge 2004). Where possible older people at risk of heat-related problems could benefit from taking cool showers/baths or air-conditioned buildings (Woolfe 2003).

Hypothermia is of greater concern in the UK due to low winter temperatures and also the age of much of the housing stock lived in by many older people (see Chapters 4 and 10). The emphasis on prevention of hypothermia within **falls** management programmes has been strongly recommended (Simpson *et al.* 1998) as mortality rates are approximately 50% in all cases of hypothermia (with those over the age of 75 five times more likely to die as a result) (Beers & Berkow [no date]).

Risk factors for hypothermia are:

- Cardiovascular disease.
- Diabetes.
- Low physical activity.
- Medications.
- Low ambient temperature.
- Poor nutrition (a high protein meal can increase the metabolic rate by 30% as opposed to a carbohydrate meal by 4%).
- General anaesthesia and surgery.

Occupational therapists need to be aware of declining thermoregulation in older people, especially those frailer and over 75. An increase in physical activity in either high or low ambient temperatures can further compromise impaired body functions that are already struggling to maintain homeostasis. Education about clothing, rehydration, and nutrition is important as well as maintenance of environmental temperatures (see Chapter 10) and dealing with inactivity such as that experienced by Mr Duffy in Chapter 5 following a **fall**.

Endocrine functions

Hormone production is essential for maintenance of circadian rhythms, energy metabolism and also dealing with intrinsic and extrinsic stressors (Morley 2003). Ageing of the endocrine system occurs to create a 'change in the smooth oscillatory release of hormones to a more chaotic pattern of release' (Morley 2003:333). A decline in efficiency of hormonal receptors and effector mechanisms also causes the endocrine system to be come sluggish and also respond less effectively to stress in older people (Bennett & Ebrahim 1995).

Hormone changes that occur with aging are:

- Decrease in insulin production and development of insulin resistance.
- Decline in thyroxine production rate.
- Reduction in production of testosterone and oestrogen – causing poorer cognitive function, loss of strength, muscle mass and bone mineral density as well as loss of fertility.

- Decline in vitamin D production – due to poor nutritional uptake and poor exposure to sunlight.

(Drake *et al.* 2000; Morley 2003).

Hormone replacement therapy has been considered and most successfully carried out with oestrogen replacement giving benefits in cognitive functioning, the reduction in bone loss and cardiovascular risk and disadvantages including the risk of breast and endometrial cancer. Testosterone replacement therapy has been shown in men to increase muscle strength and mass as well as libido, bone density and cognition; however supplementation can increase the risk of **stroke** with long-term risks not known. Vitamin D supplements are also given, but more successfully for the housebound and those in residential care are a 30-minute a day exposure to sunlight (outdoors) to restore levels (Reid *et al.* 1986).

Even though endocrine function may seem far removed from the sphere of occupational therapy, endocrines impact on all body functions. The simple supplementation of vitamin D, for example, is one that an occupational therapist can encourage in older clients to prevent **osteoporosis**.

The genito-urinary systems

Urinary system

Ageing processes within the kidneys not only impact on renal function in the excretion of urine, but also on the cardiovascular system in the control of blood pressure. The kidney is said to shrink from 400 g to 300 g by the age of 90, with a 50% loss in the number of nephrons by the age of 70. The filtration rate of the glomeruli more importantly steadily declines from the age of 40 and is associated with a rise in blood pressure. There is also a declining ability for the loop of Henlé to reabsorb sodium causing a reduced ability to concentrate urine during periods of water depletion. This has serious consequences for older people, potentially leading to more rapid dehydration in hot weather, and the need to for night-time micturition (Bennett & Ebrahim 1995). A slowing glomerular filtration rate also slows the clearance of many medications through the kidney, causing drug toxicity if they accumulate (Mangoni & Jackson 2003).

Involuntary loss of urine from the body (incontinence) causes misery for many older men and women, being seen as a social and hygiene problem. More than 20% of older people have urinary incontinence and this figure rises above 50% for those older people living in long-term residential care. More women than men suffer from incontinence of urine (Thakar & Stanton 2000).

Continence of urine (or voluntary control) requires a well-functioning lower urinary tract, with central nervous system inhibition and facilitation by the basal ganglia, frontal cortex and cerebellum, as well as good cognitive functioning, motivation, mobility and manual dexterity. Incontinence should not be accepted as a normal part of growing older but is associated with disease processes and problems that commonly occur with ageing such as **stroke** and **dementia**.

Incontinence can either be transient or established, with transient incontinence being more common in older people. Causes of transient incontinence are:

- Delirium.
- Urinary tract infection.
- Urethritis and vaginitis.
- Alcohol and drug use.
- Mental health problems such as **depression**.
- Excessive output due to high fluid intake.
- Use of diuretics (including caffeine).
- Restricted mobility.
- Impacted stools.

(Beers & Berkow [no date]).

There are three main types of established incontinence – detrusor overactivity, stress incontinence and outlet obstruction which are caused by structural and functional problems within the bladder and urethra, or due to CNS control. In older people the capacity and contractility of the bladder decrease with age, as does the ability to postpone voiding. Bladder contractions are increasingly uninhibited by CNS control and residual volumes within the bladder after voiding increase. Both the urethral length and sphincter strength decline with age in women and the prostate enlarges in men (Abrams 1995; Thakar & Stanton 2000).

Management of established incontinence varies – with detrusor overactivity responding to bladder retraining, by emptying the bladder on a regular 2–3 hourly basis. This is especially useful for those older people after stroke and also with **dementia**. Weight loss (where appropriate) and treatment of the precipitating cause of outlet incompetence (e.g. cough) can be sufficient, but otherwise the use of pelvic floor exercises is said to be successful in all age groups. Medication to alleviate the symptoms of outlet obstruction may be sufficient but otherwise resection of the prostate is carried out (Abrams 1995; Thakar & Stanton 2000).

Occupational therapists are involved in more behavioural approaches to the management of urinary incontinence. A reminder for regular use of the toilet can be necessary and more importantly an assessment of dressing ability to establish whether the client can easily manage clothing when going to the toilet. Access to the toilet may be difficult because of poor mobility and a risk assessment may be necessary to eliminate or reduce any environmental hazards for both day and night time usage. Ensuring that clients can manage pads if supplied with clothing may also be necessary as part of a dressing assessment.

Sexual functions

There has been an assumption both within the literature and by most professionals that older people do not have intimate sexual relationships and this is explored in more detail in Chapter 9. For many older people the physical changes to sexual functions make coitus more difficult and few may seek advice about these impairments, perhaps perceiving them as an inevitable part of ageing.

Reduction in hormones already discussed impact on sexual functioning, as well as cardiovascular insufficiencies, diabetes and some medications. The presence of disease processes such as **arthritis** or **respiratory conditions** may cause pain, reduced physical capacity and an increase in discomfort. Such problems may also reduce desire as a result. Women experience less sexual dreaming as they get older and this is associated with a reduction in testosterone levels, which also causes loss of libido in men (Miracle & Miracle 2001). A reduction in oestrogen levels in women with the menopause causes physical changes such as atrophy of the uterus, contraction and shortening of the vagina with loss of elasticity, thinning of the epithelium and reduction of vaginal lubrication. All of these cause discomfort during penetration and reduce desire (Bennett & Ebrahim 1995).

Older men have a more gradual decline in sexual functioning and structures, maintaining fertility almost throughout their lives. However, secretion of testosterone declines by approximately 30% by the age of 80, with decreased production of sperm, seminal fluid and greater need for stimulation to achieve an erection and a shorter time for ejaculation to occur. Erectile dysfunction occurs in 50% of men aged 40–70 years, and this increases with age. However ageing does not cause erectile dysfunction, which is more likely to be caused by vascular, neurological, endocrine or iatrogenic factors. Vascular disorders are the most common cause of erectile dysfunction in older men; especially arterial disease, with this being an early symptom of atherosclerosis. Many other factors influence sexual functioning:

- Post-event anxiety (after a cardiovascular event or **stroke**). However intercourse should not be hazardous if blood pressure is controlled.
- **Stroke** – can reduce erectile function, vaginal lubrication and sensation.
- **Arthritis** – inflammation of joints, fatigue, weakness, pain, restricted range of moment (especially hips).
- Alcohol – long-term cumulative affect; can inhibit libido.
- Surgery – long-term effects are rare, even after hysterectomy or prostatectomy.
- Medications – corticosteroids reduce libido; tranquillisers, anti-depressants and beta blockers cause impotence.
- **Diabetes** – causes erectile dysfunction.
- Incontinence of urine and catheterisation.
- Sexually transmitted diseases – AIDs has increased by 22% in older people in the last 10 years, as older people equate the use of condoms with fertility rather than 'safe sex'.

(Read 1999; Miracle & Miracle 2001).

Occupational therapists should not avoid advising older people about their sexual activity and may have to deal with their own beliefs and attitudes and be explicit about the boundaries of the therapeutic relationship. The need for advice on alternative positioning or energy conservation may be necessary as well as a health promotion role of 'safe sex' education. Miracle & Miracle (2001) describe the PLISSIT intervention model, with the acronym meaning – Permission, Limited Information, Specific Suggestions, Intensive Therapy. For the majority of occupational therapists the first two aspects of permission and limited information may be within their scope, with referral for more specific help or therapy by a more experienced colleague. However, like any other aspect of daily life it is crucial that the occupational therapist acknowledges the need for help by the most appropriate professional and the older person is dealt with sensitively and professionally at all times.

Summary

This chapter has attempted to discuss those body functions and structures involved in the integumentary, cardiovascular, respiratory and immune systems, neuromusculoskeletal system, digestive, metabolic and endocrine system and genito-urinary and reproductive systems in relation to normal ageing and also those pathological processes that occur during older age. The consequences of impairments in body functions and structures have been related where possible, to occupational performance and the role of the occupational therapist has been discussed.

References

Abrams P (1995) Fortnightly Review: Managing lower urinary tract symptoms in older men. *British Medical Journal* 310, 1113–1117.

Allen SC (1998) *Medicine in Old Age*, 4th edn. Edinburgh: Churchill Livingstone.

Bassey EJ (2001) Exercise for prevention of osteoporotic fracture. *Age and Ageing* 30 (Supplement 4), 29–31.

Bateson MC (1999) Gallbladder disease. *British Medical Journal* 318, 1745–1747.

Beers MH & Berkow R (no date; updated contantly) *The Merck Manual of Geriatrics*, 3rd edn. Accessed 21.05.2004. http://www.merck.com/mrkshared/mm_geriatrics/home.jsp

Bennett G & Ebrahim S (1995) *The Essentials of Health Care in Old Age*, 2nd edn. London: Edward Arnold.

Bonder BR & Wagner MB (2001) *Functional Performance in Older Adults*, 2nd edn. Philadelphia: FA Davis.

British Heart Foundation Statistics Web Site (2004) Accessed 26.05.2004. http://www.heartstats.org/temp/HFSsptabsp4.1spweb03.xls

Crepeau EB, Cohn ES, Boyt Schell BA (2003) *Willard & Spackman's Occupational Therapy*, 10th edn. Philadelphia: Lippincott Williams & Wilkins.

Drake EB, Henderson VW, Stanczyk FZ et al. (2000) Associations between circulating sex steroid hormones and cognition in normal elderly women. *Neurology* 54(3), 599–603.

Harridge SDR & Young A (1998) In: Pathy MSJ (ed.) *Principles and Practice of Geriatric Medicine*, 3rd edn. Chichester: John Wiley, pp. 897–905.

Herbert R (1991) The normal ageing process reviewed. *Nursing Standard* 5(51), 36–39.

Horan MA & Ashcroft GS (1997) Ageing, defence mechanisms and the immune system. *Age and Ageing* 26 (Supplement 4), 15–19.

Horwath CC (1989a) Marriage and diet in elderly Australians: results from a large random survey. *Journal of Human Nutrition and Dietetics* 2(3), 185–193.

Horwath CC (1989b) Socio-economic and behavioural effects on the dietary habits of elderly people. *International Journal of Biosocial and Medical Research* 11, 15–30.

Horwath CC (2002) Nutrition and aging. In: Mann J & Truswell AS (eds). *Essentials of Human Nutrition*. Oxford: Oxford University Press, pp. 551–565.

Kamm MA (1998) Faecal incontinence. *British Medical Journal* 316, 528–532.

Keatinge WR (2004) Death in heat waves. *British Medical Journal* 327, 512–313.

Keller HH (1993) Malnutrition in institutionalised elderly: how and why? *American Geriatric Society* 41(11), 1212–1218.

Kiecolt-Glaser JK, Marucha PT, Malarkey WB, Mercado AM, Glaser R (1995) Slowing of wound healing by psychological stress. *Lancet* 346, 1194–1196.

Kirkwood TBL & Ritter MA (1997) The interface between ageing and health in man. *Age and Ageing* 26 (Supplement 4), 9–14.

Knies RC (1996). Geriatric trauma; what you need to know. *International Journal of Trauma Nursing* 2(3), 85–91.

Krondl M, Lau D, Yurkiw MA, Coleman PH (1982) Food use and perceived food meanings of the elderly. *Journal of the American Dietetic Association* 80(6), 523–529.

Leslie P, Carding PN, Wilson JA (2003) Investigation and management of chronic dysphagia. *British Medical Journal* 326, 433–436.

Lovallo WR (1997) *Stress and Health: Biological and Psychological Interactions*. London: Sage. Publications.

Mangoni AA & Jackson SHD (2003) Age-related changes in pharmacokinetics and pharmacodynamics: basic principles and practical applications. *British Journal of Pharmacology* 57(1), 6–14.

Margetts BM, Thompson RL, Elia M, Jackson AA (2003) Prevalence of risk of undernutrition is associated with poor health status in older people in the UK. *European Journal of Clinical Nutrition* 57(1), 69–74.

Michelozzi P (2003) A warning system to prevent heat health effect in Rome. *British Medical Journal* 327, 512–513.

Ministry of Agriculture, Fisheries and Food and the Department of Health (1998) *Report of the Diet and Nutrition Survey*, Volume 1. London: HMSO.

Ministry of Health (New Zealand) (1996) *Food and Nutrition Guidelines for Healthy Older People: A Background Paper* – online. Accessed 26.05.2004. http://www.moh.govt.nz/moh.nsf/ae8bff4c2724ed6f4c256669006aed56/fa6df710fdfea794cc256df70070539f?OpenDocument#Introduction

Miracle AW & Miracle TS (2001) Sexuality in late adulthood. In: Bonder BR & Wagner MB (eds). *Functional Performance in Older Adults*, 2nd edn. Philadelphia: FA Davis, pp. 218–235.

Morley JE (2003) Hormones and the aging process. *Journal of the American Geriatrics Society* 51(7), s333–s337.

Phillips F (2003) Nutrition for healthy ageing. *Nutrition Bulletin. British Nutrition Foundation* 28, 253–263.

Read J (1999) Sexual problems associated with infertility, pregnancy and ageing. *British Medical Journal* 318, 587–589.

Reid IR, Gallagher DJA, Bosworth J (1986) Prophylaxis against vitamin D deficiency in the elderly by regular sunlight exposure. *Age and Ageing* 15(1), 35–40.

Royal College of General Practitioners, the Office of Population Censuses and Surveys, and the Department of Health (1995) *Morbidity Statistics from General Practice*, 4th National Study, 1991–1992. London: HMSO.

Royal College of Physicians (2002) *Nutrition and Patients: A Doctor's Responsibility*. London: Royal College of Physicians.

Simpson JM, Marsh N, Harrington R (1998) Managing Falls among elderly people. *British Journal of Occupational Therapy* 61(4), 165–168.

Spurgeon B (2003) French government announces new plans for elderly care. *British Medical Journal* 307, 465.

Thakar R & Stanton S (2000) Management of urinary incontinence in women. *British Medical Journal* 321, 1326–1331.

Tortora GJ & Grabowski SR (2003) *Principles of Anatomy and Physiology*, 10th edn. New York: John Wiley.

Trombly CA & Radomski MV (2002) *Occupational Therapy for Physical Dysfunction*, 5th edn. Philadelphia: Lippincott, Williams and Wilkins.

Walker D & Beauchene RE (1991) The relationship of loneliness, social isolation, and physical health to dietary adequacy of independently living elderly. *Journal of the American Dietetic Association* 91(3), 300–304.

Wilmshurst P (1994) Temperature and cardiovascular mortality. *British Medical Journal* 309, 1029–1030.

Woodruff-Pak DS (1997) *The Neuropsychology of Aging*. Malden, USA: Blackwell Publishing.

Woolfe RW (2003) Beware of fans. *British Medical Journal* 327, 512.

World Health Organisation (2001) *The International Classification of Functioning Disability and Health*. Geneva: WHO.

Worfolk J (1997) Keep frail elders warm! *Geriatric Nursing* 18(1), 7–11.

Chapter 8

ACTIVITY AND PARTICIPATION: PART 1

Anne McIntyre, with contributions from Wendy Bryant

The WHO (2001) considers the concepts of activity and participation as crucial elements of functioning and disability alongside **body functions** and **structures** (discussed in Chapters 6 and 7), interacting with the **personal** and **environmental context** of an older person. This chapter and Chapter 9 will discuss the activity and participation issues of older people, which could be considered the key elements of **occupational performance**.

Within the ICF, the WHO (2001) provides the following definitions:

- Activity – The execution of a task or action by an individual.
- Participation – The involvement in a life situation.

With

- Activity limitation – Difficulties an individual may have in executing an activity.
- Participation restriction – Problems an individual may experience being involved in a life situation.

The WHO (2001) also differentiates between **capacity** and **performance** of activities in the ICF, with capacity being what an individual can do as opposed to performance – what they do do.

The promotion of health and wellbeing through engagement in occupation has been discussed in Chapter 2. How we engage in occupation is taken further in this chapter and Chapter 9. Even though the terms 'activity' and 'occupation' are used interchangeably in practice, both Creek (2003) and Harvey & Pentland (2002) consider that there is a task–activity–occupation hierarchy, with tasks and activities only being meaningful when placed in a personal and environmental context.

Whereas 'occupation' may be unfamiliar terminology outside the profession, the use of the term 'activities of daily living' (ADLs) is familiar to many. However, universal agreement of the concept and definition of ADL has been problematic – with subdivision of ADL into basic or personal ADLs (BADL, PADL) and instrumental or extended ADLs (IADL, EADL). The inclusion and exclusion of activities within these subdivisions can vary between professions, organisations, and geographical boundaries. It could be argued that the concept of ADL ignores the contexts of individuals, and therefore such performance has no meaning, lacking client-centredness. Therefore, the consideration of the contextual factors for an individual on their activity and participation in the ICF (WHO 2001) is to be welcomed, as is the meeting of two opposing models – the medical and social model of disability into a bio-psycho-social model. However, the introduction of universally agreed domains within the ICF, do not always fit seamlessly with established occupational therapy use.

Occupational therapy practice is not only influenced by the conceptual understanding of activity and occupation but also by the health and social traditions of the workplace. Such traditions influence the way we work, the outcome measures and the interventions we carry out. It may also influence the evidence base and research methodologies we use.

Occupational therapy research has identified age-related deterioration in ADL in older people (Hayase *et al.* 2004) and more so in all older people with **dementia** (Oakley *et al.* 2003). These researchers concentrated on motor and processing skills in activity capacity, rather than considering actual performance. However, such evidence can provide us with baseline information to inform our practice. Also of interest is work of Fricke and Unsworth (2001), which highlighted the different perceptions of important IADLs, with older people listing use of telephone, transportation (including driving) and reading as most important, because of the high value of leisure activities, with occupational therapists listing use of telephone, medication management and snack preparation. Such evidence reinforces the need for client-centred practice, the importance of meaningful occupation by considering the participatory reliance on activity, and appropriate outcome measures to enhance our evidence base.

Many outcome measures are presented in Chapter 5, with some using the traditional concepts of ADL. Increasingly more occupational therapy specific outcome measures are being devised to address client-centred practice and engagement in occupation. The reader is directed to Unsworth (2000) and also Law et al. (2001).

Of the nine domains listed in the ICF, five domains, which could be considered the more 'traditional' activities of daily living and related to 'doing,' are discussed in this chapter and the remaining four in Chapter 9. The domains discussed in this chapter are summarised in Box 8.1.

Box 8.1 Domains within the Activity and Participation components of the ICF (WHO 2001).

Learning and applying knowledge

- Purposeful and sensory experiences
- Basic learning
- Applying knowledge

Box 8.1 (*cont'd*)

General tasks and demands

- Undertaking single tasks
- Undertaking multiple tasks
- Carrying out daily routine
- Handling stress and other psychological demands

Mobility

- Changing and maintaining body position
- Carrying, moving and handling objects
- Walking
- Climbing stairs

Self-care

- Washing oneself
- Caring for body parts
- Toileting
- Dressing
- Eating
- Drinking
- Looking after one's health

Domestic life

- Acquisition of necessities
- Household tasks
- Caring for household objects and assisting others

Learning and applying knowledge

Defining learning and applying knowledge

The first domain of the Activities and Participation component classified by the ICF is learning and applying knowledge. Without the ability to learn and the skill to apply that learning, activity is limited. Assessment of potential for rehabilitation usually involves consideration of these aspects. It is important to acknowledge that learning and applying knowledge applies equally to the occupational therapist working with older people, at every stage of involvement. Clinical reasoning involves active consideration of each experience, identification of learning needs and application of existing knowledge (Mattingly & Fleming 1994). It is important to have a sense of how decisions emerged, especially in the complex settings encountered when working with older people.

Box 8.2

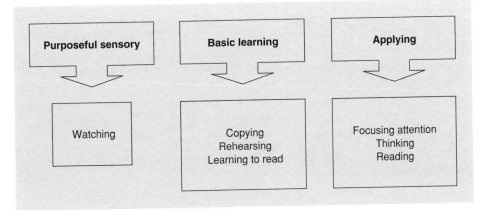

Purposeful sensory experiences

Sensory experiences require the body structure to receive the sensory input, and the body function to process it (as already discussed in Chapter 6), with the environment having equal significance as a provider of stimuli.

Mr Adams (Box 8.3) had hearing and mobility difficulties and **dementia**, which caused him difficulty in using his senses to process new information. Auditory and tactile input was difficult for him to access because of his hearing and mobility problems, and all stimulation difficult for him to understand because of his **dementia**. The occupational therapist had identified these difficulties in an initial assessment. The group he attended was carefully planned and structured to be predictable for those involved, to maximise the possibility of recognition. The media used were easily manipulated, to maximise opportunities to be active and to communicate. Mr Adams responded to this carefully structured **environment** by participating and making a spontaneous contribution, demonstrating that he could process sensory information and communicate with others. In this setting, the occupational therapist's key role was to provide opportunities for the residents to participate in meaningful occupations (Bryant 1991).

Box 8.3 Mr Adams, who saw the snow.

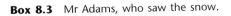

Mr Eddie Adams lived in a continuing care unit for people with dementia. He was unable to mobilise independently, had hearing difficulties and an expressive dysphasia. He participated in a group led by an occupational therapist and music therapist, which used sensory stimulation to promote meaningful occupation and communication. Initially in the group, Mr Adams was withdrawn and did not take an active part. However, as he grew familiar with the media used, he enjoyed throwing a ball to other group members and showed some signs of recognition. One day, Mr Adams became particularly animated. He succeeded in communicating his excitement about the snow falling outside to all the group.

It is important to establish that an individual is able to receive and process sensory experiences prior to attempting to learn new skills or apply knowledge. Practical strategies such as ensuring the use of hearing aids or glasses when required can have a defining impact on the success of an intervention. However, even when these strategies are used, a person may still have difficulty recognising sensory input and compensatory strategies may need to be developed, using the other senses to trigger an appropriate response. For example, a person may not recognise a hot drink when it is placed in front of them, but the sound of the drink being stirred with a spoon or the first assisted taste of the drink could be enough to stimulate unassisted feeding on each occasion.

Basic learning

Whilst this category is titled 'basic learning', it actually encompasses the range of learning from imitation to mastery of complex skills. Learning takes place from the start of therapy, as names are exchanged and the purpose explained. The prescription of equipment involves a learning process: the occupational therapist demonstrates how to use equipment and ensures that this is understood by observing its use by the older person. The use of **products and technology** may be contraindicated if it is not possible for the person to acquire the skills required to use it.

Applying knowledge

Age holds conflicting preconceptions in relation to learning: on the one hand, experience and acquisition of knowledge increases with age (Woodruff-Pak 1997), but there is a widespread belief that it is more difficult for older people to adapt and learn new skills and this is considered in this chapter alongside undertaking tasks.

Being sensitive to beliefs and values of all concerned enables the occupational therapist to structure the experience of therapy in a way that maximises opportunity for learning and applying knowledge.

General tasks and demands

Undertaking single and multiple tasks

What is a task? Interpretations vary between dictionary definitions, which consider a task to be a piece of work or a chore and the interpretation of the WHO and the occupational therapy literature. The ICF considers a task as a component of an **activity** carried out by an individual (WHO 2001). Performance of a task is dependent upon its complexity and meaning, our motivation, past experience, knowledge and capacity. Therefore task performance is highly dependent upon the performance skills (or **body functions**) we have available to us, our ability to learn new skills and tasks as well as the **environment** and the **personal context**, in which the task is carried out. In occupational therapy, we use tasks in a multitude of ways – with many of our assessments involving observation – either to consider the task's component performance skills, or which element of an activity the client finds problematic. The use of tasks will depend on the frame of reference we adopt.

Analysis of tasks is useful when considering intervention, as tasks can be structured and used within a programme of rehabilitation to facilitate (re)acquisition of skills and abilities, enhancing performance by giving meaning and value to the intervention as a 'means to an end.' Tasks will also form the target of a programme in that they are what the client needs/wants to be able to do and are therefore the goal of intervention.

Tasks are also considered in terms of their complexity, but interpretations of this vary. In the ICF the WHO (2001) considers that reading a book is a simple task, but even though this may involve relatively simple motor skills it also requires complex cognitive and perceptual functions. Reed & Sanderson (1999) suggest that the number of steps, sequences, can determine the complexity of a task or patterns within it, as well as the amount of structure, flexibility, or creativity allowed.

Tasks may be 'closed' with a definite beginning and end, such as opening a door, or 'open' such as cycle riding or knitting. Multiple tasks may involve the simultaneous and sequential performance of both simple and complex tasks, for example holding and speaking into a telephone whilst searching for pen and paper to write a message.

Our success at carrying out tasks – especially complex and multiple tasks is highly dependent on the amount of sensory input, the speed at which we can process and respond appropriately to such input (Turner 2002). This ability to process sensory input has been discussed in Chapter 6 as being the function of the attentional system and working memory.

It has been accepted in the past that older people's speed and performance of tasks have deteriorated as part of the normal ageing process. However recent research questions these preconceptions and is exploring whether change in task performance is related to normal ageing or to the onset of pathological processes.

Much of the research on task performance has involved 'laboratory' tests such as those involving executive functions rather than 'real world' tasks; however, the **Large Allen's Cognitive Level Screen (LACL)** devised by Allen et al. (1992) and described in Chapter 5, uses everyday tasks and activities to assess cognitive functioning.

Even though much of the research does not involve 'real world' tasks, it does provide useful evidence on task performance and implications for occupational therapy practice in Table 8.1.

Carrying out multiple tasks has also been under scrutiny, with recent research considering dual task performance. Therapists are aware that older people who are able to converse whilst carrying out daily living tasks are likely to be more successful and safer in their performance. Studies have been carried out to establish which tasks are the more demanding and these have implications not only for intervention but also in assessment, as a client may marshal extra attentional capacity because they are being assessed, but are unable to sustain this during actual performance in 'real' situations. Recent evidence suggests:

Table 8.1 Summary of research evidence on task performance.

Research evidence	Implications for practice
Chronological age does not necessarily predict performance in complex tasks (Martin & Ewert 1997).	People age at differing rates because of genetic programming, life experiences, as well as the skills and information accumulated.
There is a greater difference in ability in task performance between the most and least able 70-year-olds than there is between the most and least able 40–50 years old (Rabbitt 1993).	Individual assessment of task performance is necessary for each older client.
Older people of a higher educational standard perform better on cognitive (or laboratory type) tasks than younger people of lesser educational experience (Steel *et al.* 2003).	Individual assessment of task performance is necessary for each older client.
Older people do as well in 'real life' and concrete tasks as younger people (Crawford & Channon 2002; Rabbitt 1997).	Individual assessment of task performance is necessary for each older client.
Practice enhances task performance in older people beyond that of younger less practiced individuals (Welford 1958).	Practice not only enhances task performance in rehabilitation but also should be considered in job (re)training programmes that have an upper age limit.
Older people can perpetuate earlier mistakes in later practice creating 'error preservation' (Hasher *et al.* 1991).	Individuals require feedback of performance at all stages of practice to reduce errors with teaching structured to minimise possibility of error.
Older people are observed to use different strategies to achieve the same complex tasks as younger people (Crawford & Channon 2002; Rabbitt 1997).	Strategies should be considered on an individual basis.
Functional plastic changes occur in different areas of the cerebral hemispheres in older people to younger people with comparative outcome. (Ward & Frakowiak 2003).	If the CNS has a finite capacity for neuroplasticity to occur, then task performance and recovery due to rehabilitation techniques such as CIMT (Taub *et al.* 1998) will be limited in older people.
Older people need to harness greater cerebral capacity to maintain task performance (Ward & Frakowiak 2003).	Task performance may require more concentration and attention.

- Motor and higher cognitive tasks can normally be performed simultaneously with little detrimental effect on either, but performance deteriorates when two similar tasks are attempted at the same time – (i.e. talking and map reading) (Haggard *et al.* 2000).
- Speed of motor tasks and accuracy of cognitive tasks does decline in dual tasking with older adults and after acquired brain injury (e.g. **stroke**) (Yardley *et al.* 2001).

- Performance in dual tasks progressively declines with clients who have increasing cognitive impairment (Hauer *et al.* 2003).
- The complexity of the task and also the length of time a task may take are also considered to impact on dual tasking (Yardley *et al.* 2001; Haggard *et al.* 2000).
- 'Stops walking when talking' – this dual task can identify those older people with postural instability and at risk of falling (Lundin-Olsson *et al.* 1997; Bowen *et al.* 2001; Verghese *et al.* 2002).

The story of Mr Crabtree, who we met in Chapter 5, helps demonstrate how his poor dual task performance was addressed by his therapy team (Box 8.4).

Box 8.4 Mr Crabtree.

Mr Crabtree's GP referred him to the local therapy team after his last check up for assessment of his mobility problems. Both the occupational therapist and physiotherapist identified that Mr Crabtree was safer at some times more than others. They carried out walking while talking tasks (WWT) (Verghese *et al.* 2002) and identified that Mr Crabtree was less stable during these dual tasks than when performing the tasks independently. The team decision was to keep verbal feedback during tasks to a minimum during intervention and also to consider the environment in which Mr Crabtree was expected to carry out and practice his daily living activities, so that it wasn't too noisy or busy. This was easy for Mr Crabtree to consider in his own home, but he had to be reminded that he needed to be more wary when walking outside in the busy street.

Carrying out daily routines

The WHO defines this within the ICF as 'carrying out simple or complex actions in order to plan manage and complete the requirements for day to day procedures or duties' (WHO 2001:130). We tend to believe that routines are necessary elements of our daily lives (Turner 2002) being occupations with established sequences (Christiansen & Baum 1997). Routines are especially important for those people with **dementia** (Alzheimer's Society 2000). Control over daily routines is said to be important in maintaining quality of life for many older people, but where routines are imposed by others or external influences (such as in institutional care) this can be confining and a negative experience (Economic and Social Research Council 2001).

Inbuilt routines such as our circadian rhythm determines when we wake up and go to sleep (Hastings 1998). Other routines are semi-automatic which can be of great benefit to us when our attentional system is compromised (Hagedorn 1996). Such routines rely on learnt habits that are subconscious and automatic. At times routines can be ritualistic with little meaning, especially where the motivator for the routine no longer exists (such as going to work). Routines can be counterproductive, especially where there is a highly rigid structure and little opportunity for problem solving, so that the individual cannot respond to contextual influences and changes (Reed & Sanderson 1999).

Handling stress and other psychological demands

Stressors identified for older people are failing senses, illness and disability of family, friends and self, pain, limited energy, fear of dependency, death of close family and friends, loneliness and isolation and deterioration in personal control and autonomy (Pfeiffer 2002).

More personal and financial resources entail responsibilities for management and maintenance. Many older people are informal carers for family members, with over 2 million people aged over 60 caring for spouses, siblings, parents, and one quarter of all grandparents regularly caring for their grandchildren. It is common in many cultures for grandparents to look after grandchildren and this has reached crisis point in Africa where many older people are the main carer for their grandchildren orphaned by the AIDS epidemic. Many of these children also have AIDS (UN 2002) and the caregiver demands and responsibilities go unrecognised. In the western world caregiver stress is well-documented (Gilliard & Rabins 1999), especially with those carers of people with **dementia** (such as Mrs Davies' husband in Chapter 5).

Even though many older people demonstrate stoicism and self-reliance in times of stress or crisis, because of past experience of war and economic depression they react to stress in different ways than younger people (see Chapter 10). Older people are more likely to seek help at a very late stage, with the Samaritans identifying that the suicide rates in older people are relatively high in the UK and the Republic of Ireland (16% of all suicides). Even though this number has declined over recent years, a worrying increasing trend of alcohol problems with older people is emerging (Age Concern 2003; Alcohol Concern 2002; Samaritans 2000).

Stress manifests itself with physical symptoms – causing deterioration in functioning and an exacerbation of existing disease processes (see Chapter 7) (Pfeiffer 2002). Therefore **health promotion** strategies are necessary for older people – not only to encourage them to maintain healthy lifestyles and wellbeing to prevent stress, but also to join appropriate self-help groups and take part in stress management programmes as part of secondary and tertiary health promotion (see Chapter 1).

Mobility

The ICF describes mobility as 'moving by changing body position or location or by transferring from one place to another, by carrying, moving or manipulating objects, by walking, running or climbing and by using various forms of transportation' (WHO 2001:138).

As occupational therapists, we are concerned about not only how safely a client moves or obtains a position but also the quality of the movement. Many factors (and team consultation) will determine whether an educational, advisory, or compensatory approach is required with a client. Traditionally physiotherapists have been involved in the re-education of walking and transfers, whereas the occupational therapists are more concerned about the relationship between the client's ability to move and their environment, to successfully perform their chosen occupations. The story of Mrs Burns who we met in Chapter 5, is quite a common one. Environmental adaptation, provision of mobility equipment (including bed, toilet and chair raisers) and the use of problem solving and learning of new skills enabled Mrs Burns to be independent with most areas of occupational performance.

How successfully a person moves is dependent on planning and programming of movement patterns through reciprocal innervation of muscle groups, sensori-motor feedforward and feedback mechanisms, as well as adequate muscle tone, bulk and strength, balance reactions, cardiovascular and respiratory efficiency and structurally sound bones and joints (discussed in Chapters 6 and 7). In older people it is important to ascertain why they have mobility problems and there is much debate about which are part of normal ageing and what are part of patho-logical processes. Mobility problems after traumatic events (such as Mrs Burns' experience) should entail short-term need for precautionary post-operative mea-sures. In other situations such as those of Mr Duffy, Mr Branch and Mrs Gopal, who are discussed later, recovery of previous levels of mobility may not be possible.

Maintaining a position

A stable position is crucial for every day functioning. Trying to carry out an activity from an unstable position would be like trying to eat jelly sitting on a bucking bronco. The ease at which an individual can adopt a position is dependent upon the balance mechanisms, muscle strength and range of movement required to maintain it. For example, lying is a very stable position with a low centre of gravity (COG) well within a large base of support (BOS), requiring little postural control or muscle activity to maintain it. Standing is less easy to maintain, with a higher centre of gravity in a narrower base of support. As one's centre of gravity rises and the base of support decreases our balance system and neuromuscular systems become more important in our ability to maintain a position from which to carry out everyday activities.

In response to a deteriorating balance system, many older people adopt a standing or sitting position that increases their stability – often at the expense of potential mobility. Mr Duffy, who we met in Chapter 5, was observed to increase his stability in standing with legs further apart to widen his base of support, slightly flexing the hips and knees to lower his centre of gravity. To carry out an activity from this position then meant that Mr Duffy had to lean slightly forward flattening out his lumbar spine, with a kyphosis of his thoracic spine and poking his chin and head forward. This stooped posture is one that many would associate with old age – especially the 'oldest old' (Trew & Everitt 2001). As this stooped posture is associated with a reduction in spinal flexibility, range of movement and muscle weakness, an older person who has been physically inactive is more likely to acquire this posture at an earlier age. Such a position may be less energy efficient to maintain, requiring more muscle activity and therefore Mr Duffy may tire more easily and be able to stand for shorter and shorter periods of time.

Box 8.5

> Many people with hemiplegia and parkinsonian problems are observed to have problems with rolling over in bed because of impairments in body functions. Whereas Mr Branch has difficulty with initiating rolling over and sitting up in bed, Mrs Gopal has difficulty in co-ordinating and utilising her right side to roll over and getting her right leg into bed at night.

Changing position

In the ICF changing position is described as 'getting out of one position and moving from one location to another . . .' (WHO 2001:138). In much of the therapy literature and assessments this would be termed as 'ability to transfer' and refers to those more active changes in position that an individual may carry out. However, the ICF relates transfers to 'moving from one surface to another without changing position' (WHO 2001:140) such as sliding transfers.

Deterioration in muscle strength, a decline in flexibility and range of movement as well as CNS reaction times and interruption of normal movement patterns, all impact on changing from one position to another. Muscle stiffness and pain both impact on flexibility at any age with a consequential change in movement strategy and speed when rolling over and getting out of bed, for example.

Getting up from the floor is an important transfer in relation to **falls** management, with more than 47% of older people at risk of falling being unable to get up off the floor (Reese & Simpson 1996). Individuals can spend many minutes or hours on the floor (like Mr Duffy), and the consequences of a 'long lie' are hypothermia, dehydration, bronchopneumonia, pressure sores as well as anxiety and **depression** (Wild *et al.* 1981). Strategies such as 'backward chaining' are useful and necessary techniques to teach an older person how to get up off the floor are recommended as a crucial part of a **falls** management programme (Simpson *et al.* 1998).

Strategies for independent standing from sitting are an important part of an occupational therapy role – whether it is teaching a client new and safer strategies using appropriate positioning of the head, body and feet and use of biomechanical principles, or environmental adaptation such as a bed or armchair raise. People use different strategies to stand from sitting dependent not only upon the intrinsic factors already mentioned, but also on extrinsic factors such as the height, depth and firmness of the seat and the presence of armrests. However 8% of over 65-year-olds are reported to have difficulty getting up out of a chair, and 9% of over 80-year-olds require assistance (Alexander *et al.* 1991).

Carrying, moving and handling objects

Our ability to carry, reach and handle objects with the upper limb is essential for all self-care activities and most occupations. The upper limb also has a protective role as part of the body's saving reactions when overbalancing (McIlroy & Maki

1994). This parachute response, a protective mechanism against injury during a **fall**, is developed in babyhood, and accounts for the occurrence of one of the most common **fractures** in older people (especially women) – the Colles **fracture** (Singer *et al.* 1998).

There is a strong relationship between the shoulder and hand, with evidence from practice of frozen shoulder (adhesive capsulitis) being associated with Colles **fracture**. With the wrist immobilised and hand function reduced in the early stages of fracture management, the client has to consciously move the shoulder through a full range of movement on a regular basis, and failure to do so can result in a painful and restricted joint. Not only can enforced immobility predispose frozen shoulder but also **diabetes, cardiovascular disease** and hyperthyroidism.

Not only are trunk and shoulder girdle stability required for upper limb activity, but the lower limbs are also involved in anticipatory postural mechanisms to provide a stable position from which reaching, carrying and hand function are carried out. As we have already considered in Chapter 6, these mechanisms are quite often affected in older people who can find themselves unable to open curtains, hang washing on a clothes line or get clothes out of a wardrobe without losing their balance.

Other impairments impact upon upper limb function with the ageing process affecting the soft tissues around the shoulder joint causing a decline in active range of movement, especially flexion, abduction, lateral and medial rotation (Desrosiers *et al.* 1995). Such decline in upper limb function can be noted over a relatively short period of time (3 years) but is not necessarily related to chronological age but previous activity levels (Desrosiers *et al.* 1999).

Carrying items also reduces postural stability by raising the centre of gravity up and out of the base of support and also putting potentially weaker shoulder and upper limb muscle groups under greater demand. However the most significant changes are noticed in manual dexterity due to reduction in muscle mass, hand–eye co-ordination, sensory loss and cutaneous changes (e.g. skin slipperiness) (Desrosiers *et al.* 1999; Ranganathen *et al.* 2001). Such ageing of the CNS increases the time taken to manipulate and grasp objects by 40% between the ages of 25 and 70 years (Shumway-Cook & Woollacott 2001). A small study by Ranganathen *et al.* (2001) also identified that older subjects had 30% less power and pinchgrip strength than that of younger subjects. Deterioration in manipulation and grip strength has impact on an older person's ability to carry out many everyday tasks such as opening jars, milk cartons, and medication bottles for example.

There are several standardised upper limb and hand function assessments; however the provision of normative data and the reliability and validity of these have not been fully explored with older people, so in many instances older people's upper limb function and activity is compared with that of younger people (Shiffman 1992). Some assessments that do consider older adults are:

- Jebsen Test of Hand Function (Jebsen *et al.* 1969), which uses ADL type tasks (e.g. writing, eating, and picking up objects).
- Jamar Dynamometer (Mathiowetz *et al.* 1985) – measuring grip strength.

- Purdue Pegboard Test (Tiffin 1968; Costa *et al.* 1963) – has normative data on manual dexterity for older adults but otherwise concentrates on factory workers.
- Assessment of Motor Skills (AMPS) (Fisher 1995).
- Rivermead Assessment of Somatosensory Performance (Winward *et al.* 2000) – assesses touch, 2-point discrimination, hot and cold modalities.

Recent studies have associated declining grip strength with both mortality rates in older women (Rantanen *et al.* 2003) and also physical activity (Brach & Van Swearingen 2002). However, it is contested within the occupational therapy literature that assessment of body functions such as grip strength and manual dexterity do not successfully relate to performance of meaningful occupation (Cooper 2003).

Upper limb activity is also affected by our ability to maintain a position independently. Where sitting balance is compromised, for example, many individuals find that they have to 'fix' their position by holding onto armrests of chairs and wheelchairs for support if they do not have adequate postural support provided within the chair. The use of **walking products** to alleviate weight bearing through the legs after a lower limb fracture or to redistribute body weight because of poor balance immediately hampers an individual from any upper limb activity such as carrying items or opening doors. Therefore, other strategies have to be considered, such as the provision of a perching stool for washing or meal preparation, and a kitchen trolley to transport meals, drinks and any other items from room to room.

Walking

The Health Survey for England (HSE) identified that more than 30% of over 65-year-olds and 50% of over 80-year-olds living in the community consider that they have mobility problems, which compares with 36% of over 70-year-olds in the US (DH 2000; Iezzoni *et al.* 2001). The HSE (DH 2001) identified that problems with walking is the most common disability in older people.

Changes in walking (or gait) in older people are recognised as part of normal ageing in much of the literature, with a reduction of walking speed, step length and step rate (Imms & Edholm 1981; Menz *et al.* 2003; Petrofsky *et al.* 2003). However, many gait changes said to be age-related are now considered to be part of a pathological process, e.g. parkinsonism and some as part of pre-clinical signs of disability (Shumway-Cook & Woollacott 2001; Brach *et al.* 2002). As changes in **body functions** and **structures** occur due to ageing, it is not surprising that this has an impact on walking which is a highly complex task. Deterioration in walking has already been discussed as an element in dual task performance. Other factors such as use of medication, pain, anxiety, fear of **falling** and the **environment** all contribute to walking problems. Iezzoni *et al.* (2001) identified that most older people who could identify a cause for their mobility problems said that they were due to **arthritis** and **musculo-skeletal problems**, followed by **heart conditions, stroke and falls** (see Figure 8.1).

Occupational therapists are concerned about walking as part of **occupational performance** – in that the client wishes to walk to perform an occupational activity

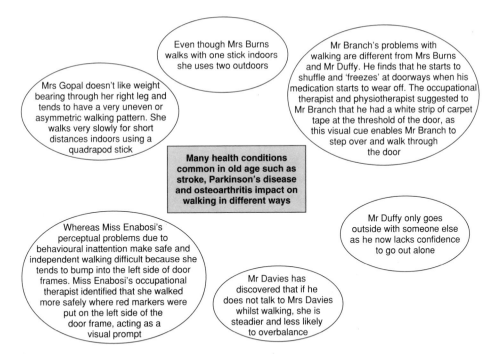

Figure 8.1 Walking difficulties caused by stroke, Parkinson's disease and osteoarthritis.

such as shopping, going to the toilet, carrying washing to the clothesline. It is therefore necessary to consider walking in the context of the activity being carried out as this will determine how far, how quickly, where and when an individual walks. Walking indoors for example has different demands of **body functions** (such as vision, balance) than walking outdoors on uneven ground (see Figure 8.2). Many assessments include mobility along with self-care items in personal activity of daily living assessments; however, these do not always discriminate between different walking demands. This is also reflected in research where determining severity of walking problems vary, with Rantanen *et al.* (2001) defining severe disability as being unable to walk ¼ mile (400 m approx), and the HSE (DH 2001) considering that an individual able to walk 200 m or more without discomfort had no disability.

Stair climbing

Falling on the stairs is the most common accident in the home, most often when descending rather than ascending the stairs (Gnanasekaran 2002); 10% of older people in England are unable to climb stairs (ONS 2002).

Stair climbing and descending use a similar movement pattern as walking with a swing through and stance phase; however stair climbing requires greater range of movement and muscle strength in the legs, either to carry the body upward on an extending knee or controlling the descent on a flexing knee. The deterioration

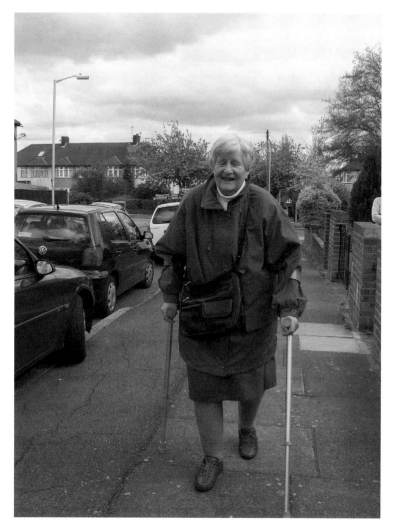

Figure 8.2 Post-operative mobility products make walking outdoors easier and safer.

in lower limb muscle strength observed in older people can make stair climbing difficult, impossible or hazardous. The reliance upon sensory input (especially visual cues) to determine an appropriate strategy when stair climbing, must also be appreciated (Shumway-Cook & Woollacott 2001).

Use of mobility products

Consideration of walking products within an **environmental context** is a very relevant part of an occupational therapist's role. An awareness of the appropriateness of the product issued within the client's context is important and an understanding of the correct and safest method of usage is crucial (see Chapter 10) as any type of walking equipment can increase risk of injury if used or maintained incorrectly. Inability to learn the new skills required with walking aid use (such as a frame or tripod) and the potential alteration to an automatic walking pattern can increase a risk of falls ands reduce mobility in an older person with cognitive and perceptual impairment.

Provision of **walking products** has been scrutinised because of reported non-use of equipment when issued to older people (Edwards & Jones 1998). It is therefore important to consider not only the impairment the client has, or may have in the future, but also their attitude and safety awareness, the **environmental context**, as well as the advantages and disadvantages of the various types of equipment. Walking products are provided to ensure greater stability and support for the individual, but in many instances requires different walking patterns.

For many the only alternative mobility product is a wheelchair – whether self or attendant propelled, or electrically powered. Wheelchair provision is not an easy option and has different performance requirements from walking; these issues are considered in Chapter 10.

Box 8.6

Consider an older person you know

- Identify what personal and external factors facilitate their mobility.
- Consider any potential barriers.
- What could an occupational therapist and/or team offer to optimise their potential?
- Is there any place for health promotion strategies for this individual and people in their situation?

Self-care

Whereas movement suggests the physical interaction between the person and their immediate **environment**, the domain of self-care is very much concerned with the person and their body. A recent survey identified that 66% of women and 58% of men in residential care experience problems with self-care (DH 2001), which can arise equally from a mental health problem as from a physical disability (such as that experienced by Mrs Davies and Mr Jones in Chapter 5). Independence in self-care (or BADL) is commonly assumed in all adults, and traditionally striving to maintain independence has been a key issue for occupational therapists. However not all older clients wish for independence; this may be due to cultural differences (Gibbs and Barnitt 1999) or due to fear and anxiety (e.g. **falling** again), having an over-protective carer or through disengagement (see Chapter 1 for ageing theories) (Sirkka and Bränholm 2003).

Washing oneself

How often do you wash? This question could be considered intrusive, and yet personal hygiene is critical to our social acceptance. It is important to recognise the significance of the cleansing process. Within the ICF washing oneself also includes showering and bathing and many recipients of occupational therapy services will emphasise the spiritual, relaxing, pain-relieving and purifying effect of immersion in water (Gooch 2003). Thus the occupation of bathing has multiple meanings: however, this is not always recognised in eligibility criteria for equipment – the emphasis on personal hygiene prevails, which causes conflict between service users and occupational therapy services.

Bathing could also be considered a dangerous activity, especially for older people, with RoSPA (2002) and Gooptu & Mulley (1994) identifying the risk of burns, **falling** (and drowning) in the bath as well as inability to get out of the bath leading to pressure sores, hypothermia and psychological consequences. The occurrence of these distressing incidences with older people demonstrate not only the impairment of body functions, but more importantly the barriers within their environments, through poor bath design, poor thermal regulation, lack or poorly positioned assistive products and alarms. However most bathing assessments are undertaken in 'dry' or simulated situations, assessing **capacity**, whereas the actual **performance** of the activity is what should be assessed in the client's own home observing a 'wet' bath (Gooch 2003).

Caring for body parts

This category separates out those body parts, which require more care than washing and drying. The absence of older people in media imagery associated with skin, hair and nail care may influence the lack of attention given to these aspects of self-care in many occupational therapy and ADL assessments. It could be argued that that skin, foot-care, and dental hygiene are not traditionally domains of occupational therapy; as already discussed in Chapter 7, these all impact both directly and indirectly on occupational performance. A prime example is the contribution of poor foot care (and long toenails) to balance problems and **falls** in older people (Burns *et al.* 2002). For clients like Mr Crabtree with **diabetes** (see Chapter 5), advice on well-fitting shoes and socks will form part of an occupational therapy assessment for both client and carer. Therefore, the occupational therapist has a responsibility to older people to ensure that these aspects of self-care are addressed.

Toileting

Toileting is a complex activity, requiring ability in mobility, transfers and dressing as well as **body functions** and **structures** to maintain continence in both urine and faeces. Some of these difficulties considered by occupational therapists in relation to toileting have already been discussed in this chapter, and the issue of urinary and faecal continence in Chapter 7. For many older people, problems with toileting can restrict their **participation** in social and leisure activities because of **environmental barriers** and poor design of public toilets for those people with mobility problems. Many older people (46%) in residential care have problems with toileting (DH 2001), and for the older person loss of independence in this activity is accompanied by a loss of privacy and dignity reminiscent of early childhood.

Dressing

The ICF describes dressing as the action of putting on clothes and footwear, and taking them off (WHO 2001). Dressing is a complex activity involving many sub-tasks and demands on **body functions** and **structures**. Choosing clothes appropriate for the **climate, culture** and time is important and will determine what is worn, the complexity and number of stages. Whereas difficulties with the physical manipulation of clothes may be easier to identify the challenge for many occupational therapists, working with older people is to unravel the problems arising from cognitive, perceptual and affective disorders. Because of its complexity, dressing involves those specific cognitive functions of sustained and selective attention as well as executive functions, which are, as already stated in Chapter 6, most noticeably impaired in clients with **Alzheimer's disease, learning disability, stroke** and **Parkinson's disease** (Bellelli *et al.* 2002). Spatial neglect, following **stroke** also impacts on successful dressing, with failure to dress the affected side and apraxia which causes problems with the sequencing of the order of dressing (Walker *et al.* 2003).

The skills of the occupational therapist will be to determine when and what type of assistance an older person may require, for example the teaching of energy-conserving techniques for those with cardiovascular or respiratory conditions, or of carers where physical or verbal assistance is required. The use of compensatory techniques involving the use of dressing products may overcome difficulties with reaching, gripping clothing and managing fastenings. For some older people changing the type of clothing worn may be acceptable, as less energy and cognitive functioning may be required to put on light stretchy clothing with fewer fastenings.

Eating and drinking

Eating and drinking are separate categories in the ICF, in contrast to other classification systems, which distinguish between eating and feeding (AOTA 2002). Eating and drinking as defined by the ICF includes a wider view of the whole process of consuming food and drink (WHO 2001). For many older people in residential care, eating and drinking are problematic (DH 2001). Jacobsson *et al.* (2000) describe the experiences of many older people after **stroke**:

- Many have fear of choking.
- Discomfort in the mouth and throat.
- Discomfort from food.
- Thirst from not being able to drink from a glass.
- Shame from their appearance – such as dribbling and facial paralysis.

- Humiliation at dependence in being fed.
- Feelings of clumsiness due to poor manual dexterity.

The need for good nutrition in later life is addressed both in this chapter and in Chapter 7, and the need for good dentition and swallowing have also been discussed in Chapter 7. Eating and feeding is an activity where many members of the interprofessional team may be working alongside each other, with the speech and language therapist and physiotherapist being concerned with the **body functions** and **structures** involved with swallowing and positioning, such as muscle tone, reflex activity and sensation; the nurse and dietician being concerned with nutritional and digestive issues; and the occupational therapist being more concerned with **activity** and **environmental issues** such as positioning, compensatory techniques and assistive equipment. Eating and drinking provides a good example of the use of the ICF as a framework in identifying different roles of team members working with an older person with the same activity.

Looking after one's health

Looking after one's health is central to the WHO's policy on **active ageing** (WHO 2002) with issues of **health promotion** being crucial. Health professionals are required to ensure the older person has opportunities to access information and resources, which promote a healthy lifestyle and live in healthy and conducive **environments** (see Chapters 1 and 10). The study by Miller & Iris (2002) (Box 8.7) indicates a broader interpretation of what constitutes a healthy lifestyle. In the past, being independent in self-care was considered an important indicator of health, even when it involved the use of **assistive products**. The three main components within the ICF of this category are:

- Ensuring one's physical comfort.
- Managing diet and fitness.
- Maintaining one's health.

What would stop an older person being able to ensure their own physical comfort? Discomfort is usually indicated by pain or altered sensation, so impairment

Box 8.7 What does being healthy involve in older age?

Miller & Iris (2002) investigated the perspectives of 45 older adults via focus groups and questionnaires. They wanted to know what the participants thought about health and wellbeing. The themes emerging suggested aspects of health in older age: 'functional independence, self-care management of illness, positive outlook, and personal growth and social contribution.' Health was much more than the absence of disease. Meaningful occupation was recognised as promoting health, and the authors recommended that health promotion programmes expand to consider aspects beyond exercise and diet.

of sensory perception, especially the sense of touch, will impair the ability to perceive discomfort. An occupational therapist will have particular responsibility for pressure care for those who are immobile for significant periods of time: this could involve interventions such as prescribing cushions for wheelchair users. Discomfort can also be experienced in terms of temperature and so heating and ventilation should comprise part of a home assessment (see Chapter 10).

The benefits of physical exercise and good nutrition are important throughout the lifespan, with McCarter & Kelly (1993) suggesting that not only do these facilitate prevention of disease, but also prolong healthier lives with an improvement in the biological age by 10–20 years. Studies show that a good diet in later years helps both in reducing the risk and in managing diseases, such as **heart disease, cancers, diabetes, stroke,** and **osteoporosis,** which are the leading cause of death and disability among older persons. This in turn can enable older people to maintain their independence. There is evidence that the nutritional status of patients has been neglected by health and social care professionals (Royal College of Physicians 2002) (see Chapter 7). Occupational therapists need to consider all aspects of access and management of a healthy diet for older clients; from planning and acquisition of healthy balanced meals, to preparation, storage, feeding and eating.

As already discussed previously, age itself is not a barrier to physical exercise and current **theories of ageing** consider that a decline in physical activity is not necessarily a part of normal ageing. However, a decline in physical activity is associated with an increase in chronic diseases and therefore an increase in or maintenance of physical activity throughout life and into old age maintains **activity** and active **participation** and decreases or slows the onset of disability (Penninx *et al.* 2001). The literature identifies that regular exercise in older adults reduces the risk of **cardiovascular disease** (Manson *et al.* 2002), **osteoporosis and non-insulin dependent diabetes** (NIDDM) (Young & Dinan 1994) and cognitive decline (Yaffe *et al.* 2001), and is said to improve **depressive** symptoms in older adults (Mather *et al.* 2002). A daily 30-minute regime of moderate exercise is recommended for older people (WHO 1998). Even though moderate exercise includes stair climbing, housework, gardening, lifting weights and wheelchair use; the most common form of exercise undertaken is walking. This is dependent on the access to safe, conducive, and **healthy environments** (WHO 2002) and many local authorities in the UK provide organised walks or dedicated ramble routes as well as physical activity programmes, as part of their health promotion initiatives. It is therefore important for the occupational therapist to consider the physical activity aspect of productivity as part of primary, secondary, and tertiary **health promotion.**

The implications of a good diet and regular exercise are not only to maintain health but also to prevent the onset of disease or disability. Many older people take medication because of disability or disease, and the usage of medication increases with age. The Health Survey for England (HSE) (DH 2000) identified that 80% of older people regularly take prescribed medication with 35% of over 75-year-olds taking four or more different prescribed medications daily (polypharmacy). Even though these treat the symptoms of disease, many risks are associated with the taking of medication in older age, especially with polypharmacy. Risks include complex dosage schedules, interactions of multiple medications, adverse drug reactions, re-admission to hospital and **falls**. Issues with medication in older people are:

- A narrower margin between therapeutic and toxic dosage due to an age-related decline in renal function.
- Adverse drug reactions (hypotension as a result of hypnotic or diuretic medication increasing risk of falls; non-steroidal anti-inflammatories (NSAIDs) causing gastrointestinal bleeding).
- Under-prescribing of medication.
- Medications are used incorrectly or underused by older people.
- Repeat prescriptions can be wasted or inappropriately used.
- Difficulty accessing general practitioner's surgery or pharmacy.
- Inability by older person to read or understand medication information or open packaging (DH 2001).

Box 8.8

As an occupational therapist it is important to appreciate what medication an individual takes, when and how often because of the impact on occupational performance. The Royal Pharmaceutical Society of Great Britain (2002) suggests that any health professional taking part in the single assessment process should consider the following:

- Can the older person get a regular supply of their medication?
- Can the older person understand and be able to take the medication as required?
- Can they open the medicine bottle or blister pack?
- Is the medication 'doing the job' required?

Consider Mr Branch (from Chapter 6) and the role of medication in the 'on–off' phenomena he experiences and how it affects his everyday activity. What are the issues for Mr Branch? How might the OT be involved?

Maintenance of health of older people should be promoted through initiatives to encourage a healthy lifestyle, regular exercise and healthy eating, cessation of smoking, control of excessive alcohol consumption, home safety and prevention of accidents, social support and welfare benefit advice, uptake of immunisations (influenza vaccinations), bereavement counselling, monitoring of blood pressure and an annual over-75 health check (British Geriatrics Society 2002). As much of this is reliant on the older person having insight and motivation to maintain a healthy and safe lifestyle, it is important that the occupational therapist can enable and facilitate their older clients to look after their own health.

Domestic life areas

Home is the setting for daily life and the base from which the wider **community and social networks** are experienced (as described in Chapter 3). The **home**

environment may have defined areas: privacy for self-care activities, refuge for rest and communal spaces. Successive governments have long accepted the importance of older people remaining in their own home for as long as possible (Elkan *et al.* 2001) and most occupational therapy with older people focuses on this. Outcome measures such as the **Westmead Home Safety Assessment** (Clemson 1997) and the Community Dependency Index (Eakin and Baird 1995) have been developed by occupational therapists to use within the home **environment**; however, the emphasis of assessment by occupational therapists differs according to the remit of their employer (i.e. health or social care). Home assessment may consider:

- A pre-discharge observation to ensure the older person's safety at home.
- Modification of the home environment to prevent further injury or disability.
- Observation of the older person's actual performance of everyday activity.

Even though these are integral parts of occupational therapy practice, their efficacy is currently being questioned with lack of strong evidence from two Cochrane reviews for modifications to the home **environment** for older clients (Gillespie *et al.* 2002; Lyons *et al.* 2004). Mountain and Pighills (2003) have also recommended that the practice of hospital pre-discharge home visits needs reappraisal as these seem to address short-term post-discharge safety and capacity to carry out certain activities rather than being in the interest of the older client or carer by considering actual performance of those activities important to them. A stronger evidence base is needed, reflecting occupational therapy values of client-centred practice, using outcome measures that can accurately reflect practice.

Acquisition of goods and services

As can be demonstrated in Chapter 4, older people are entitled to an overwhelming array of public services, and both the service and eligibility criteria can change at an alarming rate. Inadequate services can lead to exclusion, forcing dependence and therefore disability onto many older people. The increasingly popular use of the Internet amongst older people (see Chapter 9) has meant that older people have greater access to information and services. The use of Internet shopping, alongside mail order shopping, for example, means that many older people who lack the capacity to shop are able to perform this activity independently, even though they may have outdoor mobility and transportation problems.

Household tasks

Preparation of meals
Nutritional requirements change as people age and an inadequate intake of food and fluid is associated with diverse symptoms. These issues have already been discussed (see Chapter 7) and it is important for the occupational therapist to consider what is being consumed as well as how it is consumed. A home-based assessment is a good opportunity to explore what routines for eating and drinking

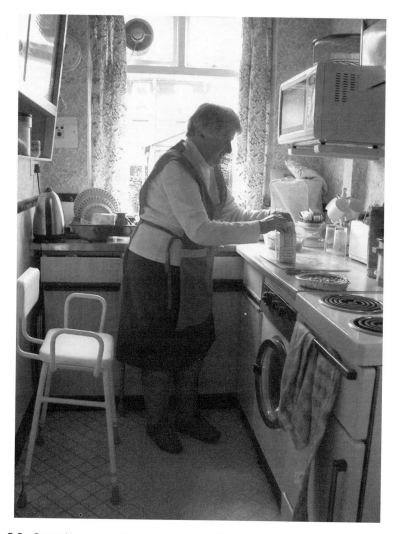

Figure 8.3 Preparing a meal involves many cognitive, perceptual and physical demands.

are established. Many routines and habits associated with meal preparation are culturally determined or will reflect a particular problem-solving strategy (Gibbs and Barnitt 1999).

In meal preparation, there are many ways of grading the complexity, which should always reflect what might realistically be expected or achieved on a long-term basis. The longer a meal takes to prepare, the more complex the preparation will be and the more demands it places on the person preparing (Figure 8.3).

Both Creek (1996) and Fair and Barnitt (1999) have studied the activity of making a cup of tea in more detail, establishing the complexity, cultural, regional and generational differences that need consideration in an assessment that occupational therapists carry out on a regular basis. Creek (1996) suggests that occupational therapists should concentrate on the process of tea-making rather than the outcome, and this principle can be applied to many everyday activities, such as dressing, where the task is complex and requires interplay between **body functions** and **structures** with personal and environmental contexts for successful completion. By considering the process of carrying out the activity, problem areas can be observed and analysed, so that problems with successful completion can be identified, or that possible future problems prevented.

Doing housework

Occupational therapy assessment will rarely involve direct observation of all these elements of housework and a client-centred approach will highlight what is a priority. Impairment of **body function** may impact on the housework required: for example, incontinence and/or feeding difficulties may result in extra laundry. Movement disorders may create difficulties in cleaning, using household appliances: for example, manoeuvring a vacuum cleaner or operating controls on cookers and disposing of rubbish. Sirkka & Bränholm (2003) identified that many older people following hip **fracture** had problems with cleaning and laundry.

Summary

This chapter has considered five domains: learning and applying knowledge, general tasks and demands, mobility, self-care and domestic life. For the older person the importance of these areas will be a personal perspective, and may alter as their situation changes. Issues may emerge over time, which were not immediately apparent at initial assessment, with assessment and outcome measurement taking into account the possible discrepancy between an older person's **capacity** and **performance** (Bootsma-van der Wiel *et al.* 2001). A partnership between the occupational therapist, the older person and their support network, with an awareness of their environment will enable the focus of therapy to be effective and meaningful. The complex nature of occupation demands this: occupation-based interventions for these domains will enable a realistic understanding of the issues to be achieved.

References

Age Concern (2003) *Age Concern's Response to the National Alcohol Harm Reduction Strategy*. London: Age Concern Policy Unit.

Alcohol Concern (2002) Alcohol misuse among older people. *Acquire* Autumn 2002.

Alexander NB, Schultz AB, Warwick DN (1991) Rising from a chair: effects of age and functional ability on performance biomechanics. *Journal of Gerontology* 46(3): M91–8.

Allen CK, Earhart CA, Blue T (1992) *Occupational Therapy Treatment Goals for the Physically and Cognitively Disabled*. USA: The American Occupational Therapy Association.

Alzheimer's Society (2000) *Maintaining Skills: An Advice Sheet for Carers*. London: Alzheimer's Society.

American Occupational Therapy Association (2002) Occupational therapy practice framework: domain and process. *American Journal of Occupational Therapy* 56(6), 609–639.

Bellelli G, Lucchi E, Cipriani G (2002) Executive dysfunction and depressive symptoms in cerebrovascular disease (Letter). *Journal of Neurology, Neurosurgery and Psychiatry* 73(4), 460–464.

Bootsma-van der Wiel A, Gussekloo J, de Craen AJM *et al.* (2001) Disability in the oldest-old: can do or 'do do'? *Journal of the American Geriatrics Society* 49(7), 909–914.

Bowen A, Wenman R, Mickelborough J, Foster J, Hill E, Tallis R (2001) Dual task effects of talking while walking on velocity and balance following a stroke. *Age and Ageing* 30(4), 319–323.

Brach JS & Van Swearingen JM (2002) Physical impairment and disability: relationship to performance of activities of daily living in community dwelling older men. *Physical Therapy* 82(8), 752–761.

Brach JS, Van Swearingen JM, Newman AB, Krishka AM (2002) Identifying early decline of physical function in community dwelling older women: Performance based and self-report measures. *Physical Therapy* 82(4), 320–328.

British Geriatrics Society (2002) *Standards of Care for Specialist Services for Older People.* London: British Geriatrics Society.

Bryant W (1991) Creative groupwork and the elderly mentally ill: a development of sensory integration therapy. *British Journal of Occupational Therapy* 54(5), 187–192.

Burns SL, Leese GP, McMurdo MET (2002) Older people and ill fitting shoes. *Postgraduate Medicine Journal* 78(3), 344–346.

Christiansen CH & Baum C (1997) Understanding occupation: definition and concepts. In: Christiansen CH & Baum C (eds). *Enabling Function and Well-Being*, 2nd edn. New Jersey: Slack.

Clemson L (1997) *Home Fall Hazards and the Westmead Home Safety Assessment.* West Brunswick, Australia: Coordinates Publications.

College of Occupational Therapists (2002) *From Interface to Integration: A Strategy for Modernising Occupational Therapy Services in Local Health and Social Care Communities.* London: College of Occupational Therapists.

Cooper C (2003) Hand impairments. In: Trombly CA & Radomski MV (eds). *Occupational Therapy for Physical Dysfunction*, 5th edn. Baltimore: Lippincott, Williams and Wilkins.

Costa LD, Vaughan HG, Levita E, Farber N (1963) Purdue pegboard as a predictor of the presence of the laterality of cerebral lesions. *Journal of Consulting Psychology* 27, 133–137.

Crawford S & Channon S (2002) Dissociation between performance of abstract tests of executive functioning and problem solving in real-life-type situations in normal aging. *Aging and Mental Health* 6(1), 12–21.

Creek J (1996) Making a cup of tea as an honours degree subject. *British Journal of Occupational Therapy* 59(3), 128–130.

Creek J (2003) *Occupational Therapy Defined as a Complex Intervention.* London: College of Occupational Therapists.

Department of Health (2000) *The Health Survey for England (HSE).* London: HMSO.

Desrosiers J, Hebert R, Bravo G, Dutil E (1995) Shoulder range of motion of healthy elderly people: a normative study. *Physical and Occupational Therapy in Geriatrics* 13(1/2), 101–128.

Desrosiers J, Hebert R, Bravo G, Rochette A (1999) Age-related changes in upper extremity performance of elderly people: a longitudinal study. *Experimental Gerontology* 34(3), 393–405.

Eakin P, Baird H (1995) The community dependency index: a standardised assessment of need and measure of outcome for community occupational therapy. *British Journal of Occupational Therapy* 58(1), 17–22.

Economic and Social Research Council (2001) *Exploring the Perceptions of Quality of Life of Frail Older People During and After their Transition into Institutional Care: Study Within The ESRC Growing Older Research Programme.* York: Economic and Social Research Council. Accessed 24.04.2004. http://www.dass.stir.ac.uk/SSP/ESRC/focus-group.htm 16/03/2004.

Edwards NI & Jones DA (1998) Ownership and use of assistive devices amongst older people in the community. *Age and Ageing* 27(4), 463–468.

Erikson E (1950) *Childhood and Society.* Middlesex: Penguin.

Elkan R, Kendrick D, Dewey M *et al.* (2001) Effectiveness of home based support for older people: systematic review and meta-analysis. *British Medical Journal* 323, 1–9.

Fair A & Barnitt R (1999) Making a cup of tea as part of a culturally sensitive service. *British Journal of Occupational Therapy* 62(5), 199–205.

Ferris AM & Duffy VB (1989) Effect of olfactory deficits on nutritional status. Does age predict persons at risk? *Annals of the New York Academy of Science* 561, 113–123.

Fisher AG (1995) *The Assessment of Motor and Process Skills.* Colorado: Three Star Press.

Fricke J & Unsworth C (2001) Time Use and importance of instrumental activities of daily living. *Australian Journal of Occupational Therapy* 48(3), 118–131.

Gibbs KE & Barnitt R (1999) Occupational therapy and the self-care needs of Hindu elders. *British Journal of Occupational Therapy* 62(3), 100–106.

Gillespie LD, Gillespie WJ, Robertson MC, Lamb SE, Cumming RG, Rowe BH (2002) Interventions for preventing falls in elderly people. *Cochrane Database of Systematic Reviews* No. 4, CD000340.

Gilliard J & Rabins PV (1999) Carer support. In: Wilcock GK, Bucks RS, Rockwood K (eds). *Diagnosis and management of dementia: a manual for memory disorders teams.* Oxford: Oxford Medical Publications, pp. 279–293.

Gnanasekaran L (2002) Performance of functional movements. In: Tyldelsley B & Grieve JI. *Muscles, Nerves and Movement in Human Occupation,* 3rd edn. Oxford: Blackwell Publishing.

Gooch H (2003) Assessment of bathing in occupational therapy. *British Journal of Occupational Therapy* 66(9), 402–408.

Gooptu C & Mulley GP (1994) Survey of elderly people who get stuck in the bath. *British Medical Journal* 308, 762.

Hagedorn R (1996) *Occupational Therapy: Perspectives and Processes.* Edinburgh: Churchill Livingstone.

Haggard P, Cockburn J, Cock J, Fordham C, Wade D (2000) Interference between gait and cognitive tasks in a rehabilitating neurological population. *Journal of Neurology, Neurosurgery and Psychiatry* 69(4), 479–486.

Harvey A & Pentland W (2003) What do people do? In: Christiansen C, Townsend EA (eds). *Introduction to Occupation: The Art and Science of Living.* Thorofare, NJ: Prentice Hall, pp. 63–90.

Hasher L, Stoltzfus ER, Zacks RT, Rypma B (1991) Age and inhibition. *Journal of Experimental Psychology: Learning, Memory and Cognition* 17(1), 163–169.

Hastings M (1998) The brain, circadian rhythms, and clock genes. *British Medical Journal* 317, 1704–1707.

Hayase D, Mosenteen D, Thimmaiah D, Zemke S, Atler K, Fisher AG (2004) Age-related changes in activities of daily living ability. *Australian Occupational Therapy Journal* 51(4), 192–198.

Hauer K, Pfisterer M, Weber C, Wezler N, Kliegel M, Oster P (2003) Cognitive impairment decreases postural control during dual tasks in geriatric patients with a history of severe falls. *Journal of the American Geriatric Society* 5(11), 1638–1644.

Iezzoni LI, McCarthy EP, Davis RB, Siebens H (2001) Mobility difficulties are not only a problem of old age. *Journal of General Internal Medicine* 16(4), 235–243.

Imms FJ & Edholm OG (1981) Studies of gait and mobility in the elderly. *Age and Ageing* 10(3), 47–156.

Jacobsson C, Axelsson K, Österlind PO, Norberg A (2000) How people with stroke and healthy older people experience the eating process. *Journal of Clinical Nursing* 9, 255–264.

Jebsen RH, Taylor N, Trieschmann RB, Trotter MJ, Howard LA (1969), An objective and standardised test of hand function. *Archives of Physical Medicine and Rehabilitation* 50, 311–319.

Law M, Baum C, Dunn W (2001) (eds). *Measuring Occupational Performance: Supporting Best Practice in Occupational Therapy*. Thorofare NJ: Slack.

Lundin-Olsson L, Nyberg L, Gustafson Y (1997) 'Stops walking when talking' as a predictor of falls in elderly people. *Lancet* 349, 617.

Lyons RA, Sander LV, Weightman AL *et al.* (2004) *Modification of the Home Environment for the Reduction of Injuries* (Cochrane Review). The Cochrane Library, Issue 3. Chichester: John Wiley.

Manson JE, Greenland P, LaCroix AZ *et al.* (2002) Walking compared with vigorous exercise for the prevention of cardiovascular events in women. *New England Journal of Medicine* 347(10), 716–725.

Martin M & Ewert O (1997) Attention and planning in older adults. *International Journal of Behavioural Development* 20(4), 577–594.

Mather AS, Rodriguez C, Guthrie MF, McHarg AM, Reid IC, McMurdo MET (2002) Effects of exercise on depressive symptoms in older adults with poorly responsive depressive disorder. *British Journal of Psychiatry* 180, 411–415.

Mathiowetz V, Kashman N, Volland G, Weber K, Dowe, Rogers S (1985) Grip and pinch strength: Normative data for adults. *Archives of Physical Medicine and Rehabilitation* 66(2), 69–74.

Mattingley C & Fleming MH (1994) *Clinical Reasoning*. Philadelphia: Slack.

McCarter RJ & Kelly NG (1993) Cellular basis of ageing in skeletal muscle. In: Coe RM, Perry HM (eds). *Ageing, Musculoskeletal Disorders and Care of the Frail Elderly*. New York: Springer.

McIlroy WE & Maki BE (1994) Compensatory arm movements evoked by transient perturbations of upright stance. In: Taguchi K, Igarashi M, Mori S (eds). *Vestibular and Neural Front*. New York: Elsevier Science.

Menz HB, Lord SR, Fitzpatrick C (2003) Age-related differences in walking stability. *Age and Ageing* 32(2), 137–142.

Miller AM & Iris M (2002) Health promotion attitudes and strategies in older adults. *Health Education and Behavior* 29(2), 249–267.

Mountain G & Pighills A (2003) Pre-discharge home visits with older people: time to review practice. *Health and Social Care in the Community* 11(2) 146–154.

Oakley F, Duran L, Fisher A, Merritt B (2003) Differences in activities of daily living motor skills of persons with and without Alzheimer's disease. *Australian Occupational Therapy Journal* 50(2), 72–78.

Office for National Statistics (2002) *Living in Britain: Results from the 2001 General Household Survey*. London: Office for National Statistics.

Penninx BW, Messier SP, Rejeski WJ *et al.* (2001) Physical exercise and the prevention of disability in activity of daily living in older persons with osteoarthritis. *Archives of Internal Medicine* 161(19), 2309–2316.

Petrofsky JS, Bweir S, Anda A, Chavez J, Crane A, Saunders J, Layman M (2003) Towards an objective method of gait analysis. *International Journal of Therapy and Rehabilitation* 10(10), 463–472.

Pfeiffer B (2002) *Understanding Older People's Stress*. Accessed 16.03.2004. http://www.outreach.missouri.edu/cmregion/thriving/archives2002/2002%20November/ Understanding%20Older%20People's%20Stress.html

Rabbitt P (1993) Does it all go together when it goes? *Quarterly Journal of Experimental Psychology* 46(3), 385–434.

Rabbitt P (1997) Ageing and human skill: a 40th anniversary. *Ergonomics* 40(10), 962–981.

Ranganathen VK, Siemionow V, Sahgal V, Yue GH (2001) Effects of ageing on hand function. *Journal of the American Geriatrics Society* 49(11),1478–1484.

Rantanen T, Guralnik JM, Ferucci L, Penninx BWJH, Leveille S, Sipila S, Fried LP (2001) Coimpairments as predictors of severe walking disability in older women. *Journal of the American Geriatrics Society* 49(1), 21–27.

Rantanen T, Volpato S, Ferucci L, Heikkinen E, Fried LP, Guralnik JM (2003) Hand grip strength and cause-specific and total mortality in older disabled women: exploring the mechanism. *Journal of the American Geriatrics Society* 51(5), 636–641.

Reed KL & Sanderson SN (1999) *Concepts of Occupational Therapy*, 4th edn. Philadelphia: Lippincott. Williams and Wilkins.

Reese AC & Simpson JM (1996) Preparing older people to cope after a fall. *Physiotherapy* 82(4), 227–235.

RoSPA (2002) *Can the Home Ever Be Safe?* Birmingham: Royal Society for the Prevention of Accidents.

Royal College of Physicians (2002) *Nutrition and Patients: A Doctor's Responsibility*. London: Royal College of Physicians.

Royal Pharmaceutical Society of Great Britain (2002) *Questions to be Asked as Part of the Single Assessment Process*. Accessed 31.03.2004. http://www.rpsgb.org.uk/nhsplan/pdfs/ oldnsfmedasstoolforms.pdf

Samaritans (2000) *Older People and Suicide*. Accessed 23.03.2004. http://www.samaritans.org.uk/know/statistics_suic_op_popup.shtm

Sirkka M & Bränholm I-B (2003) Consequences of a hip fracture in activity performance and life satisfaction in an elderly Swedish clientele. *Scandinavian Journal of Occupational Therapy* 10, 34–39.

Shiffman LM (1992) Effects of ageing on adult hand function. *American Journal of Occupational Therapy* 46(9), 785–792.

Shumway-Cook A & Woollacott MH (2001) *Motor Control: Theory and Applications*, 2nd edn. Baltimore: Lippincott, Williams and Wilkins.

Simpson JM, Marsh N, Harrington R (1998) Managing falls among elderly people. *British Journal of Occupational Therapy* 61(4), 165–168.

Singer BR, McLauchlan GJ, Robinson CM, Christie J (1998) Epidemiology of fractures in 15 000 adults: the influence of age and gender. *Journal of Bone and Joint Surgery* 80(2), 243–248.

Steel N, Huppert FA, McWilliams B, Melzer D (2003) Physical and cognitive function. In: Marmot M, Banks J, Blundell R, Lessof C, Nazroo J (eds). *Health, Wealth and Lifestyles of the Older Population in England. The 2002 English Longitudinal Study of Ageing.* London: Institute for Fiscal Studies.

Taub E, Crago JE, Uswatte G (1998) Constraint-induced movement therapy: a new approach to treatment in physical rehabilitation. *Rehabilitation Psychology* 43(2), 152–170.

Tiffin J (1968) *Purdue Pegboard Examiner Manual.* Chicago: Science Research Associates.

Trew M & Everitt T (2001) *Human Movement: An Introductory Text,* 4th edn. London: Harcourt.

Turner A (2002) Occupation for therapy. In: Turner A, Foster M, Johnson SE. *Occupational Therapy for Physical Dysfunction: Principles, Skills and Practice,* 5th edn. London: Churchill Livingstone.

United Nations (2002) *Building a Society for all Ages: HIV/AIDs and Older People.* Accessed 16.03.2004. http://www.un.org/ageing/prkit/hivaids.htm

Unsworth C (2000) Measuring the outcome of occupational therapy: tools and resources. *Australian Journal of Occupational Therapy* 47(4), 147–158.

Verghese J, Buschke H, Viola L, Katz M, Hall C, Kuslansky G, Lipton R (2002) Validity of divided attention tasks in predicting falls in older individuals: A preliminary study. *Journal of the American Geriatric Society* 50(9), 1572–1576.

Walker CM, Walker MF, Sunderland A (2003) Dressing after stroke: a survey of current occupational therapy practice. *British Journal of Occupational Therapy* 66(6), 263–268.

Ward NS & Frackowiak SJ (2003) Age-related changes in the neural correlates of motor performance. *Brain* 126(4), 873–888.

Welford AT (1958) *Ageing and Human Skill,* 1st edn. Oxford: Oxford University Press.

Wild D, Nayak US, Isaac B (1981) How dangerous are falls to older people at home? *British Medical Journal* 282, 266–268.

Winward CE, Hallgan PW, Wade DT (2000) *Rivermead Assessment of Somatosensory Performance.* Bury St Edmunds: Thames Valley Test Co.

Woodruff-Pak DS (1997) *The Neuropsychology of Aging.* Malden, USA: Blackwell Publishing.

World Health Organisation (1998) *The Role of Physical Activity in Healthy Ageing.* Geneva: World Health Organisation Ageing and Health Programme.

World Health Organisation (2001) *The International Classification of Functioning Disability and Health.* Geneva: World Health Organisation.

World Health Organisation (2002) *Physical Activity Through Transport as Part of Daily Activities.* Geneva: World Health Organisation Regional Office for Europe.

Yaffe K, Barnes D, Nevitt M, Lui L, Covinsky K (2001) A prospective study of physical activity and cognitive decline in elderly women. *Archives of Internal Medicine* 161(14), 1703–1708.

Yardley L, Gardner M, Bronstein A, Davies R, Buckwell D, Luxon L (2001) Interference between postural control and mental task performance in patients with vestibular disorder and healthy controls. *Journal of Neurology, Neurosurgery and Psychiatry* 71(1), 48–52.

Young A & Dinan S (1994) ABC of Sports Medicine: Fitness for older people. *British Medical Journal* 309, 331–334.

Chapter 9

ACTIVITY AND PARTICIPATION: PART 2

Lesley Wilson

This chapter will introduce and consider the remaining four domains identified by the World Health Organisation's (WHO) International Classification of Function (ICF) (WHO 2001) from an occupational therapist's perspective in relation to older people.

The four domains are concerned with communication, interpersonal relationships, major life areas in later years and being part of community and civic life. Essentially, this chapter is about older people 'being' and 'doing' in relationship to others rather than 'being done to'.

For clarity, the four domains and their subsections are summarised in Box 9.1 (p. 188).

Within these subsections, as already described in the previous chapter, the two dimensions, **activity** and **participation** are used as lenses to focus on the occupational aspects of each category. In other words, the innate capacity of a person to engage in these life skills is viewed alongside their actual performance in a real situation. At the risk of stating the obvious, it is not always sufficient to have the ability and the will to do something if barriers in the **environment** or other restrictions will not allow for a successful outcome.

This is true for all people but is especially pertinent for older people who are living longer. Potentially there will be more restrictions, both seen and unseen, due to the ageing process itself and due to the way in which our society regards old people (Shaw 1991). As already explored in previous chapters, stereotypes abound and occupational therapists have an obligation to alleviate wherever possible these restrictive circumstances with and on behalf of older people (College of Occupational Therapists [COT] 2000).

The reality of what all this means for older people will be explored, using case examples from the previous chapter to illustrate the text. The role of the occupational therapist as a facilitator and enabler will be highlighted where appropriate.

Communication

As outlined in Chapter 3, communication is an essential part of maintaining **social networks**. Various **products and technology** (see Chapter 10) can enable older

Box 9.1 The ICF domains and summarised sub-sections (WHO 2001).

- **Communication**
  Receiving spoken messages
  Receiving non-verbal messages
  Speaking
  Producing non-verbal messages
  Conversation

- **Interpersonal interactions and relationships**
  Basic interpersonal interactions
  Complex interpersonal interactions
  Relating with strangers
  Formal relationships
  Informal relationships
  Family relationships
  Intimate relationships

- **Major life areas**
  Informal education
  School education
  Higher education
  Remunerative employment
  Basic economic transactions
  Economic self-sufficiency

- **Community, social and civic life**
  Community life
  Recreation and leisure
  Religion and spirituality
  Human rights
  Political life and citizenship

persons to communicate effectively. A recent survey has highlighted that within Europe the United Kingdom has the highest percentage of the so-called 'silver surfers'. Furthermore the Internet use by people aged 55 and over in the UK increased by nearly 90% between March 2001 and February 2002 (Net Value 2002). Older people and their carers are also using the Internet to find health information (Metcalf *et al.* 2001). However, it is important to remember that not all information available on the Internet is accurate (Shepperd *et al.* 1999).

Occupational therapists also require excellent communication skills and strategies to manage psychological issues and to deliver client-focused services. However there is evidence that professionals encounter difficulties communicating with clients (Corner & Wilson-Barnett 1992; Georgaki *et al.* 2002; Sasahara *et al.* 2003). This in turn can impact upon client care as there is evidence that poor communication can influence the client's perceptions of the disease, their psychological adjustment and possible survival outcomes (Freedman 2003). Research by Kruijver *et al.* (2000) found that when ward nurses interacted with **cancer** patients they predominantly employed instrumental communication, mostly consisting of giving information about medical topics. Consequently an imbalance occurred regarding the amount of effective communication.

Box 9.2 Mr Clarke who lived on a farm.

> Mr Clarke, who was recovering from a depressive illness was unable to communicate the importance of being part of the annual asparagus picking on his farm to the ward staff. However, once he was in his own environment during the home visit, the context enabled him to fulfill his wishes and communicate this to the occupational therapist. Thus, his capacity to communicate which had been temporarily impaired by his depressive illness and the ward environment, returned once the performance aspects were more favourable to his participation. The occupational therapist was able to draw on this as a motivating occupational factor for Mr Clarke's recovery.

The components of communication have been broken down into subsections by the ICF, which helps to define the term itself (see Box 9.1). Communication is about general and specific features of communicating by language, signs and symbols, including receiving and producing messages, carrying on conversations, and using communication devices and techniques (WHO 2001:133). The capacity of an individual to communicate (**activity**), depends on some or all of these subsections and insight may be gained by asking the 'what' and 'how' questions. The performance (**participation**) is more complex and may be better understood by asking the 'why', 'when' and 'where' questions.

Receiving spoken and non-verbal messages

The task of receiving spoken messages involves complex sensory, neurological and cognitive functioning as well as psychological processes. The **body structures** needed include the ears, eyes and brain. Hearing and seeing are vital functions for receiving spoken messages. Spoken messages may occur using various media such as face-to-face, or indirectly via for example, the telephone, radio, television, tape recorder or computer. Comprehension is a pivotal part of processing incoming information, which in turn, calls upon the powers of thought and memory to impart meaning. There is a normal decline in the speed of information processing skills with age, but a corresponding increase in the amount of accumulated knowledge to draw on.

Non-verbal behaviour includes facial expression, gesture, posture, touch, appearance and smell. It is dependent on the context of a situation as well as being culturally determined. It serves as an accompaniment to or replacement of speech but also provides a means for the expression of emotion and attitude. It is highly reliant on the interpretive abilities of the recipient. In everyday interactions, both the sending and receiving of non-verbal messages is mostly conducted at a subconscious level. The exchange of non-verbal messages is therefore more subtle than a spoken exchange and requires the brain to function with advanced mental acuity, processing and making sense of additional visual clues.

Touch is an important part of communication, although it has become imbued with negative connotations due to its connection with physical abuse. Occupational therapists need to be especially careful when touching older people and ensure that they have permission before invading their personal space, both literally and metaphorically. Equally, therapists should remain vigilant for any signs of mal-treatment, which often goes unrecognised and unreported. For many older couples, hugging and caressing provide a sense of intimacy and lovemaking in their relationship when coitus no longer takes place (see Chapter 7) (Miracle & Miracle 2001).

The activity in Box 9.3 illustrates some of the factors to consider with respect to older people's personal space.

Box 9.3 What is personal space?

> Draw an outline of the human body, both front and back. Mark the areas which would be acceptable to touch in an everyday social situation, say a lunchtime meal in a pub.
>   Now think about the following questions and perhaps discuss them with a colleague:
>
> - What factors came to mind when you were considering this exercise?
> - Why should they be any different for an older person?
> - Where you surprised by how few areas were acceptable to touch?
> - Why might this be so?

Simply receiving a message is not effective enough if it is not understood. This can be compared to, for instance, first learning a foreign language. The sounds can be heard, but not what they mean. For those older people whose first language is not English, or for those who are used to a different dialect, ensuring that a message has been understood is an important aspect to bear in mind for health professionals (The Open University 1993). Equally, disease processes such as **dementia** or **stroke** can alter a person's ability to understand the spoken word. Furthermore, unfamiliar surroundings add to feelings of disorientation which further impair the capacity for receiving spoken messages.

If an older person has difficulties with their hearing, these non-verbal signs become especially significant. Reading and writing including braille, are forms of non-verbal communication and may be used as a way of interacting, but are significantly slower processes than the use of speech; consequently much of the pleasure may be lost with the lack of fluency. However, those that are skilled in these forms of non-verbal communication can convey subtleties of expression not always found in the spoken word (Box 9.4).

Box 9.4

> Mr Adams, who we previously met in Chapter 8, living in his continuing care unit for people with dementia, had both hearing difficulties and expressive dysphasia.
>   In therapy sessions led by an occupational therapist and music therapist he was withdrawn and non-participative. Nonetheless, one day, he was able to communicate to the group members, his excitement about snow falling outside the window.
>   This shows that even when it appears that the capacity to communicate is adversely affected by impairments, participation can still occur spontaneously, given the right circumstances and motivating factors.

For the deaf community, sign language and/or lip reading replaces speech with impressive efficiency, but the language also needs to be learnt by hearing people to have meaning in everyday communications. However, it may have limited use to older persons who become deaf in later years, for whom it would mean learning a whole new language.

Speaking and conversation

The articulation of words, or speaking, is still the principal means of expression for most of the population, despite rapid advances in electronic technology. The voice is an important part of a person's identity and a vehicle for making specific needs immediately known. It can be a useful indicator of the state of someone's health and mood. Conversation is the coming together of all these communication skills in a co-operative spoken interaction between two or more people. Impairment caused by a brain or neurological injury, such as a **stroke** or motor neurone disease can directly affect the ability of a person to articulate. Speech can also be altered due to the effect of drugs or as a result of shock and confusion. In addition, even when the activity of forming the words poses no barriers, the ability to express verbally may be impaired by the inability to mentally organise and access thoughts coherently, thus precluding participation.

Engagement in conversation is by its nature participatory. It can be affected greatly by the status of the participants, which influences the power balance of the exchange. For older people, who are already likely to be vulnerable in a health-care situation and whose status is therefore compromised, it is a vital dynamic for occupational therapists and of others to be aware. Even for those older people whose health is not in question, age itself confers a change in status, one that is not always viewed favourably in western societies (McEwen 1990). **Participation** may be further precluded by the **environment** an older person finds himself or herself in, for instance a day room with the television turned up full volume. Even the company can affect **participation** in speaking. If someone, of any age, is intimidated by others or simply does not wish to speak, **participation** stops. Age does not mean the right to remain silent should be foregone.

In the absence of disease or **pathology**, old people are not cognitively disadvantaged in their innate ability to engage in the activities associated with communication, apart from a natural slowing down, perhaps needing more time and fewer distractions to maximise the processing of information. However, disease associated with old age and the decline of functional abilities, do have an impact upon the communication process.

From an occupational therapist's perspective, the very first interaction with an older client is crucial for establishing rapport and forming the basis of an ongoing therapeutic relationship. Occupational therapists need to ensure that they utilise at all times their observation skills to assess non-verbal communication, for example the mood of the client and their feelings. Furthermore, older persons will also observe and respond to the therapist's non-verbal and verbal behaviour. Consequently occupational therapists have a role, both in the way they conduct their own interactions and in building the older person's narrative. This requires sensitive attunement to an individual's needs and the offering of any necessary reassurance. The pressured pace of life is not an excuse for these important skills not to be practised.

On a practical note occupational therapists need to ensure that communication aids are working effectively and that they are switched on, and that when older persons receive information, that they have understood it. Consequently therapists need to consider how, why, where and when they communicate. Various **products and technology** can be used to assist the therapist as discussed in Chapter 10. Indeed, occupational therapists collaborate closely with speech and language therapists. As occupational therapists interested in the clients' perspective on life, it is worth bearing in mind that although the ability of an older person to hear may be impaired by age, the capacity to listen and to be heard is not inevitably diminished.

Why, where and when older people communicate are questions to be addressed carefully by occupational therapists, as part of the overall assessment, within the **context** of their clients' and carers' lives. Occupational therapists need to ensure that communication occurs in an environment in which older persons feel confident and comfortable. Privacy and confidentiality should be maintained at all times. Communication should not be rushed, and the principles of client-centred practice should be maintained at all times. **Participation** is largely dependent on a willingness and inclination to engage with others and is usually socially motivated, as it would be for anyone.

Interpersonal interactions and relationships

Basic interpersonal interactions involve asking for what is wanted; making one's needs known and following simple instructions as already discussed in the previous communication section. Complex interpersonal interactions include the ability to conduct in-depth, reasoned discussions based on the sharing of experiences and knowledge, as well as the ability to pick up contextual clues and nuances and act on them appropriately.

The ability of older people to engage with others is largely dependent on the communication skills already described, with the additional emotional and cultural factors that inevitably come into play as soon as a personal interaction takes place. The personality and social skills developed over a lifetime are important attributes as are **contextual** and **environmental factors**. Eriksons's (1950) concept of the life tasks of old age being 'ego integrity versus despair' highlights the importance of social contact for psychological wellbeing. His later book (Erikson *et al.* 1986) gives a portrait of the experience of old age based on interviews with octogenarians and a review of the life cycle from the perspective of old age. Participating actively in mature interpersonal interactions is crucial to self-development. For example, it might be observed in some health and social care settings that staff interact with older people in an over-familiar way. This approach, while intended to be friendly and reassuring, can diminish the quality of interpersonal relationships and prevents appropriate performance in this important area of functioning. More importantly, it reinforces a 'pervasive cultural strategy of infantilisation' (Hockey & James 1993: 173). Equally, the expectations of older people are shaped by their own experiences and thus a cycle of decreasing activity and performance can be unwittingly reinforced.

Consequently occupational therapists need to ensure that they determine in the first instance how the older person wishes to be addressed. It is important to remember that at first meeting, you are a stranger to the older person. Relating with strangers is potentially an activity that older people may have some difficulty with, as new situations and unknown contexts may cause anxiety and confusion. An older person may be vulnerable in terms of their safety, although the experience that comes with age could improve their judgement.

Life experience and personality are more prescient indicators of **capacity** and **performance** than age per se. Indeed, some older persons may wish to form a formal relationship with the therapist where roles are clearly defined, with more structure, clear boundaries or even a contractual agreement like those that they would have with, for example their solicitor, bank manager or doctor.

In some **cultures**, certain family relationships may have a formal element, with the expectation of particular behaviours within that interaction. The informality of many institutions is a relatively recent phenomenon. Hence, even in situations where the roles could be expected to be less formal, older people might find a more formal approach reassuring initially, until they become more familiar with the person. Occupational therapists would come into this relationship category and an attitude of 'mutual respect' is an important and helpful starting place to build up rapport.

Informal **social relationships** and **family relationships** as discussed in Chapter 3 depend very much on an individual's circumstances. An area that occupational therapists often fail to address is that of intimate relationships. Intimate relationships including the sexual life of older people have been taboo topics until relatively recently, despite evidence that the capacity to enjoy intimacy persists often until very advanced old age (Masters and Johnson 1970; Parkin 2003).

Old people, for the past 50 years, have been be assigned an asexual identity which remains little changed in today's society (Ginn & Arber 1998) with women in particular seeming to become 'invisible' beyond a certain age in terms of expressing themselves as sexual beings (Bernard & Meade 1993). Occupational therapists have colluded with the ambivalence that characterises this aspect of personhood. In the limited amount of occupational therapy literature that explores issues of sexuality, there are general expressions of discomfort and unease when addressing them, in particular with respect to older or disabled people (Couldrick 1998, 1999).

Where sexuality is discussed, there is an assumption of heterosexuality. There is very little acknowledgement of the needs of gay, lesbian and bisexual older people (Bancroft 1989). Older lesbians in particular, are further marginalized as the taboo of ageing is not restricted to mainstream society (McDonald & Rich 1984; Adelman 1986).

However, evidence from numerous studies, usefully summarised by Spence (1991) show that the physiological changes that occur as people age, including the progress of conditions such as **heart disease** or **arthritis** do not, in themselves cause a cessation of sexual activity (see Chapter 7). Other factors, such as bereavement, societal attitudes and repression in earlier life are more likely to impact on intimacy in later life.

Indeed, intimacy in the older age group is often viewed with a certain amount of disapproval and distaste by younger people. Thus the choice to remain sexually active in old age is complicated by a number of factors, not least the availability of a partner as well as physical and mental fitness.

The choice may be taken away by the death of a spouse, ill health or admission to long-term care. Additionally, staff looking after older people experience tension in their roles between caring for and controlling the sexual behaviour of those in their care. There is very little written about sexuality in nursing homes. It seems that it is rarely discussed, which effectively removes the choice completely and also precludes a realisation of the effects on older people.

When providing services or facilities for older people, occupational therapists should ensure that close relationships are encouraged rather than ignored, if the older person so wishes, enabling the formation and continuation of emotional and physical companionship.

A starting point would be to include this area of activity in the assessment process, bearing in mind that it requires particular sensitivity. Even just offering the opportunity for an older person to express their views about intimacy and close-ness would be progress. Bor & Watts (1993) have found that older patients and clients are willing to respond to personal questions about their sexuality provided that they are not teased or judged.

From this, the therapist can determine, in consultation with the older person, how best to meet their needs, either by providing opportunities to meet like-minded people, advocating on their behalf or involving more specialist help, depending on the individual situation.

Due to the general assumption that older people are not sexually active, the risk of acquiring and therefore giving advice on the prevention of sexually transmitted diseases is frequently not openly addressed. However, there are small but significant numbers of people over the age of 55 contracting HIV in the UK and the need to practice safe sex is as important in later life as it is in earlier years (Centre for Communicable Diseases Surveillance and Communicable Diseases and Environmental Health Unit 1994; Rickard 1995). As further evidence of an active seeking of intimacy and sexual contact in later life, a 78-year-old proclaimed in his Internet dating application, 'I'm retired, not tired' (Parkin 2003:16).

Box 9.5

Consider one or two of the case studies in this book and think about how, as an occupational therapist you would go about discovering and addressing issues of intimacy or the sexual needs of the people presented.

- Do you find it hard to imagine what they might be?
- How comfortable are you dealing with this topic?
- Do you think it comes into the domain of occupational therapy?

Major life areas: education, work and employment

While the older population may generally be thought to have completed its education and indeed retired from remunerative employment, the current demographic shift towards increased numbers of people over the age of 85 has meant that life-long learning and delaying the age of retirement have become realistic options for many older people. Additionally, the spending power of older people is frequently overlooked by advertisers who neglect to target this substantial group in favour of pursuing a more youthful audience.

Despite the government's culture of promoting lifelong learning and widening **participation**, little has actually been known about older people's experiences of learning and education over the course of their lives until relatively recently. The findings of a study by Withnall & Thompson (2003), which aimed to explore the issues in depth, found that a wide range of different influences impact on people's learning activities in later life. These show that older people are interested in a wide variety of topics and define learning as an informal **activity** that is associated with a range of positive outcomes, including self-satisfaction, intellectual stimulation, pleasure and enjoyment. Additionally, older people continue to learn in a variety of ways, including the discussion of radio and television programmes with friends and family, participating in social and voluntary activities and attending classes and courses. School education is obviously no longer applicable to the older age group, but older people in increasing numbers are pursuing both informal education and higher education. Indeed, the United Nations World Assembly on Ageing (1982) endorsed the view that lifelong learning is not merely the acquisition of knowledge, but also a means of acquiring the ability to participate in the events of daily life. There is also evidence that continued learning reduces the risk of social isolation and loneliness. The University of the Third Age, which was founded in France in 1973 specifically to serve the needs of the older learner now has numerous branches world-wide. The Open University also offers an extensive range of formal courses for people to choose from and has a flexible approach well-suited to those from the older age group. Further education offered by local authorities, also offers numerous day and evening classes to suit all interests and aptitudes.

The innate capacity to learn as an **activity** is dependent on cognitive factors and need not be diminished by age, although older learners may need more time to process new knowledge. However, as already indicated, the simple acquisition of new knowledge is not perceived as being a high priority by older people who rate enjoyment and enhanced quality of life through participation as being more important. Participation in learning, however, is not just influenced by the availability of opportunities but also by social issues such as class, culture and past experience. These factors will affect the expectations and attitudes of older people towards ongoing education. Inequalities in this respect continue into old age. Recent research has demonstrated that older people can be taught information skills. A study by Trentin (2004) found that older people continued to use the Internet after completing a course about e-learning, enabling them to socialise and form relationships through email and chat rooms. Similar findings have been reported by Malcolm et al. (2001).

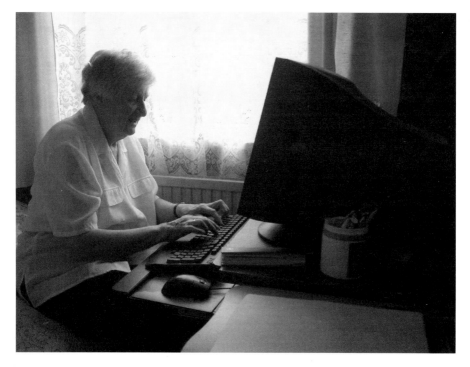

Figure 9.1 Silver Surfer at work!

From an occupational therapist's perspective, the life-enhancing potential of ongoing learning and education is self-evident. Furthermore, the wide variety of ways older people engage in learning activities are of relevance when planning intervention strategies. However, perhaps the term intervention in this context implies too active an involvement in a process that should be more subtle. The presentation of learning opportunities and provision of gentle guidance within an acceptable and enjoyable social environment would be a more appropriate and less intrusive approach. Nor should it be forgotten that older people have much to offer fellow learners and that the rich potential of this teaching role can be used by occupational therapists in arranging the exchange of learning opportunities for their clients.

The following story (Box 9.6) is an unusual but inspiring example that life is for learning and that the ability and commitment to learn can transcend age.

Many older people wish to remain economically productive not just for financial gain, but also for the dignity and purpose that work confers. As outlined in Chapters 2 and 3, older people **participate** both in paid and unpaid work which can enhance life satisfaction. (Robertson *et al.* 2003). In particular older volunteers can make a vital economic and social contribution to society by sharing skills and knowledge. Equally important, is the impact volunteering has on providing opportunities for older persons to maintain their self-respect and dignity through continued active **participation** in society (Alakija-Capeling 2002). Furthermore, contribution can include socially valued products such as mentoring, child-care,

Box 9.6

Reverend Edgar Dowse has just become the oldest person in the world to gain a PhD. At the age of 93, the father of two, who does not own a computer and dictated his thesis, already has six other degrees. He does not drive and used the bus to get to the London School of Theology whose degrees are validated by Brunel University.

'After my wife, Ivy, died in 1999, I felt the need for intense study' he said. 'As I am 93, it was a slightly unusual occurrence and I'm delighted they came to this decision'.

The principal noted that 'to gain a PhD at any age is a great achievement. To gain it at the age of 93 is remarkable'.

The previous record was held by American Elizabeth Eichelbaum who was 90 when she received a PhD from the University of Tennessee in 2000, according to the Guinness Book of Records (Brunel News 2004:1).

community leadership, political involvement or role model figures (United Nations Volunteers 2003).

Despite moves to increase the age of retirement, the majority of older people an occupational therapist encounters are pensioners rather than being in remunerative employment. This might change as the move for occupational therapists to become more active in **health promotion** as an adjunct to being reactive in **health** and **social service** arenas becomes a reality. Economic self-sufficiency confers status and security at any age, but is particularly pertinent for older people. The current and future pensions shortfall means that many future older people are likely to be denied this financial security unless they are fortunate enough to have considerable additional resources. Occupational therapists take financial status into consideration during assessment as this increasingly has a bearing on the services that can be offered. The expertise of a social work colleague or welfare rights advisor might also be sought, if felt to be appropriate in order to maximise an older person's potential income.

Community, social and civic life

A community may be thought of as a network of people (Ewles & Simnett 2003). The people in the network share common interests and experiences. The links may include neighbourhood, language, religion, ethnic background, leisure interests or other factors people may have in common, such as age. However the concept of community in old age is difficult to define as age alone does not confer conformity.

The term community is further complicated by current UK **government policies** that stress the importance of 'care in the community', implying that it is both a resource and provision as far as **health** and **social care services** are concerned (DH 1990). In a survey exploring older people's views on their quality of life, some of the main factors forming the foundation for a good life include the engagement in a large number of social, leisure and voluntary activities and living in a neighbourhood with good community facilities and services, including transport (Bowling *et al.* 2003).

Box 9.7 What is a community?

Think about your own immediate community. Draw an outline map of your local area and mark on it all the services and places you visit that on a regular basis. For instance, these could include the shops or local supermarket, library, park, playground, church, mosque or temple, coffee shop or pub, gym etc. Once you have done this, share the map with a colleague or partner and consider the following questions:

- How do you get to these places?
- How important is it to you that you use these amenities? Why?
- Do you see older people using the same facilities?
- Where do the older people in your area live?
- How would you be able to find out what they do in the community?

Interestingly, in the same survey, wider society and political issues were mentioned most as taking quality away from the lives of older people (e.g. pensions, the **environment** and foreign policy).

From a practical point of view, transport has been identified as a crucial factor in accessing facilities, without which participation in community activities is largely precluded. Despite its importance, surprisingly few studies have addressed the issue (Gilhooly *et al.* 2003).

Illness or **impairment** in old age will affect the roles taken as part of community life and these may shift in phases from being able to contribute actively, through to needing help to contribute and eventually to being recipients of others' contribution in the community. Since maintaining independence and control over one's life are key to ensuring continued quality of life, these transitions in community activity can be difficult to negotiate.

The ICF classifies all aspects of community social life in this section such as engaging in informal associations, formal associations and ceremonies. The actual ability to take part in community life is not diminished by age and relies to some extent on an individual's predisposition to do so. Engagement in the community can also be through the political process, which may involve being elected onto both national and community councils. The political power of old people has increased in line with demographic changes, with one in four voters now being over the age of 65 (Dean 2003). Trades Unions in particular have been active in promoting social justice for older people and have successfully influenced politicians by organising rallies and marches which have been well-attended (Trade Union Congress 2004). From an occupational therapist's perspective, the roles of advocacy and empowerment are important to enable **activity** and **participation** in these areas, roles that are supported by **social policy** (Dunning 1995).

However the interdependence of many factors such as good health, financial security and access to transport should be acknowledged. The availability of, contact with, and even access to, resources are not in themselves always enough to include an older person as part of a community. Firstly, there needs to be the desire to be

Box 9.8 Mr and Mrs Davies.

The example of Mr and Mrs Davies to whom we were introduced in Chapter 5 shows how the community occupational therapist assisted the couple through a series of living transitions within the community to accommodate both Mrs Davies' increasing dependence due to her memory problems and Mr Davies' need for help to look after her. This was achieved whilst also enabling both of their occupational needs and interests to be addressed. In Mr Davies' case this was play bowls and in Mrs Davies' to continue with singing in the church choir.

involved and secondly the choices to be available before **participation** can occur. An old person, like anyone, needs to feel welcomed rather than isolated. The value western society places on an older person's contribution in general needs to be enhanced, and occupational therapists are useful allies and advocates in this ongoing debate.

Occupational therapists are also well-placed to ease the transition towards increased dependence within a community and can work both with the older person and with those in the community who are able to offer care, supplementing this by arranging **statutory** and **voluntary services** where appropriate. Additionally, occupational therapists recognise the occupational changes that older people face and can use this knowledge to maximise the potential of these changes (Jonsson *et al.* 2000).

Occupational therapists working in the community have access to a wide variety of support networks, both formal and informal that they can use to link people who want to join the networks and equally those who would benefit from receiving help. Most of the major charities also operate local support networks and occupational therapists often work in collaboration with representatives from these groups.

Recreation and leisure

Engaging in any sort of play or sports, relaxation, going to art galleries, museums or theatres, doing anything for enjoyment and amusement, hobbies and travelling for pleasure are all included in this section of the ICF (WHO 2001).

The beneficial effects that leisure pursuits have on **health** and **wellbeing** make them particularly pertinent to occupational therapists working with people in the older age group. Indeed the philosophical and practical bedrock on which occupational therapy is based acknowledges the connection between occupation and health (Wilcock 1998). Paradoxically, those who pursue meaningful activities into their advancing years independently have no need of the services of an occupational therapist but where they do, the ultimate aim is in returning occupational resources to the individual to enable self-sufficiency, rather than to create dependence. Increasingly, the role of the occupational therapist may expand into this **health-promoting** arena.

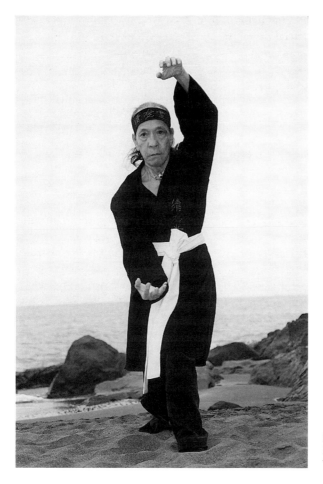

Figure 9.2 Master Dan Phu Nguyen, founder of Viet Vo Thanh Long, age 89.

Leisure and recreation become more central to people's lives after retirement (Hersch 1990) and are important potential areas for life satisfaction (Griffin & McKenna 1998). However, the choice of leisure activity is an individual one and maintaining activity levels just for the sake of it does not necessarily confer beneficial effects. Having said that, the establishment of routines involving leisure is generally linked to improved health and life satisfaction (Marino-Schorn 1986; Parker 1996).

The concept of occupational balance within occupational therapy and occupational science literature is still being researched, although Meyer (1922) introduced the notion of balance early in the philosophy of occupational therapy, advocating a balance between work, rest, play and sleep.

Westhorp (2003) explores the concept of lifestyle balance in terms of occupations in considerable detail and proposes a dynamic cycle of change within which control is a vital element for the maintenance of health and wellbeing. However, there is an acknowledgement that the topic has not been well researched by occupational therapists to date. One definition of occupational balance, such as it is, is based on a belief that balanced occupations can contribute to health and well-being but this belief is not substantiated by research (Christiansen & Baum 1997). What does emerge clearly, however, is the strong perceived effect of occupational balance on health and this also applies to older people.

Religion and spirituality

The terms religion and spirituality are often bracketed together, as they are here by the ICF, although they are by no means synonymous. The precise meaning of the terms is still poorly understood and definitions remain elusive. The unique personal or transpersonal nature of the inner experience is perhaps too nebulous to set down clearly in words, although many have tried to do so (Jewell 2004).

Occupational therapists value the spiritual dimension of occupation and also acknowledge the importance of spirituality as part of their holistic, client-centred approach. However, much of the literature on this topic has come from Canada and America (e.g. Egan & Delaat 1994, 1997; Christiansen 1997; Enquist et al. 1997). The small number of UK studies show that there is still much uncertainty amongst occupational therapists, about how to address spiritual matters in practice (Udell & Chandler 2000; Belcham 2004).

The ICF (WHO 2001) focuses on the active doings associated with religious and spiritual practice, such as going to places of worship or praying and chanting. However, the contemplative and intangible aspects of acknowledging a power beyond the human that do not reveal themselves in obvious activity are equally important. Recent studies have shown that those older people with strong religious convictions have higher levels of life satisfaction, are less likely to be depressed and more likely to be at ease with their personal past and the prospect of death (Ayele et al. 1999; Coleman et al. 2002).

In the health domain, spirituality and religion have traditionally been seen to be the responsibility of the hospital chaplain, although the medical profession and occupational therapy, amongst others, have also recognised the importance of faith in healing.

From a practical perspective, occupational therapists can assist older people in carrying out the occupations associated with their spiritual needs in many ways. Some examples include ensuring access to places of worship, including transport and ramped wheelchair entrances, by recommending or designing comfortable seats and even suggesting larger and clearer print for songsheets or religious texts. Many churches are now fitted with loop systems to enhance hearing, which community occupational therapists can recommend if appropriate.

Spiritual leaders are also willing to visit people in their own homes or in a residential setting and it may fall to the occupational therapist to arrange this if the need is not identified by others in the care team. Additionally, occupational therapists may become involved in running groups to meet the spiritual needs of older people as part of a team approach as described in Box 9.9.

Box 9.9

An example of the occupational therapist and chaplain working together is described by Bryant & Law (1990). A teamwork project was set up to meet the spiritual needs of elderly mentally ill people in hospital. Weekly services were conducted in the hospital chapel and themes were identified and presented to reflect the liturgical and seasonal patterns of the year. In this way, the spiritual side of the patients' lives, which is often ignored in institutional settings, was acknowledged and nourished. Interestingly, the team also looked after its own spiritual needs, by having a day away once a year. This aspect of looking after oneself in order to care for others is often overlooked in healthcare practice.

Summary

The four domains and the subsections of the ICF concerned with communication; interpersonal relationships; major life areas and community, social and civil life have been considered in this chapter in relation to older people and the role of the occupational therapist. The potential for activity and participation has been discussed and the impact of the effects of ageing explained. Occupational therapists working with older people have the added responsibility and privilege of recognising, respecting and integrating the richness and individuality of a person's longer lifespan.

References

Adelman M (ed.) (1986) *Long Time Passing: Lives of Older Lesbians*. Boston: Alyson Publications.

Alakija-Capeling S (2002) *United Nations Volunteer Statement. Second World Assembly on Ageing*. Madrid, Spain 8th–12th April. Accessed 17.05.2004. http://www.un.org/ageing/coverage/unvE.htm

Ayele H, Mulligan T, Gheorghiu S, Reyes-Ortiz C (1999) Religious activity improves life satisfaction for some physicians and older patients. *Journal of the American Geriatric Society* 47(4), 453–455.

Bancroft J (1989) *Human Sexuality and Its Problems*. London: Churchill Livingstone.

Belcham C (2004) Spirituality in occupational therapy: theory in practice? *British Journal of Occupational Therapy* 67(1), 39–46.

Bernard M & Meade K (1993) *Women Come of Age*. London: Edward Arnold.

Bor R & Watts M (1993) Talking to patients about sexual matters. *British Journal of Nursing* 2(130), 657–660.

Bowling A, Gabriel Z, Banister D, Sutton S (2003) *Adding Quality to Quantity: Older People's Views on their Quality of Life and its Enhancement*. Sheffield: Economic Social Research Council (ESCR) Growing Older Programme. Accessed 17.05.2004. http://www.shef.ac.uk/uni/projects/gop/index.htm

Brunel News (2004) Brunel validates oldest PhD student in the world. *Staff Newsletter of Brunel University*, Feb/March, No 67. Middlesex: Brunel University.

Bryant W & Law M (1990) A spiritual lift from a world of confusion. *Therapy Weekly* February 1.

Centre for Communicable Diseases Surveillance and Communicable Diseases and Environmental Health Unit, Scotland (1994) *Quarterly Surveillance Table no. 20* (unpublished). Mesmac Tyneside Report 1993/4.

Christiansen C (1997) Acknowledging a spiritual dimension in occupational therapy practice. *American Journal of Occupational Therapy* 51(3), 169–180.

Christiansen C & Baum C (eds). (1997) *Occupational Therapy: Enabling function and Wellbeing*. Thorofare, NJ: Slack.

Coleman P, McKieran F, Mills M, Speck P (2002) Spiritual belief and quality of life: the experience of older bereaved spouses. *Quality and Ageing – Policy, Practice and Research* 3(1), 20–26.

College of Occupational Therapists (2000) *Code of Ethics and Professional Conduct for Occupational Therapists*. London: College of Occupational Therapists.

Corner J & Wilson-Barnett J (1992) The newly-registered nurse and the cancer patient: an educational evaluation *International Journal of Nursing Studies* 29(2), 177–190.

Couldrick L (1998) Sexual Issues within occupational therapy, Part 1: Attitudes and practice. *British Journal of Occupational Therapy* 61(12), 492–496.

Couldrick L (1999) Sexual issues within occupational therapy, Part 2: Implications for education and practice. *British Journal of Occupational Therapy* 62(1), 26–30.

Dean M (2003) *Growing Older in the 21st Century*. Swindon: Economic and Social Research Council.

Department of Health (1990) *The NHS and Community Care Act*. London: HMSO.

Dunning A (1995) *Citizen Advocacy with Older People: A Code for Good Practice*. London: Centre for Policy on Ageing.

Egan M & Delaat D (1994) Considering spirituality in occupational therapy practice. *Canadian Journal of Occupational Therapy* 61(2), 95–101.

Egan M & Delaat D (1997) The implicit spirituality of occupational therapy practice. *Canadian Journal of Occupational Therapy* 64(1), 115–121.

Enquist D, Short-DeGraff M, Gliner J, Oltjenbruns K (1997) Occupational therapists' beliefs and practices with regard to spirituality and therapy. *American Journal of Occupational Therapy* 51(3), 173–180.

Ewles L & Simnett I (2003) *Promoting Health A Practical Guide*, 5th edn. London: Bailliere Tindall.

Erikson E (1950) *Childhood and Society*. Middlesex: Penguin.

Erikson E, Erikson J, Kivnick H (1968) *Vital Involvement in Old Age*. New York: Norton.

Freedman TG (2003) Prescriptions for health providers. *Cancer Nursing* 26(4), 323–330.

Georgaki S, Kalaidopoulou O, Liarmakopoulos L, Mystakidou K (2002) Nurses' attitudes towards truthful communication with patients with cancer. *Cancer Nursing* 25(6), 436–441.

Gilhooly M, Hamilton K, O'Neill M, Gow J, Webster N, Pike F (2003) *Transport and Ageing: Extending Quality of Life via Public and Private Transport*. Sheffield: Economic Social Research Council (ESRC) Growing Older Programme. Accessed 18.05.2004. www.shef.ac.uk/uni/projects/gop/index.htm

Ginn J & Arber S (1998) Gender and older age in Bernard M, Phillips J (eds). (1998) *The Social Policy of Old Age*. London: Centre for Policy on Ageing.

Griffin J & McKenna K (1998) Influences on leisure and life satisfaction of elderly people. *Physical and Occupational Therapy in Geriatrics* 15(4), 1–16.

Hersch G (1990) Leisure and aging. *Physical and Occupational Therapy in Geriatrics* 9(2), 55–73.

Hockey J & James A (1993) *Growing up and Growing Old*. London: Sage.

Jewell A (ed.) (2004) *Ageing, Spirituality and Well-being*. London and New York: Jessica Kingsley.

Jonsson H, Borell L, Sadlo G (2000) Retirement: an occupational transition with consequences for temporality, balance and meaning of occupations. *Journal of Occupational Science* 7(1), 29–37.

Kruijver IP, Kerkstra A, Fancke AL, Bensing JM, van de Wiel HBM (2000) Evaluation of communication training programs in nursing care. A review of the literature. *Patient Education and Counselling* 39(1), 129–145.

MacDonald B & Rich C (1984) *Look Me in the Eye*. London: The Women's Press.

McEwen E (ed.) (1990) *Age: The Unrecognised Discrimination*. London: Age Concern.

Malcolm M, Mann WC, Tomita M, Frass L, Stanton K, Gitlin G (2001) Computer and internet use in physically frail elders. *Physical and Occupational Therapy in Geriatrics* 19(3), 15–32.

Masters WH & Johnson VE (1970) *Human Sexual Inadequacy*. Boston: Little Brown.

Metcalf MP, Tanner TB, Coulehan MB (2001) Using the internet for health care information – and beyond. *Caring* 20(5), 42–44.

Marino-Schorn JA (1986) Morale, work and leisure in retirement. *Physical and Occupational Therapy in Geriatrics* 4(2), 49–59.

Meyer A (1922) The philosophy of occupational therapy. *Archives of Occupational Therapy* 1, 1–10. (Reprinted 1997 in *The American Journal of Occupational Therapy* 31(10), 639–642.)

Miracle AW & Miracle TS (2001) Sexuality in Late Adulthood. In: Bonder BR & Wagner MB (eds). *Functional Performance in Older Adults*, 2nd edn. Philadelphia: FA Davis, pp. 218–235.

Net Value (2002) *'Silver Surfers' Continue to Join the Internet Revolution*. Press Release, London, 28th March. Accessed 19.05.2004. http://www.net4nowt.com/news_archive/arc2–2002.htm

Parker M (1996) The relationship between time spent by older adults in leisure activities and life satisfaction. *Physical and Occupational Therapy in Geriatrics* 15(4), 1–16.

Parkin S (2003) Growing old disgracefully. *The Guardian Newspaper* 29.1.03, p. 16.

Rickard W (1995) HIV/Aids and older people. *Generations Review* 5(3), 2–6.

Robertson I, Warr P, Callinan M, Bardzil P (2003) *Older People's Experience of Paid Employment: Participation and Quality of Life*. Sheffield. Economic and Social Research Council (ESRC) Growing Older Programme.

Sasahara T, Miyashita M, Kawa M, Kazuma K (2003) Difficulties encountered by nurses in the care of terminally ill cancer patients in general hospitals in Japan. *Palliative Medicine* 17(6), 520–526.

Shaw M (ed.) (1991) *The Challenge of Ageing*. NSW: Churchill Livingstone.

Shepperd S, Charnock D, Gann B (1999) Helping patients access high quality health information. *British Medical Journal* 319, 764–766.

Spence S (1991) *Psychosexual Therapy: A Cognitive Behavioural Approach*. London: Chapman and Hall.

Squire A (2002) *Health and Well-being for Older People*. London: Balliere Tindall.

The Open University (1993) *Language and Image: An Equal Opportunities Guide*. Milton Keynes: The Open University.

Trade Union Congress (2004) *Pensions*. Accessed 17.05.2004. http://www.tuc.org.uk/pensions/

Trentin G (2004) E-learning and the Third Age. *Journal of Computer Assisted Learning* 20(1), 21–30.

Udell L & Chandler C (2000) The role of the occupational therapist in addressing the spiritual needs of clients. *British Journal of Occupational Therapy* 63(10), 489–495.

United Nations (1982) *Vienna International Plan of Action on Ageing.* Accessed 18.05.2004. http://www.un.org/esa/socdev/ageing/ageipaa.htm

United Nations Volunteers (2003) *Voluntary Action by Older Persons.* Accessed 17.05.2004. http://www.unv.org/infobase/articles/2002/02_02_25USA_ageing.htm

Westhorpe P (2003) Exploring balance as a concept in occupational science. *Journal of Occupational Science* 10(2), 99–106.

Wilcock AA (1998) *An Occupational Perspective of Health.* Thorofare, NJ: Slack.

Withnall A & Thompson V (2003) *Older People and Lifelong Learning: Choices and Experiences.* Sheffield: ESRC Growing Older Programme. Accessed 17.05.2004. http://www.shef.ac.uk/uni/projects/gop/index.htm

World Health Organisation (2001) *International Classification of Functioning, Disability and Health.* Geneva: World Health Organisation.

Chapter 10

ENVIRONMENTAL IMPACTS, PRODUCTS AND TECHNOLOGY

Anita Atwal, Alex Farrow and Marcus Sivell-Muller

The Ottawa Charter (WHO 1986) has strongly influenced occupational therapy practice. Wilcock (1998, 2002) and the College of Occupational Therapists (COT 2002) draw extensively on this document to promote the role of occupational therapy in **health promotion**. The Ottawa Charter (WHO 1986) recognises factors such as peace, shelter, education, food, income, a stable ecosystem, sustainable resources and social justice and equity as pre-requisites for health. The Charter suggests that persons that are involved within **health promotion** should act as advocates – ensuring the conditions favourable to health are in place, as enablers to facilitate all people to achieve their fullest health potential and mediators – to arbitrate between differing interests in society for the pursuit of health (Scriven & Atwal 2004). The terms advocate, enabler and mediator are already engrained within occupational therapy practice and reflect the profession's commitment to client-centered practice (Chapter 4). Furthermore the terms reflect the spirit and purpose of occupational therapy. Perhaps what is needed is a deeper understanding of how factors such as war, famine, and poverty impact upon the occupational being of older people.

The ICF (WHO 2001:171) makes a significant step in emphasising that loss of independence is not only related to **body functions** but, also **environmental factors**. The term 'environmental factor' is used to describe factors that 'make up the physical, social and attitudinal environment, in which people live and conduct their lives.' Environmental factors can interact with a health condition to create either a disability and or restore functioning, depending on whether the environmental factor can be regarded as a **facilitator** or **barrier**. Consequently, disability can no longer be regarded as a feature of the individual, but rather as the outcome of an interaction of the person with a health condition and the environmental factors. This in turn has meant that the recognition of the central role played by environmental factors has changed the locus of the problem and, hence, focuses of intervention, from the individual to the environment in which the individual lives (Schneidert *et al.* 2003).

This chapter will discuss the natural and human made environment. Physical barriers and facilitators have not been discussed here but the reader is directed to Chapters 2 and 4. However other aspects of the natural and human made environment not commonly discussed in relation to older people are introduced here – climate, air quality, natural disaster and human conflict. The principles of assistive technology will be discussed with greater reference to communication, mobility products and technology. This chapter will not focus upon individual types of products or technologies, as this information can be obtained from sources such as the Disabled Living Foundation (www.dlf.org.uk), Ricability (www.ricability.org.uk), or the Foundation for Assistive Technology (www.fastuk.org) and many other Internet web pages.

Climate

Substantial changes in the degree of heat or cold such as high and low temperature can impact upon the health and wellbeing of older people. They are at high risk of developing potentially life-threatening disturbances of temperature regulation due to normal age-related changes (see Chapter 7). Mortality in Britain is lowest when the mean daily temperature is 17–18°C (Keatinge 2004). Indeed in the United Kingdom, cold spells usually bring with them a substantial increase in the number of admissions to Accident and Emergency departments. This results in substantial costs to health and social care services, for it is estimated that the NHS spends an estimated 1 billion a year treating illness caused by inadequate heating. Furthermore discharge can be delayed if the home is unfit to return to. Most winter deaths can be attributed to cardiovascular conditions, **strokes**, **respiratory** infections and **asthma** (Press 2003). Likewise, heat stress causes increases in coronary and cerebral thrombosis (Keatinge *et al.* 1986). Although in the United Kingdom annual heat-related deaths are far fewer than cold-related deaths (Donaldson *et al.* 2001). In France a heatwave in August 2003 resulted in nearly 15 000 deaths, when temperatures rose to over 40°C in the day and over 24°C at night for several days (Spurgeon 2003). Indeed it has been suggested that heat-related deaths most occur in the first day or two of a period of high temperature (MacFarlane & Waller 1976).

What can be done to prevent deaths from climate changes? One study has identified a direct correlation between people dying and the age of their homes. Properties built before 1850 are less energy efficient and require more fuel to keep warm (Wilkinson 2001). In contrast Healy (2003) found that homes in Scandinavia have the highest efficiency ratings in Europe. In order to promote the importance of keeping homes warm in the UK the government introduced a Fuel Poverty Strategy (Department of Trade and Industry 2001).

Indoor environments and older people

People spend much of their time indoors (Farrow *et al.* 1997; Manuel 1999) and the very young, older people and those whose health is compromised in some way may be in an indoor environment virtually all of the time. Many known environmental risk factors such as exposure to tobacco smoke, allergens, mould and dampness are found in the indoor environment and this may therefore be important with respect to health outcomes. While previous research supports the need for quality housing and has demonstrated the effects of vehicle emissions on older peoples' health (Department of the Environment, Transport and Regions [DETR] 1999), there is little or no research on older people that has investigated the influences of indoor air pollutants. For instance a review by Stuck in 1999 found no studies analysing the physical environment as a predictive factor for functional status decline.

The physical environment of a dwelling includes age, housing status, structure (building materials), furniture, fittings, electrical equipment, humidity, temperature, ventilation, sanitation and crowding. These in turn contribute to indoor air quality. The importance of maintaining a warm home in winter may result in reduced ventilation. Newer properties built with synthetic materials and double-glazing may be energy efficient, but may have features that have been linked to sick building syndrome. The characteristics of this syndrome include both sensory and acute neurotoxic effects including headaches and lethargy (US Environmental Protection Agency 1991). Specific constituents associated with sick building syndrome have been studied over the past 20 years. Some of these constituents known to contribute to poor indoor air quality are also found in household chemical products. While an individual has little control over the structure of the dwelling and housing status (semi-detached, terraced, flat etc.), the presence of chemical household products is under the control of the occupier. This issue may be particularly important for the older person.

Over the past two decades, consumption of household cleaning products has risen sharply in the UK (Office for National Statistics [ONS] 2000). Consumption expenditure on household cleaning materials (other than soap) since 1994 has increased by 60% in real terms. Such increased expenditure and usage will result in a significant change to the chemical constituents of the indoor air environment. It is therefore important to establish whether these products are associated with either triggering or exacerbating underlying health problems such as respiratory ill health or contributing to a reduction in cognitive function. Thus, while the home should be fitted to the physical and psychological characteristics of the older person and designed to promote familiarity and orientation with the environment, other factors such as the levels of indoor chemical pollutants should be considered. In addition, those who suffer from incontinence may be more fastidious and conscious of odours, and in turn may purchase and use products such as air fresheners in greater quantity. Chemical cleaning sprays or aerosols are used in homes to reduce bacteria or moulds and improve odours due to damp or unclean environments. The rooms in which these products are used may also be less well-ventilated in order to maintain a constant warm temperature. Thus there is the potential for a build-up chemical cocktail with unknown health effects.

The evidence from studies of the health effects of constituents of household products such as cleaning agents, comes mainly from occupational research or more rarely cohort studies of children and their parents. There have been few, if any, where the target population is older people or those who are confined to their own homes for much of the time.

Common health problems relevant to older people

In some susceptible individuals, the development of respiratory hypersensitivity or presentation of asthmatic symptoms has been related to the indiscriminate use of different household products, specifically where there is exposure to compounds such as diisocyanates, organic acid anhydrides, formaldehyde, styrene and hydro-quinone (Becher *et al.* 1996). Moorman & Mannino (2001) have reported on the increasing asthma mortality rates in the United States between 1979 and 1996 with respect to details of rates of change for different demographic subgroups. The ana-lysis is limited to death certificates that specified asthma as the underlying cause of death. Black people, females, and people aged 65 and older had the largest increases in age-adjusted asthma mortality rates between 1979 and 1996. Overall, the increase in asthma mortality rates between 1979 and 1996 was due primarily to increased mortality rates in the population subgroup aged 65 years and older. Efforts to develop strategies to reduce overall mortality from asthma should concentrate on middle-aged and older women.

Formaldehyde, frequently investigated in epidemiological studies of occupational asthma, has consistently shown association with allergic respiratory response and both acute and chronic health problems (Delfino 2002). It is ubiquitous in the indoor environment as it is a common constituent of a large number of products owing to its bactericidal action; these include carpets, wallpaper, furniture, cosmetics and cleaning chemicals. An indoor air quality survey in Louisiana found levels of air-borne formaldehyde from 53 houses (419 samples) to range from non-detectable to 6.60 mg/m^3. There were 74% of samples with detectable amounts of airborne formaldehyde and of these, 312 positive samples (~60%) exceeded the American Society of Heating, Refrigeration, and Air Conditioning Engineers guideline of 0.123 mg/m^3. A high level of formaldehyde could thus be a potential upper res-piratory irritant (Lemus *et al.* 1998).

In older people problems carrying out everyday **activities** are most strongly associ-ated with short-term memory loss and worsening orientation. Research has shown mood impairment amongst chronic solvent exposed workers, with or without psy-chomotor alteration that may reflect possible over-exposure (Campagna *et al.* 1995). Isopropanol, a common constituent of many aerosol products, was tested on young healthy volunteers. It was shown that breathing in isopropanol at the maximum allowable concentration affects postural balance. No conclusions about safety risks were possible from this study on young healthy adults (Sethre *et al.* 2000).

The negative effects of exposure to solvents may interact with the normal ageing process and affect cognitive performance. This hypothesis was tested on floor lay-ers exposed to organic solvents and a comparison group, who were not exposed. The study was carried out with workers over a period of 18 years. The results partly supported the hypothesis of greater cognitive deterioration in the exposed group, but primarily at heavy exposure (Nilson & Bach 2002).

A large non-occupational prospective cohort study of the health of infants and their parents in Bristol that began in pregnancy (ALSPAC), has reported on the use of a variety of products in the home and the health outcomes. Results indicated that air fresheners and aerosols were associated with high levels of measured volatile organic compounds in the home (TVOCs). This study, able to control for many known confounders, also found the use of both products to be associated with an increased reporting of symptoms in women, including headache and depression (Farrow *et al.* 2003).

Occupational exposure to various neurotoxic chemicals has been shown in many investigations, both toxicological and epidemiological, to impair colour vision including a recent study of toluene-exposed rubber workers and a group of non-exposed controls (Cavalleri *et al.* 2000). Dick *et al.* (2000) have also shown neurocognitive deficits and impaired colour acuity in painters who have been exposed to a mixture of solvents. Toluene is a common constituent of non-water based paint and is found in many insecticides that are used commonly in and around the home.

This evidence is relevant to older people as all of the health problems mentioned above are common in an older population: **asthma**, general respiratory ill health, impaired cognitive function such as **dementia**, and loss of visual acuity. The largest and most representative study of the causes of vision loss in older people in Britain has confirmed the major burden of age-related macular degeneration (AMD) in people 75 years and older. This problem will get worse as the population ages (Evans *et al.* 2004). In a representative Swedish population, ($n = 958$), decreased visual acuity was found in 20% and 80% of subjects at ages 82 and 97 years, respectively. 'Low' folate status, smoking, 'high' BMI and low physical activity were found to be potential risk factors (Bergman *et al.* 2004). Apart from smoking, other environmental factors have not been investigated.

It is difficult to assess the influence of indoor air pollutants on older people's health. In the case of respiratory symptoms and asthma the evidence in young people is quite strong and it would seem reasonable to expect there also to be an effect in older people. With regard to loss of cognitive function this is established in younger people if they are exposed to high levels. Few studies have measured volatile organic compounds (VOCs) in the home and it is unlikely that they would reach levels that have been found in occupational exposure. The association with loss of visual acuity from occupational studies is also established at high exposure levels. Given the importance of visual acuity and cognitive function in older people it is surprising that so little work has been carried out to establish VOC levels in the indoor environment. While it is not possible to conclude that VOCs are contributing substantially to older people's ill health, it is certainly the case that there needs to be further investigation of this important risk factor.

Natural and human-caused events

Pestilence, famine, plague and war; scholars of the Bible will recognise these events as the Four Horsemen of the Apocalypse. To fit a more contemporary frame of reference the International Classification of Functioning (ICF) (WHO 2001) has developed a refined definition that promulgates two categories – natural and human caused events. Natural events are those extremes of nature that can cause dramatic change to the physical environment. Natural events can occur regularly or irregularly, such as earthquakes and severe or violent weather conditions such as tornadoes, hurricanes, typhoons, floods, forest fires and ice storms. Human-caused events are those that owe nothing to nature but are the creation of humankind and also bring disruption, displacement and destruction. As a result of conflict or environmental disaster, these events affect more than land and homes but also the social infrastructure. Both the ICF categories affect the individual's or the community's wellbeing, in some cases right to the point of denying life and even extinction.

Occupational therapists are nurtured in the understanding of the person and their inter-relation with the environment. Added to this, therapists are knowledgeable and sensitive to the context of any **activity**, occupation or event and its immediate significance to the individual.

Occupation and conflict

Human beings have sought environments in which to live in and develop that support their existence. Without water or a regular food source, we would simply fail to thrive. Nonetheless humans are found living in accommodation with the environment in some of the harshest climatic regions of the globe. Of course, those living in Siberia have long adapted to the harshness of the winter and the need to prepare and employ strategies with which to manage not mere survival, but to maintain an ability to continue with work and other productive activities. Since the beginning of time, human beings have demonstrated the desire to engage in leisure, or to seek opportunities from which pleasure and enjoyment are gained. Whether it is in the cold of Siberia or the heat of the Ethiopian desert, games and socialising leisure activities form the basis of social life. In such communities cultural modes have established practices that compensate and support those older members of the community who find increasing barriers to not only social interaction, but to mere survival. The restrictions on **activity** are recognised and long-established strategies, and customs loaded with relevant **cultural** meaning are applied to ensure the impairment or restriction is limited.

For the peoples of these extreme climatic environments, there is a habituation in the way the individual and the group undertake their occupational performance. In common with this learnt collective understanding and an acceptance of these events, those peoples who live in regions affected by typhoons and hurricanes, demonstrate habitualised modes by which they prepare for and individually address the trauma and wreckage wrought after the storms have passed. By so doing both the individual and community, old and young are able to form strategies by which as near normal a lifestyle is maintained.

For peoples accustomed to living for several months in freezing temperatures or searing heat, extreme elements exist that in temperate regions are often perceived as barriers to participating in an **activity**. However where they are the norm, these conditions but fail to take on the significance that prevents **participation**.

War on the other hand is the most obvious manifestation of a human-caused event that leads to disruption and dislocation of people from their everyday lives; the destruction of material, the pollution of land, water and air and the subsequent effects on established social infrastructure are part and parcel of conflict in its many guises. Health conditions are directly and indirectly exacerbated. Affected individuals' functioning is decreased and disability is commonplace; in fact, some commentators suggest that is a major objective of war and conflict. Depending on the nature of the conflict it is very possible that normal day-to-day **participation** in **activity**, whether employment, leisure or depending on proximity, aspects of **activities** of daily living are restricted, whether by direct events or the overall environmental context.

Given modern media, details of high intensity wars, characterised by the pooling of huge resources into vast combined coalitions, like those of the world wars and more recently in Afghanistan and Iraq, are broadcast throughout the world, and the impact upon the individual is recognised. Alternatively, those marked out by intermittent guerrilla tactics, as in the case of Palestine and East Timor, bring not just possible death and injury, but have significant effects on normal day-to-day activities upon both the individual and the wider group. Major industrial accidents, like that at the Union Carbide plant in Bhopal in 1984 and the meltdown in April 1986 of Chernobyl in the Ukraine are human-caused events. These have had an immense impact upon the wellbeing of many people who have been, and in innumerable cases still are, affected by such an incident.

Whilst noting the success of individual and community coping strategies in dealing with catastrophic events, these have been shown to be dependent upon earlier experiences and previous exposure to crisis, in particular events of the same or similar nature. For those peoples who inhabit regions of the world where extremes of climate are the norm, we know a habituation is formed to cope with demands of existence amongst the elements. Equally, it is possible to recognise the role of previous experience in developing strategies to cope with human-made events.

Humanitarian interventions have been criticised for neglecting older people, failing to address gender, social and cultural issues, using systems to discriminate against them and even undermining their ability to support themselves (HelpAge International 2000).

A suitable illustration of how the use of a meaningful occupation amongst older people proved to have much broader and greater reaching therapeutic consequences than first thought is that of a knitting group established among a group of older Bosnian women refugees. Notwithstanding other factors, there was no disguising the fact that for many individuals in this community this was the third time in their living memory that conflict had touched them directly. Their apparent fatalism and preparedness, demonstrated by the possessions they still maintained and their attempt to adapt to this perceived temporary dislocation were commented on by many observers and relief workers. This differentiated older people not as a prescribed 'vulnerable group' but in fact as individuals that coped better with the chan-

Box 10.1 Older people in disasters and human conflicts.

Help Age International (2000) has issued guidelines for best practice when working with older people in disaster or conflict situations. It provides a vulnerable individual checklist and tackles issues that the global community needs to solve to ensure older people's wellbeing is best served.

ging realities. The narrative in Box 10.2 comprises excerpts from a diary, which one of the authors maintained working as a relief worker in the former Yugoslavia. The excerpts demonstrate the value of context, the older person experience and overcoming the trauma of community and individual brutalisation and loss.

Box 10.2 Occupation and conflict.

'Whilst working as a relief worker with a United Nation High Commission For Refugees (UNHCR) implementing partner I spent time at numerous collective centres throughout this region. In September 1993, I was working with 180 to 200 Bosnian refugees at a town called Posusje on the Bosnian/Croatian border. The displaced persons, as they were labelled, were accommodated in a derelict secondary school. They had split themselves into extended family groups and occupied the classrooms and offices as their accommodation. As is often the norm amongst refugee communities throughout the globe, the majority of this group were women and children. A further breakdown of the population revealed some 29 older men and just three men over the age of 16, but younger than 70. The rest were either children or women. At first sight, the families appeared large. Traditionally relief work is built on a number of tenets. As a rule, these principles follow a Maslow hierarchy in addressing displaced persons needs. Furthermore, there is an acknowledgement that 'vulnerable groups' have particular issues and these require seeking out and addressing. Finally, where at all possible, empower and encourage both user and host population to discuss, work together and come to mutually beneficial decisions and outcomes. Besides the obvious grouping of young children and pregnant women, the older people and those with health conditions and disability were focused upon. At this stage is important to note that two months before the creation of this collective centre, European newspapers had carried stories of widespread atrocities, concentration camps and the brutalisation of the civilian population by armed militias. Of particular note were the rumours of systematic rape of the female population including young girls. In between creating activities for the displaced youth of the centre and ensuring continual dialogue between the local town council and the refugees on the various issues that could cause problems, I would spend time taking a short walk along the main track with several of the older women. At that time my local language was limited, but it did not stop these rural mountain people attempting to communicate with me and give me advice. They were very much interested in London and in particular the knitted wool jumper that my Grandmother had sent me to keep out the Balkan winter. After a number of weeks, it became apparent that the older women sought some wool and needles in order to undertake a similar project. The necessary equipment was found through a charitable organisation and passed on to the women. I visited the main assembly area where I found several older women sitting comfortably, knitting away and drinking coffee. I was sufficiently smug to think that through providing them with the materials to engage in a meaningful occupation, I had enabled what were often considered as 'forgotten vulnerable victims' and thus contributed to an improvement in their wellbeing.

Over the next few weeks, the relief team noticed that after the collective domestic activities of daily living were complete the majority of the women appeared to head for the assembly hall and remain there for much of the day. On one occasion, I noticed a young woman leaving the assembly hall tearfully. I asked of another what was the problem and she explained that I should come along and see how useful the knitting group had become. Of course, in my ignorance, I thought I was going to see all the women knitting useful jumpers as it had become cold. I was astounded to sit amongst the 70 or so women and watch as some knitted and drank coffee whilst one woman spoke animatedly. It became apparent that one older woman was talking about the effects the war had had upon her and her family, but not the current conflict; she was

Box 10.2 *(cont'd)*

> referring to a war some 50 years previously. Another older woman offered similar ex-
> periences and as I tried to discern words I still had yet to master, a younger woman in
> her late twenties began to cry and talk emotively. It was explained to me that she was
> describing what had had been done to her by armed men who had come to her home.
> More women spoke and there was a considerable out-pouring of grief. I was not the
> only man in the room; there was a very old man who sat playing with his moustache
> throughout. Before I left the room, I noticed an older woman, without tears give
> matter-of fact-advice.'
>
> Marcus Sivell-Muller

It appeared that with the introduction of an **activity**, whose focus was primarily to offer some meaningful and realistic occupation for the older women, those
younger had found a therapeutic **environment** in which to discuss and bring up
the events that had been done to them in their eviction and forced migration. At
the same time the older women, often seen by external observers as a vulnerable
group, were able to reflect upon their own experiences and offer not mere empathy and solace but also strategies and a living model of coping with events.

Products and assistive technology

Occupational therapists are in a unique position in that they are the only professionals with expertise in occupation but also in the **environment, assistive technology**
and older people. The Canadian Association of Occupational Therapists (2003)
strongly advocates that occupational therapists need to be able to enable clients to
select, educate and use assistive technology to support their **occupational performance**. The ICF (WHO 2001:173) defines assistive products and technology as
'product, instrument, equipment or technology adapted or specially designed for
improving the functioning of a disabled person.' This definition therefore incorporates a broad and diverse range of products from simple devices such as grab
rails to sophisticated video surveillance products.

Assistive technology and products are of particular relevance to occupational therapists as they are used to enhance all aspects of **occupational performance**. Despite
having a key role in assessment, education provision and evaluation of assistive
technology and products, there is evidence that occupational therapists have a very
narrow focus of assistive technology. A survey by OTOP (Occupational Therapy for
Older People 2002) found that over 60% of its members had never used electronic
assistive technology. Reasons for not using these products were related primarily
to funding problems with multiagency provision, and lack of demand. An issue of
lack of demand provokes an interesting debate, since this could be attributed to
therapists' lack of skills and knowledge about assistive technology. Another reason could be the fact that the installation of assistive products can be extremely
disruptive for an older person and their family, and there is also fear of potential

failure. How can we enable older people to trust in assistive products and technologies when occupational therapists may themselves have reservations and doubts?

Funding and provision of assistive technology and products

In England the National Health Service and local authorities, including **social services** and **housing**, provide most assistive technology. The National Service Framework for Older People (DH 2001), The Report of the Royal Commission on Long Term Care (1999) and the National Strategy of Carers (DH 1999) have acknowledged the importance of assistance technology in promoting wellbeing and independence, supporting carers.

Commercial suppliers and industrial design engineers have an important role both in developing, designing and selling affordable assistive technology products to older people. The Department for Trade and Industry (DTI 2000) has published a useful study of the difficulties disabled people have using everyday products.

Some suppliers have been criticised for using unethical marketing tactics. Age Concern commissioned Ricability to investigate companies selling products such as stairlifts, powered scooters and armchairs and beds (Age Concern 2002).

The key issues relating to products sold to older people in their own homes as opposed to shops were:

- Influential advertisement.
- Detrimental effects on cancellation rights of invited home visits.
- Over forceful selling practices.
- Products unsuitable for person's abilities and needs.
- Poor demonstration.
- Large deposits required.
- Dramatic price reductions to induce purchases.
- Verbal agreement not written into the final contract.
- Restricted consumer rights when products made to personal specification.
- Pressurised selling of expensive maintenance contracts.
- Poor after-sale services.

Assistive technology is an important aspect of ensuring that intermediate care works effectively, can reduce length of stay, and avoid admission into hospital. There are also cost benefits, with assistive technology being considered an inexpensive alternative to hands on care (Audit Commission 2004). Indeed assistive technology can be introduced and then gradually withdrawn or vice versa according to the older persons rehabilitation, functional and diagnostic needs. Miller Polgar (2001) advocates that assistive technology can enable a person to carry out meaningful occupations which in turn offers choices and can facilitate integration and full **participation** within the community. Mann *et al.* (1999) investigated the effectiveness of assistive technology and environmental interventions in maintaining independence and reducing home care costs for the frail older people and found that assistive technology could reduce the rate of function decline, which in turn meant that older people stayed at home longer. Likewise Hoenig *et al.* (2003) found that among older people with a disability assistive technology was associated with use of fewer hours of personal assistance.

User acceptance among older people is an essential feature of ensuring older people will use assistive technology. Wielandt *et al.* (2001) carried out an audit of the use of bathing products by 64 people, eight weeks after discharge. Where a product was not being used, the most frequent reason given was that it was no longer required or that they did not know how to use the product. It seemed that products were much more likely to be used if family members were present during training. Likewise a study by Mann *et al.* (2002) suggested that almost half of the reasons for not using assistive products related to perceived lack of need. It is essential that occupational therapists choose the solution that best suits client and the carer needs, rather than on what is available. Whilst the inclusion of the carer is an integral part of occupational therapy practice, little research has been conducted regarding the involvement of the caregiver (Chen *et al.* 2000).

It is suggested however that if society adopts a primary **health promotion** approach to housing (namely the concept of lifetime homes) then home modifications will no longer be needed. Lifestyle homes are designed to meet the flexible and changing needs occurring throughout one's family life and to meet the varying needs of numerous changes of the occupier in the same house (Habinteg Housing Association 2003). It is considered that investing in lifestyle homes is cost effective as it reduces the need for assistive technology within the home. Lifestyle homes can also incorporate the principles of smart housing. This term is often used to describe the electronic and computer controlled integration of assistive technology and products in the home during its construction and can also be built into older homes. Smart homes enable an older person to maintain their independence and autonomy from one easily installed control box with core functions being control of emergency help, temperature monitoring, water and energy use monitoring, automatic lighting, door surveillance, cooker safety, water temperature control, window, blind and or curtain control, home security and online links (Fisk 2001).

Assistive technology may be associated with the dehumanisation and anonymity of care, since it could be argued that assistive technology focuses primarily on physical needs, rather than psychosocial needs. Consequently before occupational therapists make any type of changes to an older person's environment they need to consider why modifications are being made, what they should do and the individual needs of the older person. Good practice in the provision of assistive technology and products would always include attention to maintenance and repair.

Mobility products and technology

More traditional products and assistive technology such as those for mobility are assessed and provided to older people on a daily basis. Mobility problems in older people can be very restrictive in their performance of everyday occupations. Their successful performance is dependent upon the **context** in which these occupations are carried out and how supportive their environment is to successful accomplishment. The use of walking products has been scrutinised by many because of reported non-use of equipment when issued to older people (Edwards & Jones 1998). It is therefore important to consider not only the **impairment** the client has, or may have in the future, but also their attitude and safety awareness, the environmental context, as well as the advantages and disadvantages of the various types of equipment. Provision of walking products has traditionally been considered the domain of physiotherapy colleagues; however, consideration of walking products within an environmental context is a very relevant part of an occupational therapist's role. An awareness of the appropriateness of the product issued within the client's context is important and an understanding of the correct and safest method of usage is crucial.

The use of mobility products such as walking sticks and wheelchairs can compensate for **impairment** or lack of confidence, promoting independence in **occupational performance** through **activity** and **participation**. Over 28% of older adults use a mobility aid, with the usage increasing with age (ONS 2002). The use of a walking stick, crutch, quadripod, rollator or walking frame, increases stability in standing and walking maintaining an individual's centre of gravity within an enlarged base of support. However successful use is dependent on adequate upper limb strength and control as well as dynamic standing balance (see Chapter 6).

Occupational therapists are often involved in the assessment and provision of wheelchairs. Wheelchair design, construction and provision has been greatly influenced over the past few years by the new technologies, lighter weight materials, improvements in medical science, sociopolitical changes, demands and expectations of users and an increasingly ageing population. Whereas the largest group of older users have arthritis and musculoskeletal problems, the largest group of younger adults are those with neurological problems (Ham *et al.* 1998). In the UK both manual and electrically powered indoor/outdoor chairs (EPIOCs) are issued to those individuals with mobility problems. However eligibility criteria for provision will vary from area to area. The imminent setting of national minimum standards for wheelchair provision will ensure that there will be no discrimination against clients on basis of age. Older wheelchair users can be considered as belonging to three groups – the permanent full-time user who needs alternative means of mobility at all times, the part-time user (for example outdoor use only) and the temporary user (post-operative), and their needs and level of provision will differ. Exploration of the older person's perception and expectation of a wheelchair as part of the assessment and prescription process is essential, as wheelchairs are often perceived by many older people prior to provision as an easy means of independent outdoor transport. However a self-propelling manual wheelchair requires 9% more energy expenditure than walking (Ham *et al.* 1998) and therefore those with energy restrictive problems may find propelling a wheelchair both fatiguing and disappointing. Good upper limb strength and range of movement are also necessary for independent mobility in a manual wheelchair.

Box 10.3 Mr and Mrs Kurtz.

Mr and Mrs Kurtz like going out every day and meeting their friends in the local town. Even though Mr Kurtz can propel his wheelchair indoors he needs his wife to push him in the chair outdoors. Mr and Mrs Kurtz were pleased with the freedom a new wheelchair gave them, but Mrs Kurtz began to find that her shoulders were particularly painful after they had been out.

The OT at the wheelchair service solved the mystery – even though the wheelchair was suitable for Mr Kurtz, the push handles were too high for Mrs Kurtz. Once this problem was addressed Mr and Mrs Kurtz could go out in comfort.

As many users will sit for long periods in their wheelchair, adequate postural support and pressure relief are crucial elements of the assessment process. Other factors for consideration are the client's method of transfer, the environment for use, access, transportation and storage, as well as when and how often the chair will be used. Many carers of older people are partners, family or friends and themselves older, with their own limitations and health problems. It is therefore crucial that carers' needs also be taken into account when considering the ease of opening and folding, the weight of the wheelchair and the occupant for pushing and also lifting into a car for transportation. Maintenance and safety issues of the wheelchair, its accessories and pressure relieving cushions are highly important and the ability of the client or carer to take responsibility for these also need to be assessed. The needs of the carer are also important as can be seen in Box 10.3.

Electrically powered chairs tend to be provided to those individuals with relatively severe physical disability. As with manual wheelchairs, cognitive and perceptual problems need to be addressed to ensure safe and accurate manoeuvering of the more powerful and heavier wheelchair. Regular maintenance and storage of these powered chairs is even more of an issue, so that the battery is recharged adequately in the appropriate surroundings. For many people, electrically powered outdoor chairs enable independent **participation** in social and routine **activities** (such as shopping), thus maintaining quality of life (Brandt *et al.* 2004). Risk assessment is very important for both the safety of the individual and also other members of the public, and maintenance and storage issues should also be considered before purchase.

Communication

As discussed in Chapter 9, communication is an important aspect of **active ageing**. There are many interactive communication devices, which can be of use to older people such as cordless telephones, memory telephone (with a photo or a symbol instead of a number for family and friends) or textphones. There are also many devices to help older persons continue watching television, for example a home loop system which enables the hearing-aid user to hear a sound system without the other sounds around, subtitling and captions, personal inductive listening devices, personal speech amplifiers. Electronic communication devices vary and can be used to convey simple messages or complex messages. They display or speak words produced by the older person touching a keyboard, screen symbol or picture and are useful for those older people with communication problems as a result of disease – for example Mr Branch from Chapter 6, with **Parkinson's disease**.

Interactive digital services through television can be of great benefit and these include connection to the Internet and e-mail, and are of use for older people without a computer. The Internet offers older people an opportunity to access and gain information about a wide range of services, including health and social care and access to consumer goods. Computers can be adapted to ensure that all older persons can use them effectively, for example big keys, high contrast keyboards and screen magnifiers for older people who read large prints. Keyboards can also be adapted for use on wheelchairs, or for single-handed use. Voice recognition and word prediction are useful devices for older persons with communication problems.

However, not all information technology and products work successfully. The Guildford **Falls** Project (2003) found that some clients were not happy with wearing fall detectors and there were many false alarms. Some problems also occurred with the bed sensors since these were fitted under the castors of beds, which caused them to be unstable. Pressure mats beside beds were found to be a hazard to the participants and were not acceptable to many people because of their appearance and could not be appropriately programmed for each individual.

Table 10.1 Assistive technology to promote independence and wellbeing.

Telecare provided at a distance using information and communication technology, for example health monitors.	Promotes confidence and reassurance
Reminder systems – e.g. electronic/speaking clocks, day planners, automated medicine reminders.	Can assist with managing short-term memory loss.
Home safety can be enhanced by the installation of video camera, automatic bedroom lights, sensors to detect intruders, gas, smoke, fire alarms and water temperature monitors.	Promotes confidence and reassurance for both older people and carers. Can be of great benefit for older people who are disorientated at night or have short-term memory deficits.
Social Alarm System. Alarms can be worn by older people or installed within home.	Promotes confidence and reassurance.
Assistive technology can promote independence in activities of daily living. For example a pressure mat can get the attention of a carer when an older person has moved from a bed or a chair for a variable and predetermined period. The change in pressure as the older person moves is identified by a control unit, which gives an audible and visual alarm (Miskelly 2001).	Promotes confidence and reassurance for both older people and carers. Can be of great benefit for older people who are disorientated at night or have short-term memory deficits

Box 10.4 Using information technology with older people.

- Consider an older person you know.
- How does (or could) information technology facilitate their activity and participation?

Summary

The natural environment and human-made changes to the environment impact upon the health and wellbeing of older people. Occupational therapists need to ensure that their assessments, treatments and interventions take into account the complex interactions that occur between the physical, social and attitudinal environment. Indeed occupational therapists need to collaborate with epidemiologists, public health workers and occupational health experts to conduct further research into this area.

With regard to the use of assistive products and technology, the challenge for occupational therapists is to be become confident and committed to the use of a wider range of assistive products and technology in practice. Occupational therapists need to consult with older people to ascertain their perceptions of assistive technology. They must ensure that each client is treated as an individual and that clients' concerns are always addressed, respected and acknowledged. Occupational therapists must collaborate with older people, carers, rehabilitation engineers, scientists, housing experts and other health and social care professionals to conduct interprofessional research regarding assistive technology and older people.

References

Age Concern (2002) *Sharp Selling Practices in the Sale of Assistive Products to Older People.* London: Age Concern.

Audit Commission (2004) *Assistive Technology.* London: The Audit Commission.

Becher R, Hongslo JK, Jantunen MJ, Dybing E (1996) Environmental chemicals relevant for respiratory hypersensitivity: the indoor environment. *Toxicology Letters* 86(2–3), 155–162.

Bergman B, Nilsson-Ehle H, Sjostrand J (2004) Ocular changes, risk markers for eye disorders and effects of cataract surgery in elderly people: a study of an urban Swedish population followed from 70 to 97 years of age. *Acta Ophthalmologica Scandinavica* 82(2), 166–174.

Brandt A, Iwarsson S, Stahle A (2004) Older people's use of powered wheelchairs for activity and participation. *Journal of Rehabilitation Medicine* 36(2), 70–72.

Canadian Association of Occupational Therapists (2003) *Position Statement. Assistive Technology and Occupational Therapy.* Ottawa, Ont: CAOT.

Campagna D, Mergler D, Picot A *et al.* (1995) Monitoring neurotoxic effects among laboratory personnel working with organic solvents. *Revue D Epidemiologie et de Sante Publique* 43(6), 519–532.

Cavalleri A, Gobba F, Nicali E, Fiocchi V (2000) Dose-related color vision impairment in toluene-exposed workers. *Archives of Environmental Health* 55(6), 399–404.

Chen C, Mann WC, Tormita M, Nochajski S (2000) Caregiver involvement in the use of assistive devices by frail older persons. *Occupational Therapy Journal of Research* 20(3), 179–199.

College of Occupational Therapy (2002) *From Interface to Integration: A Strategy for Modernising Services in Local Health and Social Care Communities – A Consultation*. London: College of Occupational Therapy.

Delfino RJ (2002) Epidemiologic evidence for asthma and exposure to air toxics: linkages between occupational, indoor, and community air pollution research. *Environmental Health Perspectives* 110 (Suppl 4), 573–589.

Department of the Environment, Transport and Regions (DETR) (1999) *Air Pollution: What it Means for your Health*. London: Department of the Environment, Transport and Regions.

Department of Health (1999) *Caring about Carers: A National Strategy for Carers*. London: HMSO.

Department of Health (2001) *The National Service Framework for Older People*. London: HMSO.

Department of Trade and Industry (2000) *A Study of the Difficulties Disabled People Have When Using Everyday Consumer Products*. London: HMSO.

Department of Trade and Industry (2001) *The UK Fuel Poverty Strategy*. London: HMSO.

Dick F, Semple S, Chen R, Seaton A (2000) Neurological deficits in solvent-exposed painters: a syndrome including impaired colour vision, cognitive defects, tremor and loss of vibration sensation. *Quarterly Journal of Medicine* 93(10), 655–661.

Donaldson GC, Kovats RS, Keatinge WR, McMitchel RJ (2001) Heat and cold-related mortality and morbidity and climate change. In: Maynard RL (ed.) *Health Effects of Climate Change in the UK*. London: Department of Health, pp. 70–80.

Edwards NI & Jones DA (1998) Ownership and use of assistive devices amongst older people in the community. *Age and Ageing* 27(4), 463–468.

Evans JR, Fletcher AE, Wormald RP (2004) Age-related macular degeneration causing visual impairment in people 75 years or older in Britain: an add-on study to the Medical Research Council Trial of Assessment and Management of Older People in the Community. *Ophthalmology* 111(3), 513–517.

Farrow A, Taylor H, Golding J (1997) Time spent in the home by different family members. *Environmental Technology* 18, 605–614.

Farrow A, Taylor H, Golding J (2003) Symptoms of mothers and infants related to total volatile organic compounds in household products. *Archives of Environmental Health* 58(10), 633–641.

Fisk M (2001) the implications of smart home technologies. In: Peace S & Holland C (eds). *Inclusive Housing in an Ageing Society* Bristol: Policy Press, pp. 101–124.

Guildford Falls Project (2003) Accessed 16.05.2004. http://www.teis.port.ac.uk/jsp/search/activity.jsp?project=1260

Habinteg Housing Association (2003) *Lifetime Homes*. Accessed 16.05.2004. http://www.habinteg.org.uk/

Ham R, Aldersea P, Porter D (1998) *Wheelchair Users and Postural Seating: A Clinical Approach*. London: Churchill Livingstone.

Healy JD (2003) Excess winter mortality in Europe: a cross country analysis identifying key risk factors. *Journal Epidemiology and Community Health* 57(10), 784–789.

HelpAge International (2000) *Older People in Disasters and Humanitarian Crises: Guidelines for Best Practice*. HelpAge International. Accessed 07.09.2004. http://www.helpage.org/images/pdfs/bpg.pdf

Hoenig H, Taylor DH, Sloan FA (2003) Does assistive technology substitute for personal assistance among the disabled elderly? *American Journal of Public Health* 93(2), 330–337.

Keatinge WR, Coleshaw SRK, Easton JC, Coter F, Mattock MB, Chelliah R (1986) Increased platelet and red cell count, blood viscosity, and plasma cholesterol levels during heat stress, and mortality from coronary and cerebral thrombosis. *American Journal of Medicine* 81(5), 795–800.

Keatinge WR (2004) Death in heat waves. *British Medical Journal* 327, 512–513.

Lemus R, Abdelghani AA, Akers TG, Horner WE (1998) Potential health risks from exposure to indoor formaldehyde. *Reviews on Environmental Health* 13(1–2), 91–8.

MacFarlane A & Waller RE (1976) Short term increases in mortality during heat waves *Nature* 264(5585), 434–436.

Mann WC, Ottenbacher KJ, Frass L, Tomita M, Granger CV (1999) Effectiveness of assistive technology and environmental interventions in maintaining independence and reducing home care costs for the frail elderly. A randomised controlled trial. *Archives of Family Medicine* 8(3), 210–217.

Mann WC, Goodall S, Justiss MD, Tomita M (2002) Dissatisfaction and non-use of assistive devices among frail elders. *Assistive Technology* 14, 30–24(1), 4–12.

Manuel J (1999) A healthy home environment? *Environmental Health Perspectives* 107(7), A353–A357.

Miller Polgar J (2001) Using technology to enable occupation. *Occupational Therapy Now* September, 23–25.

Miskelly FG (2001) Assistive technology in elderly care. *Age and Ageing* 30(6), 455–458.

Moorman JE & Mannino DM (2001) Increasing US asthma mortality rates: who is really dying? *Journal of Asthma* 38(1), 65–71.

Nielsen J, Bach E (1999) Work-related eye symptoms and respiratory symptoms in female cleaners. *Occupational Medicine* 49(5), 291–297.

Occupational Therapy for Older People (OTOP) (2002) *Are OTs Turned on to Technology. Paper Handout at the Turned on to Technology Conference.* London: College of Occupational Therapists.

Office for National Statistics, UK (2000) *Consumer Trends.* Data for the fourth quarter, no. 19. London: Office for National Statistics.

Office for National Statistics (2002) Living in Britain. *Results from the 2001 General Household Survey.* London: Office for National Statistics.

Press V (2003) *Fuel Poverty and Health. A Guide for Primary Care Organisations and Public Health and Primary Care Professionals.* London: National Heart Forum.

Royal Commission on the Funding of Long Term Care (1999) *With Respect to Old Age: Long Term Care-rights and Responsibilities.* London: HMSO.

Sethre T, Laubli T, Berode M, Krueger H (2000) Neurobehavioural effects of experimental isopropanol exposure. *International Archives of Occupational and Environmental Health* 73(2), 105–112.

Schneidert M, Hurst R, Miller J, Ustun B (2003) The role of environment in the International Classification of Functioning, Disability and Health (ICF). *Disability and Rehabilitation* 25(11–12), 588–595.

Scriven A & Atwal A (2004) Occupational therapists as primary health promoters: opportunities and barriers. *British Journal of Occupational Therapy* 67(10), 424–429.

Shepperd S, Charnock D, Gann B (1999) Helping patients access high quality health information. *British Medical Journal* 319, 764–766.

Spurgeon B (2003) French government announces new plans for elderly care. *British Medical Journal* 307, 465.

Stuck AE, Walthert JM, Nikolaus T, Büla CJ, Hohmann C, Beck JC (1999). Risk factors for functional status decline in community-living elderly people: a systematic literature review, *Social Science and Medicine* 48(4), 445–469.

US Environmental Protection Agency (1991) *Indoor Air Facts No. 4 (revised): Sick Building Syndrome (SBS)*. Office of Radiation and Indoor Air 6609J, April.

Wielandt T, McKenna K, Tooth L, Strong J (2001) Post discharge use of bathing equipment prescribed by occupational therapists: what lessons to be learned? *Physical and Occupational Therapy in Geriatrics* 19(3), 47–63.

Wilcock AA (1998) *An Occupational Perspective of Health*. Thorofare USA: Slack.

Wilcock AA (2002) *Occupation for Health, Volume 2: A Journey from Prescription to Self Health*. London: College of Occupational Therapists.

Wilkinson P, Armstrong B, Landon M (2001) *Cold Comfort. The Social and Environmental Determinants of Excess Winter Death in England, 1986–96*. Bristol: The Policy Press.

World Health Organisation (WHO) (1986) *Ottawa Charter for Health Promotion*. Geneva: WHO.

World Health Organisation (2001) *International Classification of Functioning, Disability and Health*. Geneva: WHO.

World Health Organisation (2003) *The Health Impact of 2003 Summer Health Waves*. Briefing note for the delegation of the fifty-third session of the WHO Regional Committee for Europe. Accessed 30.04.2000 http://www.euro.who.int/document/Gch/HEAT-WAVES%20RC3.pdf

USEFUL RESOURCES

Statutory and non-statutory agencies and organisations providing support and advice to older people on:

Support, relationships and attitudes

Carers National Association: provides information on benefits and how to access support services.
www.carersonline.org.uk/

The Princess Royal Trust for Carers: provides comprehensive carer support services in the UK.
www.carers.org/home/

Action on Elder Abuse: aims to prevent the abuse of older people by raising awareness, education, research and disseminating information.
www.elderabuse.org.uk/

Services for the production of consumer goods

Disabled Living Centres Council: provides information about the network of Disabled (independent) Living Centres in the UK that give help and advice about assistive technology.
www.dlcc.org.uk/

RICA (Research Institute for Consumer Affairs): a national research charity dedicated to providing independent information on products and services to disabled and older consumers.
www.ricability.org.uk.

Housing Services

Care and Repair England: www.careandrepair-england.org.uk

Elderly Accommodation Council: www.housingcare.org/

Housing and Older People Development Group:
www.housing.opdm.gov.uk/information/olderpeople/index.htm

Utilities services and systems

Home Energy Efficiency Scheme: grants for insulation and heating improvements.
www.firesafetytoolbox.org.uk/ncfsc/targetaudience/olderpeople/
homeenergyefficiencyscheme.htm

Winter Fuel Payments: www.thepensionservice.gov.uk/winterfuel/home.asp

National Energy Action: campaigns for affordable warmth and improved energy
efficiency for those who are vulnerable to the cold.
www.nea.org.uk/

Solid Fuel Association: information and advice on all forms of solid fuel heating.
www.solidfuel.co.uk/frame/800index.html

Transportation Services and systems

Department of Transport: provides advice and assessment for older drivers via MAVIS
(Mobility Advice and Information Service) and also on public transport issues through
the Mobility and Inclusion Unit.
www.dft.gov.uk

Associations and organisational services

AARP (formerly the American Association of Retired Persons): now an international
organisation, dedicated to enhancing quality of life and leading social change for
and by older people.
www.aarp.org/

Age Concern: branches across UK. Age Concern is the UK's largest organisation
working with and for older people.
www.ageconcern.org.uk/

British Society of Gerontology: promotes research and education of human ageing and later life, fostering application of the evidence base to improve quality of
life for older people.
www.britishgerontology.org/

Centre for Policy on Ageing: informs, investigates, formulates and influences social
policy for older people. It also aims to promote awareness of the needs of older
people, encouraging good practice.
www.cpa.org.uk/index.html

Citizens Advice Bureau: provides general advice on benefits and heating.
www.nacab.org.uk/

Dial UK: UK network and disability information and advice services run by people with direct experiences of disability.
www.dialuk.org.uk/

Disabled Living Foundation: information and advice to assist with all aspects of daily living.
www.dlf.org.uk/

Help The Aged: provides information and advice for older people and their carers about welfare and disability.
www.helptheaged.org.uk/

Mental Health in Later Life: a service set up by the Mental Health Foundation to encourage older people to look after their mental health, and services provided are useful and available.
www.mhilli.org/index.html

RoSPA (Royal Society for the Prevention of Accidents): provides information and advice on safety issues within the home.
www.rospa.com/CMS/index.asp

Royal British Legion: provides financial, social and emotional support to ex-service men and women.
www.britishlegion.org.uk/

Social Security services and systems

Benefit Enquiry Line: www.guide-information.org.uk/guide/

British Pensioners and Trade Unions Action Association: for advice on welfare rights.
www.seniorsworld.co.uk/bptuaa/

The National Pensioners Convention (NPC): Britain's biggest pensioner organisation.
www.natpencon.org.uk/

The Pension Service: part of the Department for Work and Pensions.
www.thepensionservice.gov.uk/

Nursing Home Fees Agency: advice and information on getting and paying for care.
www.ucarewecare.com/nursing-home-fees.php

War Pensions Welfare Service: advice and practical help to war disablement pensioners and war widows, or widowers and their dependants.
www.veteransagency.mod.uk/welfare/wpws.htm

General Social Support services and systems

Women's Royal Voluntary Service: provides practical help to older people, families in crisis, those affected by disaster and to the housebound.
www.wrvs.org.uk

Health systems and services

Department of Health: provision of health and social care policy, guidance and publications in England.
www.dh.gov.uk

NHS Direct: a confidential telephone service that offers information and advice.
www.nhsdirect.nhs.uk

NHS Gateway: www.nhs.uk/

World Health Organisation (WHO): www.who.int

Education services and systems

Third Age Trust (U3A): represents the University of the Third Age in the UK, promoting lifelong learning for older people. Member of **AIUTA:** the International Association of Universities of the Third Age.
www.u3a.org.uk/ and www.worldu3a.org/aiuta/

Labour and Employment services and systems

Age Positive: promotes and encourages employers to recruit older people and prepare for age discrimination in employment legislation in 2006.
www.agepositive.gov.uk

Political services and systems

Better Government for Older People (BGOP): a movement of organisations working in partnership to change attitudes and services in order to achieve an improved society for older people across the UK.
www.bgop.org.uk

Directgov: UK government portal. www.direct.gov.uk/Homepage/fs/en

UK parliament: www.parliament.uk/

Government office for London: go-london.gov.uk/

London assembly: go-london.gov.uk/

Northern Ireland assembly: www.niassembly.gov.uk/

Scottish executive: www.scotland.gov.uk/Home

Scottish Parliament: www.scottish.parliament.uk/home.htm

National Assembly for Wales: www.wales.gov.uk/index.htm

European Union: europa.eu.int/

Australian government: www.australia.gov.au/

Government of Canada: canada.gc.ca/main_e.html

U.S. government: www.firstgov.gov/

United Nations: www.un.org/

INDEX